Culture, Diversity and Health in Australia

Australia is increasingly recognised as a multicultural and diverse society. Nationally, all accrediting bodies for allied health, nursing, midwifery and medical professions require tertiary educated students to be culturally safe with regards to cultural and social diversity. This text, drawing on experts from a range of disciplines, including public health, nursing and sociology, shows how the theory and practice of cultural safety can inform effective health care practices with all kinds of diverse populations.

Part 1 explores key themes and concepts, including social determinants of health and cultural models of health and health care. There is a particular focus on how different models of health, including the biomedical and Indigenous perspectives, intersect in Australia today. Part 2 looks at culturally safe health care practice focusing on principles and practice as well as policy and advocacy. The authors consider the practices that can be most effective, including meaningful communication skills and cultural responsiveness. Part 3 examines the practice issues in working with diverse populations, including Indigenous Australians, Culturally and Linguistically Diverse Australians, Australians with disabilities, Australians of diverse sexual orientation and gender identity, and ageing Australians. Part 4 combines all learnings from Parts 1–3 into practical learning activities, assessments and feedback for learners engaging with this textbook.

Culture, Diversity and Health in Australia is a sensitive, richly nuanced and comprehensive guide to effective health practice in Australia today and is a key reference text for either undergraduate or postgraduate students studying health care. It will also be of interest to professional health care practitioners and policy administrators.

Tinashe Dune is a multi-award-winning Senior Lecturer in the areas of health sociology and public health and is also a clinical psychology registrar. At Western Sydney University Dr Dune teaches in the Interprofessional Health Science program. Her research and teaching focuses on marginalised populations. This includes the experiences of culturally and linguistically diverse people, those living with disability, ageing populations, LGBTIQ-identifying people and Indigenous populations. Dr Dune utilises mixed-methods approaches and interdisciplinary perspectives, which support multidimensional understandings of the lived experience, health outcomes and empowered ways to improve wellbeing.

Kim McLeod is Senior Lecturer in the School of Social Sciences at the University of Tasmania. Kim is known for her expertise in philosophically informed and arts-based health research. Much of Kim's work explores the social change that contributes to health equity and population-level wellbeing. Kim's approach to understanding health as ongoing processes of change is presented in her single authored book, *Wellbeing Machine: How Health Emerges from the Assemblages of Everyday Life*. Kim brings a multidisciplinary approach to her research practice. She commonly collaborates with researchers from the Health Sciences, Humanities and Social Sciences on health-related research projects. Kim's teaching expertise is introducing health profession students to cultural safety and the social context of health. She leads collaborative research projects to explore best teaching practice in this area.

Robyn Williams has nursing and education qualifications and has over 37 years of experience of working with Indigenous peoples, primarily in the Northern Territory but also all over Australia. Her fields of expertise include cultural safety, effective communication, curriculum development and program implementation, evaluation of community-based programs, and qualitative research in Indigenous and rural and remote health issues and culturally safe practitioners.

Culture, Diversity and Health in Australia

Towards Culturally Safe Health Care

Edited by
Tinashe Dune, Kim McLeod and Robyn Williams

Routledge
Taylor & Francis Group
LONDON AND NEW YORK

First published 2021
by Routledge
2 Park Square, Milton Park, Abingdon, Oxon OX14 4RN

and by Routledge
605 Third Avenue, New York, NY 10158

Routledge is an imprint of the Taylor & Francis Group, an informa business

British Library Cataloguing-in-Publication Data
A catalogue record for this book is available from the British Library

Library of Congress Cataloging-in-Publication Data
A catalog record has been requested for this book

ISBN: 978-0-367-68676-5 (hbk)
ISBN: 978-1-760-52738-9 (pbk)
ISBN: 978-1-003-13855-6 (ebk)

Typeset in Bembo
by SPi Global, India

I dedicate this book to my children, Naya, Yarran and Burnum Lawson—so the world will be ready for you.

Love
Tinashe

I dedicate this book to my partner Joanne, and Biscuit, our Golden Retriever. Your companionship sustains me every day. This book is also for all the students who are embarking on a journey in relation to culturally safe health care. Thank you for the contribution you will make towards more equitable health for us all.

All the best
Kim

I dedicate this book to my partner Mick for your years of patience with my windmill tilting, and my two adult sons Stephen and Joseph—you give me hope for a future that has caring, compassionate and critical thinkers. I also dedicate this book to the students past, present, and future that have, do and will embrace the challenge of negotiating culturally safe practice.

Robyn

Contents

Figures

Tables

Boxes

Contributors

Stewart Alford is an Associate Lecturer in Health Services Management and Academic Course Advisor in Postgraduate Health at Western Sydney University. Stewart holds undergraduate and postgraduate qualifications in Health Services Management, Aged Care, Therapeutic Recreation and Mental Health. Stewart has recently submitted his PhD surrounding the facilitation of self-determination and personal resilience in consumers with an enduring mental illness through the therapeutic recreation intervention "Recovery Camp". Stewart is passionate about supporting individuals from vulnerable populations to access both equitable and efficient health care services. Stewart's developing research interests are in the areas of self-determination theory, resilience, volunteerism and consumerism in health care.

Amit Arora is a multi-award-winning academic in public health with an outstanding track record in research, teaching and knowledge translation. Amit teaches in the undergraduate and postgraduate health science programs at Western Sydney University with a focus on social determinants of health, public health and minority health and wellbeing. Amit's research expertise includes health equity, chronic disease prevention, early childhood nutrition, mixed methods research and community engagement. His interdisciplinary work has had direct translational outcomes in health service delivery.

Rob Atkinson began his nursing career in 1986 in Gympie General Hospital as an Assistant in Nursing, before studying to obtain an Enrolled Nurse qualification in 1987. Robert began his remote Nurse career in Palm Island Hospital, before moving to Bamaga Hospital in 1995, where he completed the "Remote Isolated Practice Endorsement". Robert's clinical and research interests include primary health care and Indigenous health care, which is influenced significantly by his work as a Remote Area Nurse for over 25 years. Robert has worked in Western Australia in rural and remote hospitals and clinics, areas of the outer islands of the Torres Strait and more recently in the Desert of Central Australia with his family.

David Ayika is a Physician, Health Project Manager, Researcher, Sessional Lecturer and Public Health Professional. Most of his work focuses on mental and social wellbeing of medical practitioners, primary health care and patient care. David's research projects focus on sexual and reproductive health, culture role in health outcome and people living with a disability, aged population health, migrants and CALD people health. His vision is in transforming health outcome through research collaboration with academia and clinical practices and ultimately effecting positive health policies in public health for better health outcomes.

Angela Brown is an experienced clinical nurse and midwife and currently works as the Midwifery Program Director at the University of South Australia. She contributes to obstetric policy and guideline development at State, National and International levels. She has a strong interest in cultural safety and equitable health outcomes for Aboriginal women and babies, refugee health and wellbeing, development of evidence-based obstetric guidelines and respectful maternity care.

Rocco Cavaleri is an academic and researcher within the Physiotherapy Department at Western Sydney University. He is passionate about investigating the mechanisms underlying chronic disease, particularly chronic pain, as well as developing safe and effective treatment methods. Rocco probes the nervous system using non-invasive brain stimulation techniques, while also appreciating the broader psychosocial determinants of health and wellbeing. He is an advocate for evidence-based practice and seeks to actively support the translation of research into clinical practice.

Liesa Clague is a descendant of the Yaegl, Bundjalung and Gumbaynggir peoples from the North Coast of New South Wales on her mother's side and on her father's side has Manx heritage from Isle of Man. Liesa did her PhD in education at Macquarie University, on *Gan'na:* Listening to the perspectives of Primary School Students on their School-Based Garden. Liesa has worked in the Aboriginal sector such as Aboriginal Health Medical Research Council of NSW and Aboriginal Medical Services (AMS) in NSW, and non-government sector with organisations such as Family Planning NSW, Family Planning NT, and Cancer Council NSW. She has worked in Darwin Hospital as a midwife and at the Centre for Disease Control in the Northern Territory. Liesa came from a leading role in the Faculty of Medicine and Human Science at Macquarie University as the Aboriginal and Torres Strait Islander health educator and worked in curriculum development for the Medical program as well as embedding Aboriginal and Torres Strait Islander health across some of Macquarie University's departments.

Cristyn Davies is a Research Fellow in the Discipline of Child and Adolescent Health, Faculty of Medicine and Health, University of Sydney. She is a board director at Twenty10 Incorporating GLCS NSW, a non-governmental organisation primarily focused on the health and wellbeing of LGBTIQA+ young people. She has expertise in gender and sexuality; child and adolescent health and development; LGBT health, discrimination and violence; sexual and reproductive health; Human Papillomavirus and HPV vaccination; vaccine delivery systems; and Knowledge Translation and Implementation Science. Cristyn is committed to using evidence-based research to close the gap between research and its translation into policy and practice.

Douglas Ezzy is a Professor of Sociology at the University of Tasmania. His research is driven by a fascination with how people make meaningful lives and respectful relationships. He is lead investigator of the Australian Research Council Discovery project "Religious freedom, LGBT+ employees, and the right to discriminate" and a second ARC project on "Religious Diversity in Australia". He is a co-investigator on the Canadian "Nonreligion in a Complex Future" project lead by Professor Lori Beaman. His books include *LGBT Christians* (2017, with Bronwyn Fielder), *Reinventing Church* (2016, with Helen and James Collins), *Teenage Witches* (2007, with Helen Berger) and *Qualitative Analysis* (2002).

Lisa Fitzgerald is an Associate Professor in the School of Public Health, University of Queensland. She is public health sociologist with research interests in the health and wellbeing of people experiencing marginalisation and the social determinants of (sexual) health.

Lisa is the course coordinator of PUBH7620 Social Perspectives and PUBH7003 Qualitative Research Methods. She is engaged in social research projects related to HIV, sexual health, young people, LGBTIQA+ health, sex worker health and teaching the social determinants of health as a threshold concept in public health teaching and learning. Amongst her current interests, Lisa has an emerging interest in social research associated with young people and climate change.

Rubab Firdaus is a Research Officer at Western Sydney University as well as a practising physiotherapist. She has expertise in migrant populations and Indigenous-centred ideologies. She is also a sessional academic in the areas of Culture, Diversity and Health within the Bachelor of Health Science and teaching cultural competence to students across ten allied health disciplines at Western Sydney University. She has also been an alumnus of the University and acts as an ambassador for International and Domestic Students in their transitions to postgraduate study.

Ellen Fraser-Barbour is a Scholarly Fellow at Flinders University. Ellen has worked in government and non-government organisations and believes in recognition of the rights of people with disability across all aspects of community. Most recently Ellen served as a member of the Health Performance Council in South Australia co-leading an audit of access to health services and health outcomes for people with disability. Before starting her PhD in 2017, Ellen worked in a range of roles across the disability sector, including as a Disability Developmental Educator (Allied Health), team leader, family support worker and therapy assistant. She has also been involved in various peer-led advocacy groups. Ellen identifies as a disabled woman who is passionate about human rights and has a particular focus on discrimination, violence, abuse and neglect and prevention, recognition and redress.

Emma S. George is a Senior Lecturer in Health and Physical Education at Western Sydney University. Emma teaches across a range of undergraduate health science subjects, and her research aims to promote lifelong physical activity, reduce chronic disease risk and improve physical and mental health outcomes. She works closely with community and industry partners to develop evidence-based community health initiatives. Emma's research expertise includes health promotion intervention design, implementation and evaluation, mixed methods research, men's health, epidemiology and physical activity measurement. Her research has involved working with middle-age men, sport fans, older adults, youth and culturally diverse populations.

Natalie Hamam is a qualified Occupational Therapist with a range of clinical experience. Natalie is currently based in Albury and works in private practice with adults and children. She has completed a Graduate Diploma in Sexual Health in 2008, a research masters on sex after stroke in 2017 and also a Graduate Certificate in teaching and learning in higher education in 2018. Natalie is passionate about all people having access to the services they need at a fair price.

Sophie Hickey is an applied sociologist who works in health service research. She currently manages a large longitudinal cohort study of Aboriginal and Torres Strait Islander mothers and children designed to provide feedback to local service providers on best practice maternity care, which has seen a profound reduction in preterm birth for women accessing the new model of care. Sophie works in a very multidisciplinary team and uses institutional ethnography, participatory action research and implementation science to improve health services for Aboriginal and Torres Strait Islander people.

Syeda Zakia Hossain has a PhD in Sociology, an academic at the University of Sydney, is a Health Sociologist and a Demographer. She is a recipient of AusAID and Rockefeller Foundation Fellowships. Her teaching is in the areas of health sociology, cultural diversity and health, health professionals and globalisation, international health and chronic diseases, research methods and statistics. Her major research is on reproductive health, teenage pregnancy, chronic diseases including breast and cervical cancer, health inequalities, migrant women's health and wellbeing, cross-cultural issues and ageing, South Asian countries. She uses mixed methods.

Kimberley Ivory is an Honorary Senior Lecturer in Population Medicine at the University of Sydney. Dr Kimberley Ivory is also affiliated with the Sydney Health Ethics, School of Public Health, Faculty of Medicine and Health, at the University of Sydney. She is a medical doctor and completed her internship and residency at Royal North Shore Hospital. She was seconded several times to the NSW Mid-North coast, where she lived and worked as a GP for over 25 years. In 2000, she assisted in setting up a skin cancer clinic in Port Macquarie, which she ran until 2008, when she moved to Melbourne to complete her Master of Public Health (Sexual Health) at the University of Melbourne.

Keera Laccos-Barrett is a proud Ngarrindjeri woman from Southern Australia who has a strong interest in areas of Indigenous feminism, social justice, equity and human rights. Keera Laccos-Barrett is a Registered Nurse with over 10 years of clinical experience, who also holds a Graduate Certificate, Graduate Diploma and is currently undertaking a Master's in Nursing.

Pranee Liamputtong is an Adjunct Professor (Public Health) in the Translational Health Research Institute (THRI), Western Sydney University (WSU). Previously, she held a position of Professor of Public Health, School of Health Sciences, WSU and Personal Chair in Public Health, School of Public Health, La Trobe University, Melbourne. Pranee has also taught in the School of Sociology and Anthropology, La Trobe University. Her particular interests include issues related to cultural and social influences on childbearing, childrearing and women's reproductive and sexual health. She has carried out a number of research projects with refugee and immigrant women in Australia and women in Southeast Asia, particularly in Thailand and Malaysia. She has also undertaken qualitative research with women living with HIV/AIDS and women living with breast cancer in Thailand. Recently, Pranee has focused her research on sexuality and sexual health issues of Asian women, refugee/immi- grant women, young people, and trans women from CALD backgrounds.

Freya MacMillan is a Senior Lecturer in Interprofessional Health Sciences at Western Sydney University. Her research focuses on the development, evaluation and translation of lifestyle interventions for health promotion and diabetes prevention in those most at risk. She uses a mix of qualitative and quantitative techniques to do this and follows community engaged processes throughout her research to ensure the interventions she develops are appropriate, more likely adopted and sustainable.

Elias Mambo Machina is an academic tutor in culture, diversity and health at the Western Sydney University in Campbelltown, and a disability support worker for Phil Terry Healthcare Services, and All About Caring Pty Ltd. His academic tutoring introduces skills for understanding and engaging effectively with culturally and socially diverse populations in healthcare contexts. Directly, in the rehabilitation and human services, his work responds to clients' needs for assistance in activities of daily living, and person-centred individualized rehabilitation plans for community living, transitions to work, and returning to work.

Virginia Mapedzahama a PhD in Sociology. She has years of experience researching diversity, difference and social cohesion—in particular, lived experiences of diversity in Australia. Her research focuses on understanding the social construction of all categories of difference: meanings attached to this difference, how it is signified and lived, as well as its implications for those assigned difference. She explores this interest in the context of subjective experiences of migration, diaspora, blackness, race, racism and ethnicity, sexuality and gendered violence. Her expertise includes new African diaspora in Australia, race and ethnicity, cross-cultural identities, black subjectivities, hybridity, African feminisms, African women diaspora and intersectionality.

Kate A. McBride has broad research expertise in epidemiology, public health and the improvement of health at a population level through the reduction of disease. Kate's research focusses on the prevention and management of chronic disease, including cancer, diabetes and obesity within high-risk, marginalised populations, which includes through the optimisation of health care access among these individuals. Kate coordinates and teaches on several population health and evidence-based medicine units in the MD degree as well the Master's of Epidemiology. Kate began working at Western Sydney University in 2013 and most recently was appointed as Senior Lecturer in Population Health with the School of Medicine and Translational Health Research Institute.

Atari Metcalf is a junior medical doctor at St. Vincent's Hospital Sydney, with over 15 years of experience in health promotion research, policy and strategy. He began his career as a youth worker before progressing to senior research roles for online youth mental health service, ReachOut, health promotion education roles with VicHealth and Curtin University and, prior to practicing medicine, worked as an analyst on national inquiries into asylum seeker, transgender and intersex health and human rights for the Australian Human Rights Commission. Atari is a board director of ACON and formerly served on the boards of Suicide Prevention Australia and Twenty10 Incorporating GLCS NSW.

Julie Mooney-Somers is an Associate Professor at Sydney Health Ethics, School of Public Health, Faculty of Medicine and Health, University of Sydney. Her research focuses on the health of sexuality and gender diverse people (primarily related to tobacco, alcohol and other substance use). Julie leads the longest running periodic survey of lesbian, bisexual and queer women's health (SWASH) in collaboration with community health promotion organisation ACON. Engagement with LGBTIQ and First Nations people has profoundly shaped her work: she is committed to working with communities to undertake meaningful research for advocacy, health promotion and service design and delivery. www.juliemooneysomers.com

Elias Mpofu is a qualified rehabilitation counsellor and recipient of multiple international research awards in rehabilitation. Currently, he is the Professor of Health Services Research at the University of North Texas. He also is an Honorary Professor of Clinical and Rehabilitation Sciences at the University of Sydney, Adjunct Professor of the Translational Health Research Institute at the Western Sydney University and Distinguished Visiting Professor at the University of Johannesburg. Formerly Professor of Rehabilitation Services at the Pennsylvania State University, he has an international reputation in the scholarship of teaching with service-learning, and research on community-oriented health interventions.

Allyson Mutch is an Associate Professor in Health Systems in the School of Public Health, University of Queensland and a Senior Fellow in the Higher Education Academy. Her research uses qualitative methods to investigate the social determinants of health and the health and wellbeing of people who are marginalised and experiencing disadvantage. Allyson's research is firmly embedded in community, with strong links to community organisations to ensure her research is firmly grounded in the needs of community.

Angelica Ojinnaka is an emerging academic and Master of Research candidate in the Translational Health Research Institute at Western Sydney University. Her multidisciplinary research is focused in the areas of psychology, public health, social policy and sociology. Angelica's thesis examines how diverse children and young people with complex, interrelated and chronic needs perceive the Australian service system, and the extent to which they are engaged in service decision making and reform. She has a multidisciplinary background and holds an undergraduate qualification in psychology from Macquarie University. Angelica is an award-winning youth leader, working with various national youth and community organisations. She has extensive expertise in research, community development, human rights and youth mental health sectors.

Rebecca E. Olson is an Associate Professor in Sociology, University of Queensland, Co-Director of the University of Queensland's SocioHealthLab, and Program Director of the Bachelor of Social Science. Funded by competitive grants (e.g., NHMRC, Cancer Australia), her research intersects the sociologies of health and emotion. As a leading innovative qualitative researcher, Olson employs video-based, participatory, reflexive, post-qualitative and post-paradigmatic approaches to inform translational inquiry. Her recent books include *Towards a Sociology of Cancer Caregiving: Time to Feel* (Routledge, 2015) and *Emotions in Late Modernity* (Routledge, 2019, co-edited with Patulny, Bellocchi, Khorana, McKenzie and Peterie).

Rashmi Pithavadian is a sessional academic, research officer and Master of Research (MRes) candidate in the School of Health Sciences at Western Sydney University. Her MRes thesis focuses on how women with the female sexual dysfunction vaginismus seek help, and its impact on their sense of self. Rashmi has a multidisciplinary background with completed and ongoing tertiary qualifications in health sciences, sociology, cultural studies and English. Her research and award nominated teaching utilises a multidisciplinary approach to support the holistic wellbeing of marginalised populations in sexual health.

Kane Race is a Professor in the Department of Gender and Cultural Studies at the University of Sydney. He joined the department in 2007, after working at the National Centre in HIV Social Research at UNSW, where he also undertook his PhD in Health, Sexuality & Culture. He is a founding member of the Association for the Social Sciences and Humanities in HIV/AIDS and has published widely on the impact of HIV antiretroviral therapies on gay cultures, practices and politics. His work has explored embodied engagements with medicine across various contexts and cultures of consumption: HIV/AIDS; sexual practice; drug use (both licit and illicit); and more recently, markets in bottled water. His current work is concerned with the ways in which online devices and technologies participate in the making of new cultures, spaces and practices.

Kerry H. Robinson is a Professor in Sociology in the School of Social Sciences at Western Sydney University. She is Director of the Diversity and Human Rights Research Centre (DHRRC) and a member of Sexualities and Genders Research (SaGR), which she led prior to her current position with DHRRC. Her research expertise includes gender and sexuality studies; sexual harassment; gender and sexuality based violence prevention; childhood, young people, gender and sexual citizenship; sexuality education; and equity and diversity in education. Kerry has published widely in her field. She was the lead researcher of the *Growing Up Queer* research (Robinson et al., 2014).

S. **Rachel Skinner** is a Professor in the Discipline of Child and Adolescent Health, Faculty of Medicine and Health, The University of Sydney. She is Deputy Director of Wellbeing, Health and Youth, NHMRC Centre for Research Excellence in Adolescent Health: a collaboration across five Australian Universities. She is also Senior Clinical Advisor in Youth Health and Wellbeing at NSW Ministry of Health. Her research addresses a broad range of public health, biopsychosocial, behavioural and ethical aspects of adolescent health. Her approach is interdisciplinary and focussed on translation of findings into real-world interventions with clear impact on health outcomes. She is also known internationally for her work on human papillomavirus (HPV) vaccine efficacy, effectiveness and school vaccination programs; and for work on sexual behaviour, contraception and early pregnancy in adolescents.

Genevieve Z. Steiner is an Associate Professor in Cognitive Neuroscience, an NHMRC Emerging Leadership Fellow and Director of Research at the NICM Health Research Institute, Western Sydney University. Her research spans the early detection, prevention and treatment of memory and thinking problems in older people with the aim of reducing dementia risk and improving quality of life. Her team examines changes in the brain's function and structure to discover mechanisms associated with dementia risk, and test novel therapeutics that can provide early intervention.

Janelle Trees, Goori descendant of the Thungutti clan, is a Fellow of the Royal College of Australian General Practice. Her Bachelor of Medicine and Bachelor of Surgery (University of Sydney), made her the first Aboriginal person awarded Honours by their School of Medicine. She earned a Bachelor of Science with First Class Honours from the University of New South Wales. Dr Trees works as the Community Doctor in the Fitzroy Valley, travelling with her wife Claudia. Editor of Diabetes Management Journal, she writes for the Illawarra Aboriginal Medical Service's Cancer Care Team and Australian Doctor.

Alexander Workman is a Criminologist and PhD student at Western Sydney University. Alex's research focuses on Intimate Partner Violence in marginalised LGBTIQ populations, primarily focusing on survivor resilience after the relationship's conclusion. Alex's background stems from law enforcement, human rights and public health, who believes all social justice issues require an intersectional lens. Furthermore, Alex both teaches and lectures in Health Sciences and Social Sciences in criminological theory, cultural diversity, human rights and peacebuilding. Based on Alex's research output and recognition as a Subject Matter Expert, Alex is now the Convener of the Intersectionality in Law Enforcement and Public Health Special Interest Group, part of the Global Law Enforcement and Public Health Association (GLEPHA).

Acknowledgements

This book was born from the desire for the world to be ready for the diversity that is inevitable when migration and globalisation become synonymous with development. As tertiary teachers, academic researchers and health practitioners, we have seen the benefits of cultural safety and shortfalls when it is ignored. It was astonishing that until this point no Australian textbook existed to teach health students about how to support cultural safety. This book started as a response to our professional experiences, our students' frustrations and our in-depth explorations of humanity and health through scholarly research. That foundation and passion has manifested into this robust collection of rigorous evidence about cultural safety and health care in Australia. While we are immensely proud of this book, this process could not have been possible without the support of a great number of people.

I, Tinashe Dune, would like to thank Nina Sharpe, whose publishing experience and guidance helped me to develop my ideas about this book and to create a compelling case for its necessity. It was also she who connected me to Kim McLeod and Robyn Williams, whose work I had envied from afar for many years. Kim and Robyn took my ideas and goals for this book and transformed them into reality. Their expert knowledge on the needs of health students and health consumers has ensured that readers are provided with multidimensional perspectives across diverse disciplines.

With the publishing expertise and tenacity of Sandra Rigby, Samantha Mansell and Elizabeth Weiss, we were able to engage collaborators to produce high-quality and meaningful learning content for the next generation of health professionals in Australia. We have also been supported by Grace McInnes and Evie Lonsdale, whose guidance and patience in the finalisation and publishing of the book has streamlined the process and made a long journey well worth the wait.

We would also like to thank Angelica Ojinnaka, our Editorial Assistant, for her tireless and expert support in pulling all the parts of the book together into one beautiful piece of work. Her assistance and passion for the topic ensured that the book looks and feels as we had hoped from day one.

This book would not have been possible without its chapter contributors, who worked diligently to produce evidence-based knowledge for health students. Their innovation in the development of interesting reflective activities and the provision of multidimensional and intersecting case studies ensures that students are exposed to a vast diversity of experience and ways to apply their new understandings of cultural safety. The passion and priority that the chapter contributors dedicated to this book demonstrates their desire for Australia's next cohort of health care professionals and providers to be some of the best in the world. With the contributors' expert knowledge, future generations are well on their way to this goal.

Thank you to past, present and future students who shape the way we share knowledge and experience about cultural safety and who challenge us to teach in new, dynamic and contemporary ways. We thank you for your willingness to grapple with the topics presented in this book and to embrace the excitement and discomfort of providing health care in an ever-changing world.

Finally, we thank our families and close colleagues/friends, who have seen us through this journey and have cheered us on along the way. From the seed of an idea this book has grown and developed. It is because of the consistent nourishment from those who care for and love us that we have been able to see this through. Following years of work, support, passion and strength, we are proud to share this book with you.

Tinashe Dune
Kim McLeod
Robyn Williams

Abbreviations

AAG	Australian Association on Gerontology
ACCHOs	Aboriginal Community Controlled Health Organisations
ACM	Australian College of Midwives
Ahpra	Australian Health Practitioner Regulation Agency
AHRC	Australian Human Rights Commission
AIDA	Australian Indigenous Doctors Association
AIHW	Australian Institute of Health and Welfare
ALO	Aboriginal Liaison Officer
AMS	Aboriginal Medical Service (AMS)
ANMF	Australian Nursing and Midwifery Federation
AWAU	African Women Australia Inc.
BMA	British Medical Association
CALD	Culturally and Linguistically Diverse
CAN	Australian College of Nurses
CATSINaM	Congress of Aboriginal and Torres Strait Islander Nurses and Midwives
CDC	Centers for Disease Control and Prevention
CHD	Coronary heart disease
COPD	Chronic obstructive pulmonary disease
COTA	Council on the Ageing
CSDH	Commission on the Social Determinants of Health
CTG	Closing the Gap
CVD	Cardiovascular disease
DSM V	Diagnostic and Statistical Manual of Mental Disorders, Fifth Edition
FGM	Female genital mutilation
HPV	Human papillomavirus
IAHA	Indigenous Allied Health Australia
ICAC	Independent Commissioner Against Corruption
ICD-11	International Classification of Diseases
LGBTIQA+	Lesbian, Gay, Bisexual, Transgender, Intersex, Queer/questioning, Asexual, and other terms
MHIRC	Men's Health Information and Resource Centre
NATSIHWA	National Aboriginal and Torres Strait Islander Health Worker Association
NESB	Non-English Speaking Background
NHLF	National Health Leadership Forum
NHMRC	National Health and Medical Research Council
NMBA	Nursing and Midwifery Board of Australia

NRAS	National Registration and Accreditation Scheme
NRHA	National Rural Health Alliance of Australia
NSW	New South Wales
PTSD	Post-Traumatic Stress Disorder
RACGP	Royal Australian College of General Practitioners
RACP	Royal Australasian College of Physicians
RFDS	Royal Flying Doctor Service
RN	Registered Nurse
SDH	Social Determinants of Health
SES	Socio-economic status
STIs	Sexually transmitted infections
UDHR	Universal Declaration of Human Rights
UHC	Universal health coverage
WHO	World Health Organisation

Part I

Understanding culture, diversity and health

1 An introduction to culture, diversity and health in Australia

Tinashe Dune, Kim McLeod and Robyn Williams

Learning outcomes

After working through this chapter, students should be able to:

1. Explore statistics related to Australia's ethnic, cultural, racial and religious diversity.
2. Reflect on the role of social determinants of health in a diverse Australian context.
3. Understand what social constructs are, and consider their role in determining experiences of health and wellbeing.
4. Consider what health and wellbeing means to people from diverse Australian perspectives.
5. Understand what is meant by cultural safety and its significance in Australia.

Key terms

Cultural safety: An environment that is spiritually, socially and emotionally safe, as well as physically safe for people; where there is no assault challenge or denial of their identity, of who they are and what they need.
Culture: The evolved human capacity to classify and represent experiences with symbols and to act imaginatively and creatively. Cultures are differentiated by the distinct ways that people, who live differently, classify and represent their experiences.
Diversity: Degree of variation of cultures, identities and other social and economic factors within a given society.
Ethnicity: A category or group of people who identify with each other, usually on the basis of presumed similarities such as common language, geography, ancestry, history, society, culture and/or social treatment.
Identity: Identity is a person's conception and expression of their individuality or group affiliations.
Intersectionality: The interconnected nature of social categorisations such as race, class, and gender as they apply to a given individual or group, regarded as creating overlapping and interdependent systems of discrimination or disadvantage.
Race: A socially constructed grouping of humans based on shared physical categories generally viewed as distinct by a society.
Social construct: A perception of an individual, group, or idea that is "constructed" through cultural or social practice.
Social determinants of health: Conditions in which people are born, grow, work, live, and age, and the wider set of forces and systems shaping the conditions of daily life. These forces and systems include economic policies and systems, development agendas, social norms, social policies and political systems.

Chapter summary

This chapter introduces students to the social and cultural diversity of Australia. It defines diversity and notes the extent of diversities across the Australian population. Students then review introductory aspects of health and wellbeing in relation to diversity in Australia and the concept of social determinants of health. In this chapter students will begin the process of self-awareness and self-reflection and be tasked with exploring their own identities within Australia's diverse context and the ways in which this may impact their health and wellbeing. The chapter finally engages students to start thinking about their role as health care professionals in Australia's multicultural society and how they can engage with the concepts presented within the book. This chapter will briefly introduce the concept of cultural safety and provide a summary of the book's three major parts.

Diversity in Australia

Australia is quickly becoming known as one of the most diverse Western nations in the world. The most recent Census indicates that Australians represent over 300 separately identified ancestries (Australian Bureau of Statistics, 2016). Australia is therefore well known for its multicultural population characterised by a vast diversity of cultural, ethnic, religious and linguistic groups. As such, a review of Australian statistics can help to orient students to a small slice of Australia's diversity.

Country of birth, ethnicity and ancestry

In the 2016 Census, Australia's Aboriginal and Torres Strait Islander people represented 2.8% of the population—an increase from 2.5% in 2011 and 2.3% in 2006. Of the 649,171 people who identified as Aboriginal and/or Torres Strait Islander in 2016, 91% were of Aboriginal origin, 5.0% were of Torres Strait Islander origin and 4.1% identified as being of both Aboriginal and Torres Strait Islander origin (Australian Bureau of Statistics, 2016).

In addition to Aboriginal and Torres Strait Islander populations, increasing net overseas migration contributes to over 60% of Australia's total population growth. Australia thus provides a particularly rich case study of a diverse country undergoing rapid transformation. For instance, over 28% of Australians were born overseas, and another 20% have at least one parent born overseas (Australian Bureau of Statistics, 2016).

The Census also revealed that two-thirds (67%) of the Australian population were born in Australia. Overseas-born Australians make up 6,163,667 of Australia's total population of 23,401,892. Of these overseas-born Australians, nearly one in five (18%) had arrived since the start of 2012 (Australian Bureau of Statistics, 2016).

Despite the common belief that most migrants to Australia arrive from non-Western nations, England and New Zealand remain the next most common countries of birth after Australia. There have also been some increases in migration from the next two most common countries of birth—China and India—since 2011 (from 6.0% to 8.3%, and 5.6% to 7.4%, respectively) (Australian Bureau of Statistics, 2016).

Geography

For Australia's overseas-born population, New South Wales was still the most popular state or territory to live in 2016 (2,072,454 people, or 34% of the overseas-born population). Further, Sydney had the largest overseas-born population, and an overall 83% of the overseas-born population lived in a capital city compared with 61% of people born in Australia (Australian Bureau of Statistics, 2016).

Language

In Australia, there are over 300 separately identified languages spoken, with more than one-fifth (21%) of Australians speaking a language other than English at home. The top languages other than English spoken by Australians were Mandarin (2.5%), Arabic (1.4%), Vietnamese (1.2%) and Cantonese (1.2%) (Australian Bureau of Statistics, 2016).

Religion

In Australia, Christianity (52%) was the main religion reported in the 2016 Census. The Islamic population made up only 2.6% of the total population and was the second-largest religion reported after Christianity. Buddhism closely followed at 2.4%. The number of Australians who indicated that they followed *No Religion* has increased from 22% in 2011 to 30% in 2016 (Australian Bureau of Statistics, 2016).

Diversifying the term diversity

When the term *diversity* is discussed, it is most often in the context of cultural, ethnic or religious diversity as discussed earlier. However, multiple aspects of diversity need to be considered, especially when working in the health sector. This diversity includes race, gender, sexuality, age, disability, socio-economic status and education—to name a few. These elements of diversity, as well as *culture*, *ethnicity* and religion, are filtered through social, political and cultural norms and expectations that determine how we experience health in Australia (Hosseini Shokouh et al., 2017). These are called the *social determinants of health* and are discussed in depth in Chapter 2.

Box 1.1 Reflection—Understanding identity and social determinants

Answer the following questions to begin exploring your identity and the social determinants that have an impact on your health and wellbeing.

1. Where were you born?
2. Where were your parents born?
3. Where were your ancestors from?
4. Where do you live? Is it urban or rural?
5. What language(s) do you speak?
6. Do you follow a religion? If yes, which one?

An introduction to social determinants of health

In the next chapter (Chapter 2), you will be introduced to the social determinants of health and the impact these determinants have on the ways that Australians experience their health and wellbeing. Generally, the social determinants of health are the conditions in which people are born, grow, live, work and age. These circumstances are shaped by the distribution of money, power and resources at global, national and local levels.

Take, for instance, age and ethnicity as important and intersecting determinants of health. As a preview to Chapter 7, the Australian Bureau of Statistics (2016) indicated that since the 1996 Census, the median age for Aboriginal and Torres Strait Islander people has been on the rise. Twenty years ago, in 1996, the median age was 20. This had increased to 21 years in 2011 and increased again to 23 years in the 5 years to 2016. The median age for non-Indigenous people was 38 in 2016.

Notably, Aboriginal and Torres Strait Islander people continue to have a much younger age profile and structure than the non-Indigenous population. In 2016, more than half (53%) of Aboriginal and Torres Strait Islander people were under age 25 years. In comparison, almost one in three (31%) non-Indigenous people were under age 25. The difference between the two populations was also marked in the 65 years and over age group. The proportion of Aboriginal and Torres Strait Islander people age 65 years and over was considerably smaller than for non-Indigenous people (4.8% compared to 16%).

Statistics indicate that Aboriginal and Torres Strait Islander people have a lower life expectancy than non-Indigenous people (Australian Bureau of Statistics, 2018). Data also tells us that Aboriginal and Torres Strait Islander people are more likely to experience a range of health concerns earlier in life than their non-Indigenous counterparts (Australian Institute of Health and Welfare, 2016).

In this book, we ask students to begin reflecting and exploring the reasons why these statistical trends exist and persist. For instance, what is behind these differences and the factors that make changing these statistics challenging? Such questions are discussed and the answers critiqued in Chapters 2 and 7—as well as throughout this book. To assist students in exploring social determinants, understanding that our social contexts provide us with guidelines on how to live and interact is needed. These guidelines are sometimes called social constructions.

What are social constructions, and why do they matter?

Social constructions are based on a theory that people develop knowledge of the world in a social context (Burr & Dick, 2017). In line with this perspective, social constructions dictate that much of what we perceive as our reality depends on shared assumptions (Burr & Dick, 2017). These assumptions are imbedded in our cultures and inform us on how we should understand and interact with ourselves, others and the world (Burr & Dick, 2017). By understanding social constructions, we can begin to explore the idea that we often take for granted or believe in an objective reality, which is in fact socially constructed and, thus, can change as societies and cultures change (Burr & Dick, 2017). Take the concept of *race*, which many people assume to be based on scientific fact and to be helpful in understanding diverse experiences and characteristics. However, research consistently indicates that the concept of race is socially constructed and provides no insights into the genetic and physiological characteristics of diverse people (Dei, 2009). Consider the following excerpts of an article published in *Scientific American* that expounds on this reality.

Box 1.2 Race is a social construct

Article 1.1: Race Is a Social Construct, Scientists Argue

Racial categories are weak proxies for genetic diversity and need to be phased out

By Megan Gannon, Live Science on February 5, 2016

More than 100 years ago, American sociologist W. E. B. Du Bois was concerned that race was being used as a biological explanation for what he understood to be social and cultural differences between different populations of people. He spoke out against the idea of "white" and "black" as discrete groups, claiming that these distinctions ignored the scope of human diversity.

Science would favor Du Bois. Today, the mainstream belief among scientists is that race is a social construct without biological meaning. And yet, you might still open a study on genetics in a major scientific journal and find categories like "white" and "black" being used as biological variables.

> It's a concept we think is too crude to provide useful information, it's a concept that has social meaning that interferes in the scientific understanding of human genetic diversity and it's a concept that we are not the first to call upon moving away from,

said Michael Yudell, a professor of public health at Drexel University in Philadelphia.

> What the study of complete genomes from different parts of the world has shown is that even between Africa and Europe, for example, there is not a single absolute genetic difference, meaning no single variant where all Africans have one variant and all Europeans another one, even when recent migration is disregarded,

Pääbo told Live Science. "It is all a question of differences in how frequent different variants are on different continents and in different regions."

In one example that demonstrated genetic differences were not fixed along racial lines, the full genomes of James Watson and Craig Venter, two famous American scientists of European ancestry, were compared to that of a Korean scientist, Seong-Jin Kim. It turned out that Watson (who, ironically, became ostracized in the scientific community after making racist remarks) and Venter shared fewer variations in their genetic sequences than they each shared with Kim.

Assumptions about genetic differences between people of different races have had obvious social and historical repercussions, and they still threaten to fuel racist beliefs. That was apparent two years ago, when several scientists bristled at the inclusion of their research in Nicholas Wade's controversial book, *A Troublesome Inheritance* (2015), which proposed that genetic selection has given rise to distinct behaviors among different populations. In a letter to *The New York Times*, five researchers wrote that "Wade juxtaposes an incomplete and inaccurate account of our research on human genetic differences with speculation that recent natural selection has led to worldwide differences in IQ test results, political institutions and economic development".

The authors of the new Science article noted that racial assumptions could also be particularly dangerous in a medical setting.

https://www.scientificamerican.com/article/race-is-a-social-construct-scientists-argue/

Box 1.3 Reflection—Theory of social constructionism

- The theory of social constructionism states that meaning and knowledge are socially created. Social constructionists believe that knowledge arises out of human relationships. Thus, what we take to be true and objective is the result of social processes that take place in historical and cultural contexts.
- Social constructionists believe that things that are generally viewed as natural or normal in society, such as understandings of gender, race, class, and disability, are socially constructed and consequently are not an accurate reflection of reality.
- Language is central to social construction as it abides by specific rules, and these rules of language shape how we understand the world. As a result, language isn't neutral. It emphasises certain things while ignoring others. Thus, language constrains what we can express as well as our perceptions of what we experience and what we know.
- Social constructs are often created within specific institutions and cultures and come to prominence in certain historical periods. Social constructs' dependence on historical, political and economic conditions can lead them to evolve and change.
- Knowledge construction is politically driven given that the knowledge created in a community has social, cultural and political consequences. People in a community accept and sustain the community's understanding of particular truths, values and realities. When new members of a community accept such knowledge, it extends even further. When a community's accepted knowledge becomes policy, ideas about power and privilege in the community become codified. These socially constructed ideas then create social reality, and—if they aren't examined—begin to seem fixed and unchangeable. This can lead to antagonistic relationships between communities that don't share the same understanding of social reality.

https://www.thoughtco.com/social-constructionism-4586374

To explore social constructions in more depth, this book asks students to consistently reflect on what role *social constructs* play in determining experiences of health and wellbeing. And in particular, what social constructions (e.g., about race, disability, sexuality, gender) make up your *identity*, as well as how various social determinants and social constructions intersect to make you who you are. These are important considerations in supporting diverse health and wellbeing needs. By engaging with difference and diversity, we can learn how to support people from various backgrounds and promote cultural safety in all the places we live, work and play. Understanding social constructions helps us to realise that we are not just one identity but many. For instance, a woman may also be Aboriginal, be over 45 and identify as lesbian. These intersecting identities have an impact on how this woman will experience life, partly because of how these identities are socially constructed and how her community and society perceive and treat people within those identities. This is where intersectionality can help us to understand why and how social determinants and social constructions can have multiple levels and complex impacts on health and wellbeing.

Health and intersecting identities: Intersectionality

Emerging from the African American feminist movement in the 1980s, the term *intersectionality* challenges the notion of a universal gendered experience for women, with Kimberlé Crenshaw, the originator of the term, arguing that we need to look at the intersection of race and gender when understanding the experience of women of colour (Crenshaw, 1989). More recent developments of intersectionality focus on the interaction and mutually constitutive nature of gender, sexual identity, race, social class, age and other categories of difference in individual lives and social practices, and the association of these arrangements with health and wellbeing (Hankivsky, Cormier, & de Merich, 2009;Vaughan et al., 2015).

This framework recognises that people from all backgrounds are characterised simultaneously by multiple and interconnected social categories, and that these categories are properties of the individual in terms of their identity, as well as characteristics of social structures (Crenshaw, 1991). Analyses of single determinants—such as gender—independently are insufficient, as social categories such as gender, race and sexuality are experienced simultaneously (de Vries, 2015; Moolchaem, Liamputtong, O'Halloran, & Muhamad, 2015).These intersections potentially expose people to multiple modes of marginalisation (Glass et al., 2011).

Intersectionality therefore recognises that people can be privileged in some ways and definitely not privileged in others. Many different types of privilege, not just skin color, impact the way people can navigate through their environments or whether and how they are discriminated against.These are all things you are born into, not things you earned, that afford you opportunities that others may not have.These include, but are not limited to, the following social determinants:

- Race: Being born with lighter skin often comes with a range of privileges that people with darker skin are not presented with.
- Citizenship: Simply being born in this country affords you citizenship privileges (such as leaving and re-entering Australia as many times as a person wants) that non-citizens will never access.
- Class: Being born into a financially stable family can help guarantee your health, safety, education and future opportunities.
- Sexual orientation: If you identify as heterosexual, every state in this country affords you privileges that non-heterosexual folks have to fight for in the Supreme Court.
- Sex: If you were born male, you will not experience sexual violence to the extent Australian women do. One in five women have experienced sexual violence since the age of 15 (Australian Bureau of Statistics, 2017).
- Ability: If you were born able-bodied, you probably don't have to plan your life around disability access, Braille or other needs based on your abilities.
- Gender identity: If you were born cisgender (that is, your gender identity matches the sex you were presumed at birth), you don't have to worry that using public toilets or change rooms will invoke public outrage.

Not to imply that any form of privilege is exactly the same as another, or that people lacking in one area of privilege understand what it's like to be lacking in other areas. For instance, race discrimination is not the same as sex discrimination. Recognising privilege simply means being aware that some people have to work much harder just to experience the things other people take for granted (if they ever can experience them at all). In this book, keeping intersectionality in mind allows us to examine these diverse, complex and interrelated social determinants in relation to cultural safety in health care (see Chapter 4).

Cultural safety, diversity and the health care system

In this book, students will be provided with in-depth and multifaceted perspectives of cultural safety and how it is applied to health and wellbeing professional practice.The concept of cultural safety will be discussed in detail in Chapter 4, which begins with the following definition of cultural safety. *Cultural safety* is defined as:

> The effective nursing practice of a person or family from another culture and is determined by that person or family. Culture includes, but is not restricted to, age or generation; gender; sexual orientation; occupation and socioeconomic status; ethnic origin or migrant experience; religious or spiritual belief; and disability. The nurse delivering the nursing service will have undertaken a process of reflection on their own cultural identity and will recognise the impact their personal culture has on their professional practice. Unsafe cultural practice comprises any action which diminishes, demeans or disempowers the cultural identity and wellbeing of an individual.
>
> (Nursing Council of New Zealand, 2012)

Why is cultural safety important?

Cultural safety provides a means to examine how people are treated in society and how they are affected by systemic and structural issues and social determinants of health. It represents a key philosophical shift from providing care regardless of who an individual is, to acknowledging that each person's identity is central to the provision of health care (Eckermann et al., 2010; Taylor & Guerin, 2019). Cultural safety takes into account peoples' unique needs and requires an ongoing process of practitioner self-reflection, cultural self-awareness and an acknowledgement of how these factors impact care (De Souza, 2008; Ramsden, 2002). Importantly, cultural safety uses a broad definition of culture that does not reduce it to ethnicity only. Instead, it includes a range of variables, such as age/generation, sexual orientation, socio-economic status, religious or spiritual beliefs, gender and ability (Cox, 2016).

Cultural safety works on the premise that professions and workplaces also have cultures (not only the clients). Cultural safety is therefore as applicable to working with colleagues as it is to actual health care. Originally based on a Māori knowledge construct, cultural safety has a crucial role to play in Australian health care as it provides a decolonising model of practice based on dialogue, communication, power sharing and negotiation and acknowledgment of whiteness and privilege (Best, 2018; Mkandawire-Valhmu, 2018; Taylor & Guerin, 2019; Wepa, 2015). These actions are a means to challenge racism at personal and institutional levels, and to establish trust in health care encounters.

The role of health professionals in promoting cultural safety

Unlike other models of health care between self and different "others", cultural safety is not about progress through certain levels of awareness and practice along a staged or linear continuum. The process is a lifelong one and does not require the study of any culture other than one's own—so as to be aware of the impacts and implication of our own cultures, open-minded and flexible in our attitudes towards others (Cox, 2016). Identifying what makes others different is simple—understanding our own culture and its influence on how we think, feel and behave is much more complex. This is particularly the case when one is a member of the dominant culture in a society, as the features of dominant cultures become social norms and the standard by which others are judged. The features of the more dominant cultures become normalised and therefore invisible. Ultimately, cultural safety is about the receiver of health services who determines if their care was culturally safe or not (McEldowney & Connor, 2011; Richardson, 2012). This book provides students with the opportunity to reflect on what this all means for themselves as consumers of health care and soon-to-be health care professionals/practitioners.

Box 1.4 Reflection—The role of health professionals in promoting cultural safety

If cultural safety is about the client/patient/consumer, does cultural safety apply to the people who provide health care?

What social determinants and social constructions about health workers might influence their experience of working in a culturally safe environment?

What social determinants and social constructions about health workers might influence their ability to provide care that is culturally safe?

Culture, diversity and health in Australia: Towards cultural safety

With the rapid changes in the diversity of Australian society, health students require comprehensive information to introduce and explain important aspects of Australia's social and cultural diversity. Importantly, this book helps students to explore the impact of their future health care practice on health and wellbeing outcomes. Central to this aim, students will be asked to conceptualise diverse populations using a strengths-based lens. So instead of thinking about what people lack, students will be encouraged to explore how diversity in social determinants and experience contribute to individual and community resilience and opportunities for improved health outcomes. In this book, we define strengths-based approaches as those that focus on individual strengths (including personal strengths and social and community networks) and not on their deficits. Strengths-based practice is holistic and multidisciplinary and works with the individual to promote their wellbeing. It is outcomes led and not services led.

To put strengths-based approaches into practice, this book challenges students to think about health and wellbeing in ways that decolonise experiences. Decolonising health and wellbeing means that we learn to see and respect the different ways that people and communities understand and express their experiences. That is, this book encourages students to consider what health and wellbeing might look like for non-Western cultures and the impact (for better and for worse) of Westernisation on diverse groups. To assist students in this sometimes confronting and challenging work, this book covers important aspects of cultural and social diversity in relation to the health and wellbeing of Australians within an Australian context.

Rationale for this textbook

Engaging with these diverse ways of thinking and understanding both health and wellbeing is of great importance to a health care professional's ability to be impactful in their work in Australia. Nationally, all accrediting bodies for allied health, nursing and midwifery and medical professions require tertiary students to be culturally safe with regards to cultural and social diversity. This textbook responds to this need for cultural safety teaching and learning to assist health professionals with their development of cultural safety perspectives and practice. As explained earlier, cultural safety is not a *tick-box* list or task-based activity. It requires professionals and practitioners to develop critical reflexivity, mutual respect and trust towards improving health outcomes for all Australians.

As such this book is relevant to a range of interprofessional health science, nursing and midwifery and medicine students including, but not limited to, those enrolled in the following courses: Paramedicine; Health Promotion; Health Services Management; Occupational Therapy; Personal Development, Health and Physical Education; Physiotherapy; Podiatry; Traditional Chinese Medicine; Therapeutic Recreation; and Sport and Exercise Science. To provide a broad and interprofessional perspective on cultural safety, this book is divided into four parts with chapters written by topic and discipline experts from around Australia and the world.

Overview of the textbook

Part I of the book contains three chapters focused on setting the foundation for learning about cultural safety. This section includes the following:

- Chapter 1 introduces students to the social and cultural diversity in Australia. It also defines diversity and notes the extent of diversities across the Australian population.
- Chapter 2 provides students with a conceptual framework for examining the role of social determinants on health within' Australia.
- Chapter 3 delves into models of health and wellbeing in Australia and internationally with a focus on the biomedical, biopsychosocial, primary health care, Indigenous, and non-Western perspectives.

Part II of the book contains three chapters specifically focused on engaging students with the concept of cultural safety in theory and in practice. This section includes the following:

- Chapter 4 formally introduces students to the concept of cultural safety in health practice, especially interdisciplinary and interprofessional health care.
- Chapter 5 focuses on how health policy and advocacy influence culturally diverse health care.
- Chapter 6 helps students to link their understandings of cultural safety to practical outcomes and objectives. It also highlights ways to engage in culturally safe practice, particularly in interdisciplinary and interprofessional settings.

Part III of this book includes seven chapters that provide context to cultural safety across diverse population groups. This section includes the following:

- Chapter 7 encourages students to apply their understanding of social determinants of health and cultures of health in relation to the experiences of Indigenous peoples in Australia.
- Chapter 8 develops students' understanding of Australia's migration history following the arrival of the first Europeans through to the present-day migration experiences of culturally and linguistically diverse (CALD) Australians.
- Chapter 9 explores religious diversity and how religion can impact delivery of health services.
- Chapter 10 explores social determinants of health in order to gain a better understanding of disability; its incidence, prevalence and impact on disadvantaged populations.
- Chapter 11 explores how social constructions of gender in Australia influence health outcomes for men and women.
- Chapter 12 explores the differences and intersections between gender, sex and sexuality and the changing use of language and discourses, including those within health, medicine and human rights, to describe these terms.
- Chapter 13 discusses the impact on Australia's population as a result of ageing and the impact that has on the health care system and social determinants of health for Australians across the lifespan.

Part IV of the book provides a comprehensive set of teaching materials for educators.

- Chapter 14 discusses the future of culture, diversity and health in Australia and provides a model for curriculum to support teaching and learning of cultural safety to undergraduate health students.

Cultural safety teaching and learning resources in this book

In addition to the knowledge content of each chapter, the book also provides readers and teachers with ways to develop required capacities and skills in line with national accreditation expectations. To do so, this book includes multimedia links to provide students with examples of culturally safe practice (e.g., developing self-awareness, enacting cultural responsiveness, culturally safe communication), and case studies to assist with tutorial discussions or used as assessment tasks. Each chapter will include learning outcomes, which are aligned with national cultural safety requirements. In Chapter 14, teachers are provided with assessment ideas, short-answer and multiple-choice questions to support engagement and assess learning with their students. Students will also find a table at the end of the book that students and teachers can use to review students' understanding of cultural safety. This table will also allow students to indicate the ways in which they have met each cultural safety requirement and is used as part of their assessment in the unit.

Conclusion

Australia is increasingly recognised for its multiculturalism and diversity. In Australia, migration accounts for 60% of Australia's population growth in addition to increasing recognition of the needs of people with disabilities, ageing populations, sexually diverse populations and non-Western health care services. With this change in Australian society, health students require a comprehensive understanding of important aspects of Australia's social and cultural diversity and the impact of diversity on their future health practice and community health outcomes.

Cultural and social diversity are complicated concepts, especially in the context of health and wellbeing outcomes. As such, this book is written in a way that introduces readers to some of the more complex concepts, while ensuring that readers receive an academic and well-rounded discussion of the topics.

By engaging with the concepts in this book students will be closer to effectively supporting cultural safety—an environment that is spiritually, socially and emotionally safe, as well as physically safe for people; where there is no assault challenge or denial of their identity, of who they are and what they need.

References

Australian Bureau of Statistics. (2016). *Census of population and housing: Reflecting Australia: Stories from the Census (no. 2071.0).* https://www.abs.gov.au/ausstats/abs@.nsf/Lookup/by%20Subject/2071.0~2016~Main%20Features~Snapshot%20of%20Australia,%202016~2.

Australian Bureau of Statistics. (2017). *Personal safety survey 2016. ABS cat. no. 4906.0.* Canberra: ABS. http://www.abs.gov.au/ausstats/abs@.nsf/mf/4906.0.

Australian Bureau of Statistics. (2018). *Life tables for Aboriginal and Torres Strait Islander Australians, 2015–2017. Cat. no. 3302.0.55.003*, ABS: Canberra.

Australian Institute of Health and Welfare. (2016). *Australian Burden of Disease Study: Impact and causes of illness and death in Aboriginal and Torres Strait Islander people 2011—Summary report. Australian Burden of Disease Study series no. 7. Cat. no. BOD 8.* AIHW, Canberra.

Beagan, B. L. (2003). "Is this worth getting into a big fuss over?" Everyday racism in medical school. *Medical Education*, *37*, 852–860.

Best, O. (2018). The cultural safety journey: An Aboriginal Australian nursing and midwifery context. In O. Best & B. Fredericks (Eds.), *Yatdjuligin: Aboriginal and Torres Strait Islander nursing and midwifery care* (2nd ed., pp. 46–64). Cambridge University Press.

Burr, V., & Dick, P. (2017). Social constructionism. In B. Gough (Ed.), *The Palgrave handbook of critical social psychology* (pp. 59–80). Palgrave Macmillan.

Cox, L. (2016). Social change and social justice: Cultural safety as a vehicle for nurse activism. In T. Rudge (Ed.), *Proceedings of the 2nd Critical Perspectives in Nursing and Health Care International Conference* (pp. 1–11). University of Sydney.

Crenshaw, K. (1989). Demarginalizing the intersection of race and sex: A black feminist critique of antidiscrimination doctrine, feminist theory and antiracist politics. *University of Chicago Legal Forum*, *1989*(1), 139–167.

Crenshaw, K. (1991). Mapping the margins: Intersectionality, identity politics, and violence against women of color. *Stanford Law Review*, *43*(6), 1241–1299. https://doi.org/10.2307/1229039.

De Souza, R. (2008). Wellness for all: The possibilities of cultural safety and cultural competence in New Zealand. *Journal of Research in Nursing*, *13*(2), 125–135. doi. https://doi.org/10.1177/1744987108088637.

Dei, G. (2009). Speaking race: Silence, salience, and the politics of anti-racist scholarship. In M. Wallis & A. Fleras (Eds.), *The politics of race in Canada* (2nd ed., pp. 230–238). Oxford University Press.

de Vries, K. M. (2015). Transgender people of color at the center: Conceptualizing a new intersectional model. *Ethnicities*, *15*(1), 3–27. doi. 10.1177/1468796814547058.

Eckermann, A. K., Dowd, T., Chong, E., Nixon, L., Gray, R., & Johnson, S. (2010). *Binan Goonj: Bridging cultures in Aboriginal health* (3rd ed.). Elsevier.

Glass, N., Annan, S. L., Bhandari, T. B., & Fishwick, N. (2011). Nursing care of immigrant & rural abused women. In J. Humphreys & J. C. Campbell (Eds.), *Family violence and nursing practice* (2nd ed., pp. 207–224). Springer.

Hankivsky, O., Cormier, R., & de Merich, D. (2009). *Intersectionality: Moving women's health research and policy forward*. Women's Health Research Network.

Hosseini Shokouh, S. M., Mohammad, A., Emamgholipour, S., Rashidian, A., Montazeri, A., & Zaboli, R. (2017). Conceptual models of social determinants of health: A narrative review. *Iranian Journal of Public Health*, *46*(4), 435–446.

McEldowney, R., & Connor, M. J. (2011). Cultural safety as an ethic of care: A praxiological process. *Journal of Transcultural Nursing*, *22*(4), 342–349. https://doi.org/10.1177/1043659611414139.

Mkandawire-Valhmu, L. (2018). *Cultural safety, healthcare and vulnerable populations: A critical theoretical perspective*. Routledge.

Moolchaem, P., Liamputtong, P., O'Halloran, P., & Muhamad, R. (2015). The lived experiences of transgender persons: A meta-synthesis. *Journal of Gay & Lesbian Social Services*, *27*(2), 143–171. https://doi.org/10.1080/10538720.2015.1021983.

Nursing Council of New Zealand. (2012). *Code of conduct for nurses*. https://www.nursingcouncil.org.nz/Public/Nursing/Standards_and_guidelines/NCNZ/nursing-section/Standards_and_guidelines_for_nurses.aspx.

Ramsden, I. M. (2002). Cultural safety and nursing education in Aotearoa and Te Waipounamu [Doctoral dissertation, Victoria University of Wellington].

Richardson, F. (2012). Editorial: Cultural safety 20 years on time to celebrate or commiserate? *Whitireia Nursing Journal*, *19*(19), 5–8.

Taylor, K., & Guerin, P. T. (2019). *Health care and Indigenous Australians: Cultural safety in practice* (3rd ed.). Red Globe Press.

Vaughan, C., Murdolo, A., Murray, L., Davis, E., Chen, J., Block, K., Quiazon, R., & Warr, D. (2015). ASPIRE: A multi-site community-based participatory research project to increase understanding of the dynamics of violence against immigrant and refugee women in Australia. *BMC Public Health*, *15*(1), 1–9. https://doi.org/10.1186/s12889-015-2634-0.

Wade, N. (2015). *A troublesome inheritance: Genes, race and human history*. Penguin Putman.

Wepa, D. (2015). *Cultural safety in Aotearoa New Zealand* (2nd ed). Cambridge University Press. https://doi.org/10.1017/CBO9781316151136

2 The social and cultural determinants of health

Rebecca E. Olson, Allyson Mutch, Lisa Fitzgerald and Sophie Hickey

Learning outcomes

After working through this chapter, students should be able to:

1. Discuss what is meant by the social determinants of health, as well as the strengths and limitations of this framework for understanding health inequalities.
2. Compare diverging explanations and theories for why inequalities in health outcomes persist.
3. Describe cultural diversity in Australia and how culture can shape health, both positively and negatively.

Key terms

Agency: Individuals' capacities to take actions, which can be constrained by social structures.
Artefact of measurement: A widely disproved explanation discussed in the historic *Black Report,* which suggests health inequalities are merely a statistical anomaly.
Assimilation: Processes of adopting the cultural practices of the dominant group in a society, often encouraged, sometimes enforced, by the majority group.
Behavioural factors: An explanation, accounting for approximately 20% of disparities in health outcomes, discussed in the *Black Report,* which attributes health inequalities to individual lifestyle choices.
Colonisation: A process of subjugating a people to gain access to their territory and its resources.
Cultural determinants of health: Ethnic, religious, racial, but also class, gender and sexuality differences that underpin behavioural patterns and social experiences leading to divergent health outcomes across minority and majority groups.
Cultural identity: Affinity with and sense of belonging to a culture or cultural group.
Culture: The evolved human capacity to classify and represent experiences with symbols and to act imaginatively and creatively. Cultures are differentiated by the distinct ways that people, who live differently, classify and represent their experiences.
Endemic: A disease that is consistently present within a population.

Ethnicity: A category or group of people who identify with each other, usually on the basis of presumed similarities such as common language, geography, ancestry, history, society, culture and/or social treatment.

Fundamental social causes of health inequalities: A theory that explains health inequalities by emphasising access to material and immaterial resources to mitigate the effects should disease occur.

Natural selection: An explanation supported by only modest evidence discussed in the *Black Report,* which suggests health inequalities are the result of the downward social mobility of people with poor health.

Midstream factors: Intermediary determinants of health, such as material resources, psychosocial and behavioural factors.

Neoliberalism: An extreme form of capitalism characterised by a political and economic ideology supporting economic growth through the privatisation of public goods and services, and most recently, through new strategies of relying on insecure and precarious forms of labour.

Othering: Practices of division and exclusion that can result when cultural groups cast outside groups as morally inferior.

Pathogenic: Conditions or factors that pose risk to health.

Psychosocial explanation: A theory that points to the higher levels of stress and anxiety experienced by those in lower positions within a social hierarchy in explaining persisting health inequalities.

Race: A socially constructed grouping of humans based on shared physical categories generally viewed as distinct by a society.

Racism: Any cognition, affective state, or behaviour that advances the differential treatment of individuals or groups due to their racial, ethnic, cultural or religious background.

Salutogenic: Conditions or factors that promote health.

Social democracy: A state, party or sovereignty that enacts policies to redistribute wealth, support primary health care and prioritise illness prevention through collaboration across sectors.

Social determinants of health: Conditions in which people are born, grow, work, live and age, and the wider set of forces and systems shaping the conditions of daily life. These forces and systems include economic policies and systems, development agendas, social norms, social policies and political systems.

Social gradient of disease: The graded relationship between social position and health outcomes, with those at the bottom experiencing the worst health outcomes, those in the middle experiencing better health outcomes, and those at the top experiencing the best health outcomes.

Social structure: The way social systems are organised and work to shape individual behaviour and life chances.

Socio-economic status: A term describing a person or group's social standing, typically assessed using a combination measure of income, occupation and education.

Structural/materialist explanation: The reason for health inequalities that gets the most support in the *Black Report*: differences in living and working conditions, material and economic resources.

Structural racism: The way social systems are organised to favour the majority group and exclude, subjugate or disadvantage minority groups.

Structural violence: The harm inflicted through social systems designed to limit opportunities and capabilities, particularly for those in minority groups.

Upstream factors: Health determinants that can be intervened in well before they pose a risk to health, such as socio-policies related to education and income.

Chapter summary

This chapter provides students with a conceptual framework for examining the role of social determinants on health within Australia. Here health sociology is used to provide a framework for understanding the social contexts of health, illness and health care. Students will be introduced to a range of topics related to health and wellbeing, including political, economic and environmental circumstances fostering ill health. Students will also explore societal forces constraining the health care system and individuals' responses to health and illness in Australia. The social determinants of health will be connected to diversity via discussion about how diverse populations have varying experience with social determinants of health. Finally, this chapter introduces students to the concept of intersectionality: how multiple kinds of difference can intersect in historically specific contexts, and how this in turn impacts on experiences of health care and health outcomes. Given that environmental concerns are increasingly impacting our health, this aspect of social determinants will receive mention here as well as receive attention throughout the text by reflection boxes.

Box 2.1 Reflection—Understanding health

Before you begin reading this chapter, let's start by thinking about your own health.

On a piece of paper, write down three or four things you think contribute to your health.

Keep the piece of paper handy; we'll revisit it again at the end of the chapter.

Introduction

Consider the following health inequalities:

- Afghanistan-born refugees living in Australia suffer from post-traumatic stress disorder (PTSD) and depression at much higher rates than the wider Australian population: approximately five and three times higher, respectively (Yaser et al., 2016).
- In the Northern Territory, Aboriginal males born between 2008 and 2012 have a life expectancy of 63.6 years, compared to 80 years for males of the broader Australian population (Georges et al., 2013).
- Black Americans are more likely to have diabetes, hypertension, strokes and heart disease than White Americans (Brown, O'Rand, & Adkins, 2012).
- In some affluent areas of Glasgow, men can have a life expectancy of 82 years compared with 66 years for men living in more disadvantaged areas (Bambra, 2016).

Overall, some population groups are likely to have lives that are shorter, experience more severe illness, and have levels of impairment more severe than the general population (Williams, 2013). Rather than attributing this to genetics, differences in lifestyle choice or cultural practices, research shows health inequalities are a consequence of broader social forces and inequities (Bambra, 2016). The *social determinants of health* refer to the social, economic and environmental forces, such as how much money a person earns, the type of job they have, and where they live, which matter more to health outcomes than individual behaviours or biomedical risk factors (Australian Institute of Health and Welfare, 2016).

Closely linked are the *cultural determinants of health*, which refer to ethnic, religious, racial, class, gender and sexuality differences that underpin social experiences leading to divergent health experiences and outcomes across some groups. Practices of exclusion, discrimination, stereotyping and *othering* at the hands of mainstream group members (including health professionals) is associated with poorer health outcomes for minority groups who experience structural discrimination and/or racism and must navigate the consequences of this, including restricted access to key resources such as health care (Dew, 2014). Despite this, is it also important to recognise that *culture*, and a strong connection to and identification with one's culture, can also improve resilience (Lowitja Institute, 2014).

This chapter offers a broad understanding of the social determinants of health, while considering culture more specifically, as a key determinant of health. We begin by briefly defining the social determinants of health, using smoking as an example, before considering culture and the impacts of culture and racism on health outcomes. We then step back in time to understand the origins of the social determinants of health and key reports investigating the relationship between social and health inequalities. We consider debates surrounding the varied explanations for understanding health inequalities provided within these historical reports. Using a sociological lens, we critically consider some of the limitations of the social determinants and current understandings of health inequalities.

Conceptualising the social determinants of health

The 2018 National Tobacco Campaign in Australia, "Don't make smokes your story", features Ted describing why he quit smoking:

> Family is everything to me. I can't imagine life without them to be honest. I've had my battles with smokes. My lungs got pretty bad. Sometimes I could hardly breathe and that was tough on everyone. I'm not sure why I smoked, I just did. My kids, Jarrah and Yani, I wanted to be there for them, so I quit. Quitting was tough, I just kept trying. Now I can keep up with them in the yard and I've got more money to spend on better things. Mum and the Aunties are pretty happy that I quit. They didn't want me to die from smokes like Dad did. My name is Ted, and family is my story. Don't make smokes your story.

Ted's story is intended to be motivating, but is motivation all that is required to improve health? Like many health promotion messages we hear encouraging us to drink less alcohol, exercise more, quit smoking and eat healthy, the underlying message suggests health is an individual choice, within our control. But contrast this message with findings from the British Medical Association (BMA) (2011, p. 7):

> [W]hile smoking is the proximal cause of illnesses such as COPD, CHD and lung cancer, it is the social, including cultural, and environmental factors, that largely determines whether an individual is more or less likely to smoke, and if they do start to smoke whether they are likely to quit successfully.

Moreover, the ill effects of cigarette smoking, in terms of mortality, are more pronounced in those who experience disadvantage. The death rate from smoking-related diseases is 1.3 times higher amongst the most, compared to the least, disadvantaged in Australia (Greenhalgh, Scollo, & Pearce, 2016). In light of this disparity, Cancer Council Victoria researchers remind us that: "it is important to note the influence and interplay of other health risk factors and social and economic deprivation across a life-course" (Greenhalgh, Scollo, & Pearce, 2016). These findings from the BMA and Cancer Council Victoria reflect a large body of evidence that demonstrates that social, environmental and cultural factors—the *social determinants of health*—are as important to health outcomes, if not more so, as behavioural or biomedical factors (Australian Institute of Health and Welfare, 2016).

There are many definitions of the social determinants, but let us start with the World Health Organisation's (WHO's) definition as presented by the Commission on the Social Determinants of Health (CSDH) (Commission on the Social Determinants of Health, 2008, prelude):

> … the circumstances in which people grow, live, work, and age, and the systems put in place to deal with illness. The conditions in which people live and die are, in turn, shaped by political, social, and economic forces.

In developing this definition, the CSDH focused on health inequalities and the negative impact of the social determinants of health, but it is important to acknowledge social determinants can also impact health in positive ways. For example, as the case study in Box 2.2 illustrates, being awarded a university-level education is linked to better employment opportunities, greater job security and higher remuneration, all of which are associated with more positive health outcomes. In comparison, a person who has not completed their high school certificate may experience limited employment opportunities, lower wages and unstable employment, which can negatively impact health (Baum, 2015). Aligned with the focus of this text, culture, in addition to education, employment and income, is another important determinant of health.

Box 2.2 Case study—Deng Thiak Adut's Australia Day speech

Extract from Transcript: Deng Thiak Adut's Australia Day speech

Deng Thiak Adut in his Australia Day speech (Adut, 2016), speaks on life in South Sudan and the impact of his childhood on his life today. He says,

> … I was born in a small fishing village called Malek, in the South Sudan. My father was a fisherman and we had a banana farm. I am one of eight children to Mr Thiak Adut Garang and Ms Athieu Akau Deng. So the parts of my name are drawn from both my parents. My given name is Deng which means god of the rain. In those parts of this wide brown land that are short of water my name might be a good omen … as a young boy, about the age of a typical second grader in Sydney, I was conscripted into an army … I lost the freedom to read and write … I came to Australia as an illiterate, penniless teenager, traumatised physically and emotionally by war. In Sudan, I was considered legally disabled, only by virtue of being black or having a dark skin complexion. As you can see I am very black and proud of my dark skin complexion. But in the Sudan my colour meant that my prospects could go no further than a dream of being allowed to finish a primary education. To be a lawyer was unthinkable. Australia opened the doors of its schools and universities. I would particularly like to thank the Western Sydney University where I received my Law degree and the University of Wollongong where I obtained my Master's degree in Law—an experience which enabled me to realise my dream of becoming a court room advocate. Australia educated me. How lucky I became ….

Box 2.3 Reflection—Understanding the definition of the social determinants of health

There are two key take away messages from the WHO's definition of the social determinants of health. The first relates to the "circumstances" in which people live. Reflecting on Deng's story (see the Case study in Box 2.2):

- What are some of the social circumstances that may be potentially important for understanding Deng's health?

The second part of the WHO's definition suggests these "circumstances" are shaped by broader political, social and economic "forces".

- Thinking about the circumstances you described, what role may broader "forces" play in Deng's life and health?

Cultural determinants of health

Like social determinants, cultural determinants can impact the health of population groups that share cultural identities, in both positive and negative ways. Cultural determinants can draw on the strengths of *cultural identities*, knowledges and practices and are key to the health and wellbeing of cultural groups (Lowitja Institute, 2014). However, negative cultural determinants stemming from the dominant culture in a society, such as racism and economic practices, can play a key role in driving inequalities, excluding and discriminating minority cultural groups. It is therefore essential to also consider both cultural and social determinants of health: the socio-cultural conditions that enable people to have good health and wellbeing (Napier et al., 2014). But, what is culture?

Understanding culture

Most definitions of *culture* focus on collective, shared understandings and practices, "customs, habits, language and geography that groups of individuals share" (Napier et al., 2014, p. 1609). Culture is dynamic, changing and adapting to a complex social world. Culture is part of our everyday lives, the understandings and practices we have about the social world around us (Fanany, 2012). Language is central to culture, providing structure to our thoughts, ideas, interpretations of the world around us, and to our ways for understanding and expressing ourselves (Fanany, 2012). Importantly, cultures influence our understandings and experiences of health (Napier et al., 2014).

It is through cultural understandings and practices that our identities are constructed and our language, lifestyles, values and beliefs signal to ourselves and others where we belong in society (Habibis & Walter, 2015). Culture is most often associated with *ethnicity* and ethnic identity; however, there are many other types of cultural groups/identities, including religious groups, and geographical groups, groups based on age, occupation, social class, gender and sexual identities (Napier et al., 2014). There is also great diversity within cultural groups; not all members of a group share common understandings and practices. Our cultural identities are dynamic and changing; they intersect with other forms of cultural identities. For example, we might embrace one culture in one setting (e.g., an ethnic *cultural identity* at home with family) and another cultural identity in a different setting (e.g., an LGBTQA+ identity with friends) (Napier et al., 2014).

Box 2.4 Reflection—Understanding culture

On a piece of paper, reflect on your own culture(s):

- What cultural groups do you belong to?
- Which do you identify with?

Write down all the cultural groups/identities you can think of and how these might impact on your health and wellbeing.

Going back to the Case study in Box 2.2:

- What are some of the cultural groups/identities that Deng was a part of?
- How might these cultural groups shape Deng's health and wellbeing?

Culture is about more than individual identity; cultural identities provide collective understandings of *us* and *them* and the perceived moral worth of different groups, which can lead to *othering*, difference and social division (Habibis & Walter, 2015). Powell and Menendian (2016, p. 17) define othering as "a set of dynamics, processes, and structures that engender marginality and persistent inequality across any of the full range of human differences based on group identities." In essence, othering involves relationships of power, of inclusion and exclusion set against cultural, racial, sexual, gender and linguistic differences.

In Australia, despite being a diverse country with 28% of all Australians born overseas (Australian Institute of Health and Welfare, 2016), we see othering discourse in debates about immigration. Some politicians argue for tougher immigration controls to curb national security risks of immigrant *others* (Udah & Singh, 2019). For example, Pauline Hanson, a Federal senator and leader of the ultra-conservative One Nation party, has called for a ban on immigration from certain cultural groups, in line with a history of immigration in Australia being based on a selective racialised policy (Udah & Singh, 2019). Discourses of otherness work to uphold systems of privilege and inequality through *racism* (Udah & Singh, 2019). Migrant populations in Australia generally experience good health, but *structural racism*, social isolation, emotional and mental health issues, and barriers to culturally appropriate health services are common experiences (Day, 2016). Refugees and asylum seekers, in particular, experience "structural vulnerabilities and discriminations that impact physical, mental and social wellbeing, leading to further exclusion, with negative long-term implications" (Lillee et al., 2015, p. 47). In this way, racism can been seen to be a social determinant of ill health (see Reflection Box 2.5).

Box 2.5 Reflection—Racism as a social determinant of ill health

Around the world, we observe racial and ethnic disparities in health outcomes. *Race* is a socially constructed label used to refer to the classification and stratification of people based on phenotype (i.e., skin colour and other physical attributes), while *ethnicity* categorises people by cultural group, which may include shared ancestry or nationality. While variations within racial groupings suggests there is no genetically meaningful basis to the concept of race (Williams, 2013), racism as a social problem is real (Smedley & Smedley,

2005). Racism refers to negative and prejudicial discrimination that can occur at individual, interpersonal and structural levels. Racism can be detrimental to a person's health. A review of 121 empirical studies found racial discrimination was significantly associated with negative health outcomes in children, with mental health being the most commonly reported (Priest et al., 2013). Other research implicates racism in experiences of chronic stress, which contributes to disparate cardiovascular health outcomes (Bowen-Reid & Harrell, 2002). These racial health disparities persist irrespective of *socio-economic status* (SES) (Geronimus, 1992; Geronimus et al., 2006).

Public discourse and media representations of racial and ethnic groups can perpetuate stereotypes that negatively impact health and wellbeing (Stoneham, Goodman, & Daube, 2014). Lauderdale (2006), for example, found that women with Arabic surnames who gave birth in California during the six months following the September 11, 2001, US terrorist attacks were more likely to experience preterm birth and have low-birth-weight babies compared to similar women who gave birth one year prior, and whose experiences mirrored the broader population. This was attributed to the rise of Islamophobia and increased harassment, violence and discriminations towards Muslim people in the United States.

Wiradjuri scholar Juanita Sherwood (2013) argues the impact of racism and *colonisation* continues to negatively affect the health and wellbeing of Aboriginal and Torres Strait Islander peoples in Australia, and Indigenous peoples around the world. Government *assimilation* policies and forced family separations have had devastating intergenerational impacts on the health and wellbeing of Indigenous peoples in Canada (Hackett et al., 2016) and Australia (Silburn et al., 2006). However, genuine local Indigenous community participation and ownership of health and social services have been found to counter the *pathogenic* effects of colonisation (Chandler & Lalonde, 1998; Smylie et al., 2016).

Explaining the cultural determinants of health: An "invisible" concept

Cultural determinants of health inequalities are embedded in institutions and social relationships, making them difficult to recognise as they are normalised from positions of privilege (Farmer et al., 2006). The term *structural violence* is used to link unequal social structures to the harm done to people and to the limiting impact of social conditions on individual opportunities and capabilities, particularly for those from minority cultural groups (Farmer et al., 2006). The high rates of chronic diseases in Pacific Island countries and territories offers an example of how this structural violence plays out.

Three-quarters of all deaths in the Pacific Island countries and territories are caused by non-communicable diseases with up to 90% of people ages 25–64 overweight or obese in some regions (Napier et al., 2014). Pacific Islander peoples have experienced over 50 years of obesity interventions, with most of these interventions focused on individual-level behaviour change (Hardin et al., 2018). However, obesity-related conditions continue to rise (Hardin et al., 2018). Alongside hereditary factors, much of the research into persistently high rates of obesity has focused on Pacific Islander peoples not engaging in "healthy eating behaviours" due to eating practices specific to Pacific Islander communities, and due to the cultural value placed on large bodies (Hardin et al., 2018). However, a minority of researchers have conceptualised the increasing rates of disease associated with obesity in the Pacific Islands as caused by cultural and social determinants, associated with rapid lifestyle changes, Westernisation, globalisation, and powerful international trade policies and market forces, which have ushered in the oversupply of inexpensive, high-energy, low-nutrition food (Napier et al., 2014). Simultaneously, obesity interventions themselves have actively shaped contemporary cultural understandings of body norms in the Pacific Islands, bringing blame, stigma, and shame to people with obesity (Hardin et al., 2018; Hawley & McGarvey, 2015). Thus, globalised trade policies alongside well-meaning public health responses can be understood as forms of structural violence that characterise the social and cultural determinants of health (Farmer et al., 2006).

Box 2.6 Reflection—Structural violence and cultural determinants of health

- Return to the Case study—can you identify any instances of structural violence in Deng's story?

Thinking back to Reflection Box 2.1 and what you wrote about your own health, did you identify any cultural determinants of health? After reading about the social and cultural determinants of health, is there anything you would add or revise regarding what contributes to your health?

In recent years, researchers have sought to consider cultural determinants of good health and wellbeing, originating from and promoting *strengths-based* cultural perspectives (Brown, n.d.). For Aboriginal and Torres Strait Islander peoples, this means connection to culture and country to build strong individual and collective identities, resilience and improved health outcomes across all determinants of health (Lowitja Institute, 2014; Sweet, 2013). Such an approach recognises the need for cultural understandings, contextualised and locally controlled culturally specific health services alongside working on broader "upstream", structural determinants of health. Inequalities in health matter, and identification of inequalities is essential to build more equitable and healthy societies. However, we must recognise that cultural systems of value are subtle and highly complex foundational determinants of health (Napier et al., 2014). To put these converging structural, cultural, government and financial forces into context, we return to the concept introduced at the start of the chapter, the social determinants of health.

History of the social determinants of health

Research supporting the idea that health is a product of broader social forces has "a long pedigree", which can be traced back nearly 200 years (Scambler, 2012, p. 131). In 1845, Fredrick Engels (financier to, and collaborator with, political and social philosopher Karl Marx) published his research investigating negative health effects of unsafe living and working conditions on the labouring class in Manchester. In 1848, Berlin-based medical physician Dr Rudolph Virchow (1821–1902) reported to the Prussian Government on his research into a severe outbreak of typhus in Upper Silesia (now Poland). Virchow found labourers' poor social conditions were to blame for their poor health and prescribed democracy, education, safer and higher paid working conditions and tax reform (Dew, 2012; Scarani, 2003).

More recently, interest in the relationship between social inequalities and health inequalities re-gained prominence in the late 1970s and early 1980s following the landmark *Black Report* in the UK. The report was commissioned in 1977 by the then Labour Government, but by the time it was released in 1980, the Thatcher Conservative Government had been elected and vowed not to support its recommendations (Bambra et al., 2011; Richmond, 2002). Despite the Thatcher Government's best efforts to quash the findings, the *Black Report* is widely cited and acknowledged for prompting a swell of research into health inequalities. It is also recognised as the precursor for a number of important studies examining health inequalities: the 1998 Acheson report on health inequalities in the UK; Wilkinson and Marmot's 1998 investigation into the 10 leading social determinants of health for the WHO, which saw a shift in focus from health gaps to health gradients; the *Commission on the Social Determinants of Health* (CSDH) (Commission on the Social Determinants of Health, 2008); and Marmot's 2010 *Fair Lives, Fair Society* report (Bambra et al., 2011).

In considering these reports, we can make a number of important observations. The first relates to the significant contribution of leading scholars Sir Michael Marmot and Richard Wilkinson, and the way their understandings of the social determinants of health have dominated the field for over two decades. The second acknowledges the central role epidemiology has played in research in this area. We will return to these observations later in the chapter. With this context in mind, we now consider how this body of scholarship, starting with the *Black Report*, seeks to explain health inequalities

Explaining health inequalities

The *Black Report* considered four explanations of health inequalities that provided the foundation for subsequent research into the social determinants of health. The first explanation put forward in the report suggests health inequalities are merely an "*artefact of measurement*"—a suggestion refuted by thousands of studies, which confirm that the persistent relationship between social and health inequalities is more than a statistical anomaly (Baum, 2015). The second explanation suggests health inequalities are the result of *natural selection*, with healthier, hardworking people achieving social mobility and longer lives (Macintyre, 1997, p. 727). Poor health may impact a person's ability to participate in social, economic and employment settings resulting in downward mobility; however, the contribution of poor health to social inequalities is described as "modest" at best (Baum, 2015, p. 310; Macintyre, 1997).

The third explanation, which warrants detailed consideration, suggests health inequalities are a consequence of *behavioural factors*. This explanation is closely connected with a significant body of research that Popay et al. (1998, p. 622) describe as "risk factor epidemiology", which emphasises the relationship between individuals' poor health behaviours and disease. There is little doubt that what we eat, whether we exercise, or if we smoke—what Nettleton (2013, p. 234) describes as the "holy trinity of risk"—has an impact on health. However, research acknowledges this is only part of the story; for example, the Centers for Disease Control and Prevention (CDC) in the USA suggests behaviour only accounts for around 20% of the differences we see in health outcomes between advantaged groups and those experiencing disadvantage (CDC, 2017).

Contesting this simplistic view of health behaviours, the *Black Report*'s authors sought to acknowledge the socially embedded nature of potentially health-damaging behaviours that are distributed inequitably across societies. In other words, they sought to challenge the belief that health-related behaviours are freely chosen, but instead argued that they exist within a social context (Macintyre, 1997; Marmot, 2001). To illustrate, Marmot (2019) describes a recent study of childhood poverty in the UK, which identified that a family in the poorest 10% of the population would need to spend 74% of their income on food to achieve current healthy eating advice. Reflecting on this, Marmot (2019, p. 1090) describes explanations that suggest "the poor are architects of their own misfortune" as "shoddy thinking".

Despite the *Black Report*'s efforts to develop a socially embedded understanding of behaviour, an individualised notion of "lifestyle choices" continues to dominate our approach to prevention, health care and policy (Nettleton, 2013). This assumption is embedded within a belief that individuals, who make poor "lifestyle choices", have access to the "time, resources, capability and motivation to change their lifestyle" (Germov, 2019b, p. 97)—a line of thought that ignores social, political, cultural, economic and other relational contexts. In many instances this results in *victim blaming*—where individuals are seen to be responsible for their own health and illness, with little consideration of social and material circumstances (Baum, 2015; Germov, 2019b).

The need to consider socio-economic circumstances is linked to the fourth explanation identified in the *Black Report*: the *Structural/Materialist explanation*. This explanation emphasises the role of economic, social and political factors in the distribution of health (Macintyre, 1997). These broad structural factors translate into differences in material resources and circumstances, including poverty, poorer living and working conditions, and material deprivation (Baum, 2015).

To demonstrate, let's start by examining the physical environments where people live. As Engels (1950) pointed out in the 19th century, poor living conditions can be *pathogenic*; that is, they can generate risks to health. Britain's poor and working classes, living in urban areas in the mid-1800s, endured damp and cramped living arrangements, in close proximity to factories and industrial pollutants. The middle and upper classes escaped the smog, preferring to reside outside of the city. These disparate living arrangements contributed to the large disparities in life expectancy. In the industrial city of Manchester, for example, the life expectancy was a mere 27 years, compared to the national average of approximately 40 years (Szreter, 1997; Szreter & Mooney, 1998).

This relationship between living conditions and health holds true today. Trachoma offers an example. Australia is the only developed country in the world with *endemic* trachoma, an eye infection spread through direct contact with discharge or indirectly by flies that can cause permanent vision loss if left untreated (Taylor & Anjou, 2013; WHO, 2017). Almost exclusively, it is Aboriginal Australians living in remote communities in central Australia who are affected (Australia Institute of Health and Welfare, 2017). Illustrating intersections across cultural, economic and environmental social forces, the high rate of trachoma in these communities is due to poverty and an undersupply of quality housing within Australia's remote areas. The main strategies for preventing transmission, facial cleanliness and environmental improvements, are less accessible (WHO, 2017); in houses that are overcrowded, without flyscreens and adequate plumbing and sanitation, the risk of (repeated) transmission increases (Taylor, Burton, Haddad, West, & Wright, 2014). Housing in remote communities frequently lacks these basic necessities (McDonald et al., 2009), though recent construction initiatives are easing some of the disparity in housing supply and quality in these areas (Shattock, Gambhir, Taylor, Cowling, Kaldor, & Wilson, 2015).

Box 2.7 Reflection—Living conditions and health outcomes

Drawing on the example of trachoma, answer the following questions:

- Why do women tend to be at a higher risk of contracting trachoma?
- How is the physical environment implicated in the spread of trachoma?
- What could a person with a high income do to reduce their likelihood of contracting trachoma?
- What social policies could be put in place to ameliorate the rate of trachoma in remote Australian communities?

Occupation and working conditions are also clearly implicated in enduring health inequalities. Historically, manual labourers in Engels and Virchow's era were exposed to dangerous working conditions; they worked directly with dangerous chemicals, used machinery in warehouses with poor visibility for long hours with little to no protective equipment or regulation. These conditions, no doubt, contributed to the short life expectancies seen in industrial cities, such as Manchester, described earlier. Today, Australia has work health and safety regulations in place to improve working conditions across all occupational settings. Work fatalities, however, do still take place, and they are not evenly distributed across all industries, but concentrated within certain sectors. Jobs in the transport, postal and warehousing industry and agriculture, forestry and fishing industry each account for a quarter of all worker fatalities in Australia. Construction accounts for 15% of worker fatalities, on average (Safe Work Australia, 2019).

Despite these risks, it may be safer to be employed (Marmot, 2004); unemployment is linked to higher rates of mortality and physical and mental morbidity (Mathers & Schofield, 1998). There are a couple of possible explanations for this relationship. Link and Phelan's (1995) *fundamental social causes of health inequalities* thesis offers one explanation. This theory argues access to resources allows people with a higher SES the capacity to avoid multiple risk factors or to mitigate the effects of disease should it occur (Phelan, Link, & Tehranifar, 2010). Material resources, like money, along with immaterial resources, such as power and education, enable people to counter the ill effects of deleterious living and working conditions. So, if a person is unemployed, their access to material resources, and thus their capacity to improve their living conditions or pay for health-generating, or *salutogenic,* things such as healthy food is compromised. In contrast, someone employed on a high income would be more able to secure newer housing in a safe part of town. Someone with an advanced tertiary qualification is more likely to be employed (Marmot, 2004), and in an industry with relatively few work fatalities.

A fifth explanation, not identified in the *Black Report*, that rose to the fore through the work of Wilkinson and Marmot (2003) is the *psychosocial explanation* (Germov, 2019a). Marmot acknowledges the role of material resources and structural factors in understanding the relationship between social and health inequalities, but also suggests one's positioning within the social hierarchy and the subjective or psychosocial effects of insecurity, stress and anxiety experienced have consequences for health (Marmot, 2004; Øversveen et al., 2017). Similarly, social relationships, networks and other sources of support will shape the ways individuals navigate stress and access the resources needed to participate in society. Marmot (2004) illustrates this proposition in the Whitehall studies, a longitudinal study of the health of public servants. In this setting, all employees are exposed to the same workplace conditions, but have different levels of authority, control and pay. What Marmot found is that those public servants with higher-ranking jobs, who have more control over their work, tend to have better health outcomes. Those who have less control over their work, particularly people in highly demanding jobs with little control over their work, tend to have poorer health outcomes: specifically, higher risk of depression and coronary heart disease (Marmot, 2004). What's more, this relationship follows an incremental or graded relationship with those at the bottom experiencing the worst health outcomes, those in the middle experiencing better health outcomes, and those at the top experiencing the best health outcomes. This graded phenomena is what Marmot has labelled the *social gradient* (Marmot, 2004; Scambler, 2012).

In presenting these five explanations of health inequality, it is easy to get lost in debates that suggest one perspective supersedes the others, but in reality each has a contribution to make and is not mutually exclusive (Macintyre, 1997). As Marmot argues (2001, p. 1168) social structures and a person's access to material resources will affect psychosocial processes, they do not operate in isolation. Models of the social determinants of health (see Solar & Irwin, 2010), present a conceptual framework that acknowledges the broader structural determinants of health—or *upstream factors*—including macro socio-economic policies and factors related to socio-economic position such as education, income, gender and class; along with intermediary determinants of health—or *midstream factors*—which include psychosocial factors, material circumstances and behavioural factors. Together these upstream and midstream factors provide a framework for the social determinants of health, informing our understanding of inequitable *downstream* health outcomes.

The social determinants of health—Critical perspectives

The social determinants of health, particularly through the work of Marmot, has been highly influential, informing recommendations made by of the WHO (2010) and governments worldwide. Despite its pre-eminence, many call for further critical assessment of the social determinants of health as a framework for understanding health inequalities. Next we consider three critiques of current approaches.

Limitations of measurement

Over the past few decades, a considerable number of epidemiological studies have demonstrated the association between a person's socio-economic position and health outcomes. Often, researchers measure this relationship by examining statistical correlations between key population health markers, such as mortality rates and life expectancy, and measures that represent a group's standing in society, such as occupation, income, education or neighbourhood. *Socio-economic status* (SES) is a common marker for relative social standing used in epidemiological and social science research. SES can be measured in many ways, but frequently draws on a combination of income, occupation and education to classify individuals or families into three categories: low, middle or high SES (Australian Bureau of Statistics, 2011).

This substantial collection of epidemiological research provides a vast body of evidence from which we can identify a relationship between social and health inequalities; however it is not as well equipped to understand the complexity of social processes, nor consider the mechanisms through which the social shapes health and illness (Popay et al., 1998; Schofield, 2007, p. 108). As Gagné and Ghenadenik (2018) argue, variables used as indicators of SES are frequently used as common practice and rarely questioned in terms of their ability to theoretically or empirically contribute to research. As a consequence, research within the field often provides a limited and overly reductionist view of the relationship between social and health inequalities that "disconnects individuals from their social context" and "falls back into the search for single causes" (Popay et al., 1998, pp. 627–628) (see Reflection Box 2.1).

Box 2.8 Case study—The limitations of epidemiological research examining health inequalities

Epidemiology is the study of the origins and patterns of disease. Social epidemiology focuses on social factors that impact health and wellbeing.

Social factors such as where we are born, how much we earn, what cultural groups we belong to can go some way towards predicting how healthy we are. We live in complex, ever-changing and dynamic social contexts. Therefore, the different ways we conduct research and analyse data can paint different stories about how this impacts our health and wellbeing. For example, an Australian longitudinal study that followed-up "Aboriginal" people living in an urban setting from birth to 30 years old found different outcomes depending on the research approach used (Hickey, 2015a, 2015b). In fact, even the way Aboriginal and Torres Strait Islander status is collected in datasets has changed over this time, with Torres Strait Islander people not explicitly being identified in the original study unless they also identified as Aboriginal (Hickey, 2015b). Statistical analysis of existing survey data focused on socioeconomic disadvantage, family dysfunction, stress, problematic alcohol use and mental illness among this group compared to non-Indigenous people, while qualitative life history interviews conducted with the same Aboriginal and/or Torres Strait Islander people focused on the strength and resilience of Aboriginal and/or Torres Strait Islander people. When provided the opportunity to co-construct their own life narratives within the research process, the Aboriginal and/or Torres Strait Islander interviewees talked about never being without, the opportunity for upwards social mobility, the importance of family as positive role models and social support, abstinence, learning from past experiences and coping through challenges. The original quantitative dataset had no variables to capture the historical impact of government policy on the lives and wellbeing of Aboriginal people, yet surviving through the generational impact of the Stolen Generations (forcible family separations supported by past racist government assimilation policies) was perceived to have considerable importance to the wellbeing of Aboriginal and/or Torres Strait Islander families. Interviewees consciously made life decisions in an attempt to minimise the impact of racism on their wellbeing (Hickey, 2016), and cultural identity was described as a positive and dynamic part of their everyday lives (Hickey, 2015a, 2015b).

Unidirectional/causal relationships

Building on our reservations about epidemiological research conducted under the umbrella of the social determinants of health, we also draw attention to the frequently unquestioned assumption that the relationship between the social determinants and health is unidirectional (Øversveen et al., 2017). Øversveen et al. (2017) acknowledge emphasis on unidirectional relationships stems from efforts to challenge the dominance of individualism and the discourse of risk; however, they argue such an approach ignores the complexity of social processes. In emphasising a casual pathway that begins at the upstream level, Popay et al. (1998) suggest we are positioning people as passive, with no capacity for *agency*. Such a critique asks us to step beyond the discussion of risk factors and lifestyle choices to consider the ways in which health practices are not only socially embedded, but also how they are produced and reproduced by agents within a social context that may be constraining or enabling (Øversveen et al., 2017; Popay et al., 1998;). In other words, can we begin to consider how "health inequalities are created by the interaction between individual action and social structure without necessarily attributing causal primacy to one of the two" (Øversveen et al., 2017, p. 108)?

Socio-political context

A final critique of the social determinants of health seeks to acknowledge the primacy of the socio-political context, particularly the dominance of neoliberal capitalism (Coburn, 2004; Scambler, 2012). In particular, Coburn (2004) argues we need to go further than examining disparities in income and in health, to consider the political economies prompting these inequities.

He gives the example of "health without wealth" countries (Baum, 2015, p. 315), such as Costa Rica and Cuba, and Scandinavian countries, such as Finland. These countries have social democratic political economies. *Social democracies* put policies in place to redistribute wealth through taxes and other initiatives, lessening the gap between those with higher and those with lower SES. Social democracies also tend to have universal health insurance and strong primary health care. That is, they prioritise illness prevention through collaboration with other sectors: housing, agriculture and water. They also prioritise basic care for all, rather than offering the most cutting-edge care to those who can afford it (Baum, 2015). As a result, these countries tend to have good health outcomes despite, in some cases, lower wealth by international standards.

Box 2.9 Case study—Costa Rica and the United States of America

A comparison of the health outcomes and health spending of Costa Rica and the United States of America (USA) provides a good example of the importance of looking at more than wealth to the distribution of wealth in understanding health outcomes. Costa Rica funds their health care clinics and hospitals publically through taxes, as well as member and employer contributions. These services are open to all of the country's inhabitants (Montenegro Torres, 2013). This system seems to work well. In 2015, Costa Ricans spent just under $930 USD per person on health. The life expectancy at birth in Costa Rica that year was a high 82.5 years for women (WHO, 2019).

Compare Costa Rica to the USA. In 2015, on average individuals in the USA paid $9,536 USD, more than 10 times the amount paid by Costa Ricans in the same year and had a shorter life expectancy of 81 years for women (WHO, 2019). This shows that wealth is not all that matters. Indeed, as Coburn (2004) argues, it is the neo-liberal political economic orientation of countries like the USA that is a primary cause of their comparatively poorer social determinants of health.

In contrast, *neoliberalism*, a more extreme form of economic liberalism, emerged following a period of moderate welfare-state capitalism in many English-speaking countries, such as the USA, UK and Australia in the decades after World War II. Neoliberalism is generally characterised by a political and economic ideology that encourages economic freedom and growth, the privatisation of public goods and services, increased individual responsibility (particularly in health and health care) and the reduction of overall costs and public spending through new organisational strategies, such as flexible (precarious) labour (Scribano, 2018).

The USA is a primary example of a neoliberal economy, particularly in relation to its health care system. The USA's neo-liberal political economic orientation means there are large inequalities between the wealthiest and the poorest members of society, in terms of material resources and health outcomes. It also means there is limited public support for primary health care and universal health care coverage, such as Australia's Medicare. Middle- and upper-class residents pay high premiums for health insurance. The very old and very poor have access to many services through government-funded schemes (called Medicare and Medicaid). Those in between who do not qualify for government schemes, and do not earn enough to pay regular health insurance premiums, are caught in the gap. Although the Affordable Care Act saw a reduction in the number of people uninsured in the USA, from 16% in 2010 to 9.1% in 2015 (Obama, 2016), a significant number of Americans remain uninsured and vulnerable to medical bankruptcy if they need to use a hospital in an emergency.

Box 2.10 Case study—Alan, a neoliberal worker

In 2016, Sir Michael Marmot visited Australia to present the Boyer Lectures series in which he discussed health inequities and the social determinants of health (Marmot, 2016). In his insightful lectures, he described stories of people across the globe impacted by the demeaning nature of contemporary work practices and the effect of this work on people's health and wellbeing. Marmot described Alan, a "picker" in a giant warehouse, working for large multinational online shopping company, working 12-hour shifts, walking 18 km a shift, grappling with the stress of receiving penalty points for failing to achieve impossible targets, packing 100 large items an hour, or a smaller item every two minutes. Marmot's contemporary example, similar to his Whitehall studies, exemplifies the health impacts of limited control in the workplace: stress and anxiety, important psychosocial aspects of health. Though this is not an emphasis of Marmot's lecture, the effects of neoliberalism on Alan's work practices and on his health are apparent. Alan's story exemplifies the pathogenic nature of contemporary work practices, brought about by neoliberalism, globalisation and technological change.

Like Coburn, fellow sociologist Scambler (2012) agrees the political economy is largely to blame for the economic social determinants of health. He sees *social structure*, the way social systems are organised and work to shape or determine individual behaviour, as key to explaining health inequalities. However, Scambler (2012) goes further, placing blame with key agents of neoliberalism: namely, the managers and chief executives who enact the ill effects through downsizing, increasing part-time and precarious work, reducing autonomy in jobs and outsourcing. He emphasises the role of people in powerful positions who enact policies and practices complicit with neoliberalism. In doing so, Scambler (2012) emphasises the importance of both structure and *agency*, or individual actions. He argues it is not just social structures to blame, but the individuals who reinforce, rather than resist, these social structures.

Box 2.11 Reflection—Understanding the political economy and health, structure and agency

Imagine you are 6 months pregnant and employed casually on a low wage. You start to develop the following symptoms: dizziness, cramping and occasional vomiting. Would you stay home or go to work? Would you make an appointment with a general practitioner (GP), or wait to see if it gets worse, and then visit the Emergency Department? How would the following structural circumstances influence your decision?

- Whether your pay would be reduced for missing work
- The cost of visiting a GP
- Whether or not you are insured
- Where you lived: Australia, Costa Rica or the USA
- Overall, how much is your decision making (your agency) shaped by social structures?

In sum, the social determinants of health provide understanding of why health outcomes are patterned, with the least advantaged in a society having fewer material resources and less autonomy, preventing them from making more salutogenic choices. But the way society is structured has a substantial impact on these choices, and thus on the social determinants of health. And health, of course, does not only follow an economic gradient. All over the world, minority groups from diverse cultural backgrounds experience worse health outcomes than those in mainstream groups (Williams, 2013). These economic and cultural forces intersect with environmental and other relational factors, such as gender, to underpin disparities in the incidence and impact of disease.

Conclusion

Health is much more than an individual choice. The social, political and economic settings in which people live and work in many ways determine health outcomes. The thinking behind the social determinants of health is not new, but neoliberal political ideology, which emphasises privatisation and individualistic thinking, encourages a focus on lifestyle and behavioural factors, over an emphasis on social, structural, material and cultural forces. While both lifestyle choices and these broader social forces work to shape health outcomes, the social determinants of health provides a framework for acknowledging upstream factors affecting health, and supporting the implementation of social democratic policies, which work to prevent health inequities. The social determinants of health framework also accommodate the positive and negative ways culture affects health outcomes, from the salutogenic effects of a shared cultural identity, to the ill effects of structural racism and discrimination. Overall, the social determinants of health offer health professionals and policymakers a useful concept for moving beyond individualistic notions of health as a lifestyle choice, towards more holistic considerations of the complex, social, cultural, political and economic forces shaping health.

Box 2.12 Reflection—Summary

At the start of this chapter we asked you to make a note of the things you thought were contributing to your health—having read through the chapter, is there anything that you might like to change or add to your list? Any qualifications you would like to make? Or is your list the same?

As you work through chapters of this book, keep your list handy, and think about what you have written.

References

Adut, D. T. (2016). *Transcript: Deng Thiak Adut's Australia day speech*. https://www.smh.com.au/national/transcript-deng-thiak-aduts-australia-day-speech-20160121-gmau63.html.

Australian Bureau of Statistics. (2011). *Measures of socioeconomic status*. (no. 1244.0.55.001). https://www.ausstats.abs.gov.au/Ausstats/subscriber.nsf/0/367D3800605DB064CA2578B60013445C/$File/1244055001_2011.pdf.

Australian Institute of Health and Welfare. (2016). *Australia's health 2016*. https://www.aihw.gov.au/getmedia/9844cefb-7745-4dd8-9ee2-f4d1c3d6a727/19787-AH16.pdf.aspx.

Australian Institute of Health and Welfare. (2017). *Indigenous eye health measures 2016*. https://www.aihw.gov.au/reports/indigenous-australians/indigenous-eye-health-measures-2016.

Bambra, C. (2016). *Health divides: Where you live can kill you*. Policy Press.

Bambra, C., Smith, K. E., Garthwaite, K., Joyce, K. E., & Hunter, D. J. (2011). A labour of Sisyphus? Public policy and health inequalities research from the Black and Acheson Reports to the Marmot Review. *Journal of Epidemiology and Community Health, 65*(5), 399–406. https://doi.org/10.1136/jech.2010.111195.

Baum, F. (2015). *The new public health* (4th ed.). Oxford University Press.

Bowen-Reid, T. L., & Harrell, J. P. (2002). Racist experiences and health outcomes: An examination of spirituality as a buffer. *Journal of Black Psychology, 28*(1), 16–36. https://doi.org/10.1177/0095798402028001002.

British Medical Association. (2011). *Social determinants of health—What doctors can do*. https://www.paho.org/hq/dmdocuments/2012/Social-Determinants-Doctors-Eng.pdf.

Brown, N. (n.d.). *Promoting a social and cultural determinants approach to Aboriginal and Torres Strait Islander Affairs [PowerPoint slides]*. https://www.checkup.org.au/icms_docs/183362_Prof_Ngiare_Brown.pdf.

Brown, T. H., O'Rand, A. M., & Adkins, D. E. (2012). Race-ethnicity and health trajectories: Tests of three hypotheses across multiple groups and health outcomes. *Journal of Health and Social Behavior, 53*(3), 359–377.

Centers for Disease Control and Prevention (CDC). (2017). *SMART: BRFSS city and county data and documentation*. https://www.cdc.gov/brfss/smart/smart_data.htm.

Chandler, M. J., & Lalonde, C. (1998). Cultural continuity as a hedge against suicide in Canada's First Nations. *Transcultural Psychiatry, 35*(3), 191–219. https://doi.org/10.1177/136346159803500202.

Coburn, D. (2004). Beyond the income inequality hypothesis: Class, neo-liberalism, and health inequalities. *Social Science and Medicine, 58*(1), 41–56. https://doi.org/10.1016/S0277-9536(03)00159-X

Commission on Social Determinants of Health. (2008). *Closing the gap in a generation: Health equity through action on the social determinants of health*. World Health Organisation. https://www.who.int/social_determinants/final_report/csdh_finalreport_2008.pdf

Day, G. E. (2016). Migrant and refugee health: Advance Australia fair? *Australian Health Review, 40*(1), 1–2. https://doi.org/10.1071/ahv40n1_ed.

Dew, K. (2012). *The cult and science of public health: A sociological investigation*. Berghahn Books.

Dew, K. (2014). Patient-centered care or discrimination? Diagnosis among diverse populations. In A. G. Jutel & K. Dew (Eds.), *Social issues in diagnosis: An introduction for students and clinicians* (pp. 93–104). Johns Hopkins University Press.

Engels, F. [1845] (1950). *The condition of the working class in England in 1844*. Allen and Unwin.

Fanany, R. (2012). Language, culture and health. In P. Liamputtong, R. Fanany, & G. Verrinder (Eds.), *Health, illness and wellbeing: Perspectives and social determinants*. Oxford University Press.

Farmer, P. E., Nizeye, B., Stulac, S., & Keshavjee, S. (2006). Structural violence and clinical medicine. *PLoS Medicine, 3*(10), 1686–1691. https://doi.org/10.1371/journal.pmed.0030449.

Gagné, T., & Ghenadenik, A. E. (2018). Rethinking the relationship between socioeconomic status and health: Challenging how socioeconomic status is currently used in health inequality research. *Scandinavian Journal of Public Health, 46*(1), 53–56.

Georges, N., Gutheridge, S. L., Li, S. Q., Condon, J. R., Barnes, T., & Zhao, Y. (2013). Progess in closing the gap in life expectancy at birth for Aboriginal people in the Northern Territory, 1967–2012. *Medical Journal of Australia, 207*(1), 25–30. https://doi.org/10.5694/mja16.01138.

Germov, J. (2019a). *Second opinion: An introduction to health sociology* (6th ed.). Oxford University Press.

Germov, J. (2019b). The class origins of health inequality. In J. Germov (Ed.), *Second opinion: an introduction to health sociology* (6th ed.). Oxford University Press.

Geronimus, A. (1992). The weathering hypothesis and the health of African-American women and infants: Evidence and speculations. *Ethnic & Disease, 2*(3), 207–221.

Geronimus, A., Hicken, M., Keene, D., & Bound, J. (2006). Weathering and age patterns of allostatic load scores among blacks and whites in the United States. *American Journal of Public Health, 96*(5), 826–833.

Greenhalgh, E. M., Scollo, M. M., & Pearce, M. (2016). Contribution of smoking to health inequality. In E. M. Greenhalgh, M. M. Scollo, & M. H. Winstanley (Eds.), *Tobacco in Australia: Facts and issues*. Cancer Council Victoria. http://www.tobaccoinaustralia.org.au/chapter-9-disadvantage/9-3-contribution-of-smoking-to-health-inequality.

Habibis, D., & Walter, M. M. (2015). *Social inequality in Australia: Discourses, realities and futures* (2nd ed.). Oxford University Press.

Hackett, C., Feeny, D., & Tompa, E. (2016). Canada's residential school system: Measuring the intergenerational impact of familial attendance on health and mental health outcomes. *Journal of Epidemiology and Community Health*, *70*(11), 1096–1105. https://doi.org/10.1136/jech-2016-207380.

Hardin, J., McLennan, A. K., & Brewis, A. (2018). Body size, body norms and some unintended consequences of obesity intervention in the Pacific Islands. *Annals of Human Biology*, *45*(3), 285–294. https://doi.org/10.1080/03014460.2018.1459838.

Hawley, N. L., & McGarvey, S.T. (2015). Obesity and diabetes in Pacific Islanders: The current burden and the need for urgent action. *Current Diabetes Reports*, *15*(5), 29. https://doi.org/10.1007/s11892-015-0594-5.

Hickey, S. (2015a). What's in a label: Social factors and health issues for a small group of Aboriginal people born in Brisbane, Australia [Doctoral dissertation, University of Queensland]. UQ eSpace. https://espace.library.uq.edu.au/view/UQ:382316.

Hickey, S. (2015b). It all comes down to ticking a box: Collecting Aboriginal identification in a 30-year longitudinal health study. *Australian Aboriginal Studies*, *2*, 33–45.

Hickey, S. (2016). They say I'm not a typical Blackfella: Experiences of racism and ontological security in urban Australia. *Journal of Sociology*, *52*(4), 725–740. https://doi.org/10.1177/1440783315581218.

Lauderdale, D. (2006). Birth outcomes for Arabic-named women in California before and after September 11. *Demography*, *43*(1), 185–201. https://doi.org/10.1353/dem.2006.0008.

Lillee, A., Thambiran, A., & Laugharne, J. (2015). Evaluating the mental health of recently arrived refugee adults in Western Australia. *Journal of Public Mental Health*, *14*(2), 56–68. https://doi.org/10.1108/JPMH-05-2013-0033.

Link, B. G., & Phelan, J. (1995). Social conditions as fundamental causes of disease. *Journal of Health and Social Behavior*, 80–94. https://doi.org/10.2307/2626958.

Lowitja Institute. (2014). *Cultural determinants of Aboriginal and Torres Strait Islander health roundtable*. https://www.lowitja.org.au/content/Document/PDF/Cultural-Determinants-RT-Report-FINAL2b.pdf.

Macintyre, S. (1997). The Black Report and beyond what are the issues? *Social Science & Medicine*, *44*(6), 723–745. https://doi.org/10.1016/S0277-9536(96)00183-9.

Marmot, M. (2001). From Black to Acheson: Two decades of concern with inequalities in health. A celebration of the 90th birthday of Professor Jerry Morris. *International Journal of Epidemiology*, *30*(5), 1165–1171. https://doi.org/10.1093/ije/30.5.1165.

Marmot, M. (2004). *Status syndrome: How your social standing directly affects your health and life expectancy*. Bloomsbury.

Marmot, M. (2016). Fair Australia: social justice and the health gap. *The 2016 Boyer Lectures*. Australian Broadcasting Corporation. https://www.abc.net.au/radionational/programs/boyerlectures/series/2016-boyer-lectures/7802472.

Marmot, M. (2019). Everything and the kitchen sink. *The Lancet*, *393*(10176), 1089–1090. https://doi.org/10.1016/S0140-6736(19)30506-9.

Mathers, C. D., & Schofield, D. J. (1998). The health consequences of unemployment: The evidence. *Medical Journal of Australia*, *168*(4), 178–182. doi. 10.5694/j.1326-5377.1998.tb126776.x.

McDonald, E., Bailie, R., Grace, J., & Brewster, D. (2009). A case study of physical and social barriers to hygiene and child growth in remote Australian Aboriginal communities. *BMC Public Health*, *9*(1), 346. https://doi.org/10.1186/1471-2458-9-346.

Montenegro Torres, F. (2013). *Costa Rica case study: Primary health care achievements and challenges within the framework of the social health insurance*. World Bank. https://openknowledge.worldbank.org/bitstream/handle/10986/13279/74962.pdf?sequence=1&isAllowed=y.

Napier, A. D., Ancarno, C., Butler, B., Calabrese, J., Chater, A., Chatterjee, H., Guesnet, F., Horne, R., Jacyna, S., Jadhav, S., Macdonald, A., Neuendorf, U., Parkhurst, A., Reynolds, R., Scambler, G., Shamdasani, S., Smith, S. Z., Stougaard-Nielsen, J., Thomson, L., … Woolf, K. (2014). Culture and health. *The Lancet*, *384*(9954), 1607–1639. https://doi.org/10.1016/S0140-6736(14)61603-2.

Nettleton, S. (2013). *The sociology of health and illness* (3rd ed.). Polity Press.

Obama, B. (2016). United States health care reform: Progress to date and next steps. *Journal of the American Medical Association*, *316*(5), 525–532. https://doi.org/0.1001/jama.2016.9797.

Øversveen, E., Rydland, H. T., Bambra, C., & Eikemo, T. A. (2017). Rethinking the relationship between socio-economic status and health: Making the case for sociological theory in health inequality research. *Scandinavian Journal of Public Health*, *45*(2), 103–112. https://doi.org/10.1177/1403494816686711.

Phelan, J. C., Link, B. G., & Tehranifar, P. (2010). Social conditions as fundamental causes of health inequalities: Theory, evidence and policy implications. *Journal of Health and Social Behavior*, *51*(S), S28–S40. https://doi.org/10.1177/0022146510383498.

Popay, J., Williams, G., Thomas, C., & Gatrell, T. (1998). Theorising inequalities in health: The place of lay knowledge. *Sociology of Health and Illness*, *20*(5), 619–644. https://doi.org/10.1111/1467-9566.00122.

Powell, J. A., & Menendian, S. (2016). The problem of othering: Towards inclusiveness and belonging. *Othering and Belonging*, *1*, 14–39.

Priest, N., Paradies, Y., Trenerry, B., Truong, M., Karlsen, S., & Kelly, Y. (2013). A systematic review of studies examining the relationship between reported racism and health and wellbeing for children and young people. *Social Science & Medicine*, *95*, 115–127. https://doi.org/10.1016/j.socscimed.2012.11.031.

Richmond, C. (2002). Sir Douglas Black. *Bristish Medical Journal*, *325*(7365), 661–662. https://doi.org/10.1136/bmj.325.7365.661.

Safe Work Australia. (2019). *Fatality statistics*. https://www.safeworkaustralia.gov.au/statistics-and-research/statistics/fatalities/fatality-statistics.

Scambler, G. (2012). Health inequalities. *Sociology of Health & Illness*, *34*(1), 130–146. https://doi.org/10.1111/j.1467-9566.2011.01387.x.

Scarani, P. (2003). RudolfVirchow (1821–1902). *Virchows Archives*, *442*(2), 95–98. https://doi.org/10.1007/s00428-002-0742-6.

Schofield, T. (2007). Health inequity and its social determinants: A sociological commentary. *Health Sociology Review*, *16*(2), 105–114. https://doi.org/10.5172/hesr.2007.16.2.105.

Scribano, A. (2018). Inroduction: The multiple Janus faces of neoliberalism. In A. Scribano, F. Timmermann Lopez, & M. E. Korstanje (Eds.), *Neoliberalism in multi-disciplinary perspective* (pp. 1–20). Palgrave Macmillan. https://doi.org/10.1007/978-3-319-77601-9.

Shattock, A. J., Gambhir, M., Taylor, H. R., Cowling, C. S., Kaldor, J. M., & Wilson, D. P. (2015). Control of trachoma in Australia: A model based evaluation of current interventions. *PLoS Neglected Tropical Diseases*, *9*(4), 1–12. https://doi.org/10.1371/journal.pntd.0003474.

Sherwood, J. (2013). ColonisationIt's bad for your health: The context of Aboriginal health. *Contemporary Nurse*, *46*(1), 28–40. https://doi.org/10.5172/conu.2013.46.1.28.

Silburn, S. R., Zubrick, S. R., Lawrence, D. M., Mitrou, F. G., DeMaio, J. A., Blair, E., Cox, A., Dalby, R. B., Griffin, J. A., Pearson, G., & Hayward, C. (2006). The intergenerational effects of forced separation on the social and emotional wellbeing of Aboriginal children and young people. *Family Matters*, *75*, 10–17.

Smedley, A., & Smedley, B. (2005). Race as biology is fiction, racism as a social problem is real: Anthropological and historical perspectives on the social construction of race. *American Psychologist*, *60*(1), 16–26. https://doi.org/10.1037/0003-066X.60.1.16.

Smylie, J., Kirst, M., McShane, K., Firestone, M., Wolfe, S., & O'Campo, P. (2016). Understanding the role of Indigenous community participation in Indigenous prenatal and infant-toddler health promotion programs in Canada: A realist review. *Social Science & Medicine*, *150*, 128–143. https://doi.org/10.1016/j.socscimed.2015.12.019.

Solar, O., & Irwin, A. (2010). *A conceptual framework for action on the social determinants of health*. World Health Organisation.https://www.who.int/sdhconference/resources/ConceptualframeworkforactiononSDH_eng.pdf.

Stoneham, M. J., Goodman, J., & Daube, M. (2014). The portrayal of Indigenous health in selected Australian media. *The International Indigenous Policy Journal*, *5*(1), 1–13.

Sweet, M. (2013). *Culture is an important determinant of health: Professor Ngiare Brown at NACCHO Summit*. Crikey. https://blogs.crikey.com.au/croakey/2013/08/20/culture-is-an-important-determinant-of-healthprofessor-ngiare-brown-at-naccho-summit/.

Szreter, S. (1997). Economic growth, disruption, deprivation, disease, and death: On the importance of the politics of public health for development. *Population and Development Review*, *23*(4), 693–728.

Szreter, S., & Mooney, G. (1998). Urbanisation, mortality and the standard of living debate: New estimates of the expectation of life at birth in nineteenthe-century British cities. *Economic History Review*, *51*, 84–112.

Taylor, H. R., & Anjou, M. D. (2013). Trachoma in Australia: An update. *Clinical & Experimental Ophthalmology*, *41*(5), 508–512.

Taylor, H. R., Burton, M. J., Haddad, D., West, S., & Wright, H. (2014). Trachoma. *The Lancet*, *384*, 2142–2152.

Udah, H., & Singh, P. (2019). Identity, othering and belonging: Toward an understanding of difference and the experiences of African immigrants to Australia. *Social Identities*, *6*, 1–17.

Williams, D. R., & Mohammed, S. A. (2013). Racism and health I: Pathways and scientific evidence. *American Behavioral Scientist*, *57*(8), 1152–1173. https://doi.org/10.1177/0002764213487340.

Williams, J. E. (2013). Biological pre-emption: Race, class and genomics. *Sociology Compass*, 7(9), 711–725.https://doi.org/10.1111/soc4.12063.

Wilkinson, R., & Marmot, M. (2003). *Social determinants of health: The solid facts* (2nd ed.). World Health Organisation. https://www.euro.who.int/__data/assets/pdf_file/0005/98438/e81384.pdf.

World Bank. (2019). *Current health expenditure per capita (current US$)*. https://data.worldbank.org/indicator/SH.XPD.CHEX.PC.CD

World Health Organisation (WHO). (2010). *The Commission on the social determinants of health, what, why and how?* http://www.who.int/social_determinants/thecommission/finalreport/about_csdh/en/index.html.

World Health Organisation (WHO). (2017). *Trachoma fact sheet*. http://www.who.int/mediacentre/factsheets/fs382/en/.

World Health Organisation (WHO). (2019). *Life expectancy for women: Data by country*. http://apps.who.int/gho/data/view.main.WOMENLEXv?lang=en.

Yaser, A., Slewa-Younan, S., Smith, C. A., Olson, R. E., Uribe Guajardo, M. G., & Mond, J. (2016). Beliefs and knowledge about post-traumatic stress disorder amongst resettled Afghan refugees in Australia. *International Journal of Mental Health Systems*, *10*(31), 1–9.

3 Cultural models of health and health care

Alexander Workman, Syeda Zakia Hossain, Pranee Liamputtong, Angelica Ojinnaka and Elias Mpofu

Learning outcomes

After working through this chapter, students should be able to:

1. Discuss different definitions of health as conceptualised or perceived through different cultural lenses.
2. Identify key principles or components of various models of health and how they interact with diverse groups of people in a society.
3. Evaluate the limitations and facilitators of diverse models of health and their role in reducing health inequalities and health inequities.
4. Analyse how diverse models of health may influence all health practitioners' engagement with cultural safety.
5. Justify the role of diverse models of health in the creation of culturally safe health care environments.

Key terms

Biomedical model of health and wellbeing: The biomedical model of health and wellbeing focuses on biological factors. In this model, health is conceptualised as the absence of disease or illness.
Eurocentrism: A cultural phenomenon that views the histories and cultures of non-Western societies from a European or Western perspective.
Ethnocentrism: Evaluation of other cultures according to preconceptions originating in the standards and customs of one's own culture.
Primary health care model: The entry level to the health system and, as such, is usually a person's first encounter with the health system.
Non-Western models of health and wellbeing: Non-Western models of health and wellbeing embrace more than just the disease or illness an individual may experience. These models also focus on developing a deep connection to the region's philosophical and spiritual values.
Biopsychosocial models of health and wellbeing: An interdisciplinary model that looks at the interconnection between biology, psychology, and socio-environmental factors.
Immigrational/emigrational experiences of health: The experiences of health over the course of immigration/emigration, including increases/decreases in vulnerability to health diseases and conditions or the development and occurrence of health problems.

Chapter summary

This chapter discusses diversity in models of health and wellbeing in Australia and internationally with a focus on the biomedical, biopsychosocial, primary health care, Indigenous, and non-Western perspectives. First, this chapter encourages students to investigate and critically analyse how these models manifest and intersect in health care settings nationally and globally and how they are used and supported. These models are then linked to health and wellbeing outcomes for diverse populations through case studies and research findings. Pedagogical features of the chapter include interactive and self-reflection activities for students to explore their "culture of health" and how it compares to models present in broader society such as Australia. By the end of this chapter, students would have developed a comprehensive understanding of the role of diverse models of health in establishing culturally safe health care environments.

Box 3.1 Reflection—Getting sick

Before you begin to read this chapter, take a few minutes to consider what happens within your own family when you are sick (for example, with a cold or the flu). After you have thought this through, record your answers to the following questions:

- Does the treatment of your illness come from traditional remedies your family uses, complementary remedies or do you traditionally seek treatment from your general practitioner (GP)?
- Do you combine a range of treatment types to address your illness?
- How closely do you follow the instructions of taking any medication, including traditional medicine or treatment protocol given by your family or health care practitioner?

Compare your answers with your peers, and examine any similarities or differences you observed with cultural influence on health. At the end of this chapter, reflect on your answers to determine if you have an approach that falls within one of the three models discussed throughout this section or is it a combination of two or more? Or, is it something completely different? The next step to this activity will be at the end of the chapter.

Introduction

Health inequalities or disparities in health statuses and services and health inequities or avoidable health care deprivations, are a global phenomenon. However, certain groups of individuals are more likely to experience inequalities at higher rates than others based on inequities associated to their visible differences and their identity (Cora-Bramble, Tielman, & Wright, 2004; Kurtz, Janke, Vinek, Wells, Hutchinson, & Froste, 2018; Liamputtong, 2019; Rose, 2018). For instance, Kurtz et al. (2018) note that some groups who experience these health inequalities stem from countries who underwent the process of colonisation, the First Nations peoples of these colonised nation-states including; *Aboriginal* and *Torres Strait Islander peoples*, Canadian *Metis*, New Zealand *Māoris*, Bangladeshis *Garos* and Alaska's *Inuit* peoples, to name a few.

Moreover, persons with varying identities, including cultural and linguistic diversity, gender, gendered identity and sexual orientation, may experience disproportionate health inequalities (Dune & Liamputtong, 2019; Liamputtong & Suwankhong, 2019; Wilkerson et al., 2011). For example, inequalities extend to those who are culturally and linguistically diverse (CALD), as well as, those who identify as lesbian, gay, bisexual, transgender, intersex and queer or questioning (LGBTIQ) (for more information pertaining specifically to this population, please see Chapter 12) and, those of different socially constructed genders (refer to Chapter 11). Individuals whose cultural identities intersect one or more of these diverse communities may receive differential treatment that contrasts from the mainstream, on the basis of these visible differences. These treatments are significantly Eurocentric and enacted by the dominant culture in these communities, affecting the cultural safety of treatment practices (Mortensen, 2010).

Culture in the context of diversity and cultural safety for this chapter includes, but is not limited by, an individual, age or generation, gender, sexual orientation, occupation, socioeconomic status, ethnic origin or migrant experience, religious or spiritual belief and disability status (Kurtz et al., 2018; Liamputtong & Suwankhong, 2019). Culture develops within a social, political, and historical context and views the world through the lens that their culture is the dominant and correct one (Liamputtong & Suwankhong, 2019; Talbot & Verrinder, 2017). Moreover, these lenses permeate all social structures and are reflective in policies and procedures that govern social systems. According to Talbot and Verrinder (2017) and Liamputtong and Suwankhong (2019), it is important to understand the social, political, and historical contexts of cultural groups in order to foster an environment where they feel safe.

This chapter will explore the nature of health inequalities and inequities that impact diverse cultural groups in Australia and globally. The chapter further investigates how diverse cultural groups that may be different to Westernised, Eurocentric cultures (Australia, Canada, USA, to new a few), vary in their conceptualisation of health (Bhopal 2007; Liamputtong & Suwankhong, 2019). The chapter considers several health models such as the biomedical model, biopsychosocial model, primary health care models, and *non-Western models of health and wellbeing* (defined later in this chapter). The chapter also provides insights into the role of health professionals in creating a culturally safe environment informed by varying models of health, which is crucial for effective client–practitioner relationships and health care practice (Ike & King, 2008; Tucker et al., 2015). Moreover, this chapter discuses a number of distinct types of health care models, and a diverse range of clients' perspectives of health, some of which fall into one or a combination of different health models. It is also critical to assess whether Australia's current models of health influence the Australian Indigenous and CALD background population's experiences with health care practitioners and health care services. Almost 30% of Australia's population are CALD, and they are a continually growing diverse population (Australian Bureau of Statistics, 2016, 2020), necessitating the use of different models of health care other than the dominant biomedical model of health care. We acknowledge that there are several types of health care practices, including modern medicine (biomedical model), traditional medicine (Chinese medicine, homeopathy) and alternative therapy for people from all walks of life; however, this chapter briefly discusses the biomedical model, the biopsychosocial model, *primary health care models*, and non-Western models of health. It is important to note that with Indigenous and non-Western models of health, there are multiple ways to doing and fulfilling health needs that go beyond the scope of this chapter. Please refer to Chapter 7 for a more in-depth discussion on Indigenous models of health care.

Before we continue with this chapter, answer the following questions.

Box 3.2 Reflection—Understanding health

How do you define health?
Point of consideration: answer the following questions before you proceed:

1. How do you define health?
2. Where does your own understanding of "health" come from?
3. How do you explain the concept of "health" to other people?
4. Think about whether "health" is something we have or something we do or both.
5. What are its essential components?
6. Who decides on these components?
7. What is a healthy person?
8. What does a person need to have to make them healthy?
9. How do we learn about "health", and how might this influence our understandings of "wellbeing"?

What is health?

The definition of *health* has remained unchanged as a narrow concept, focusing on physical wellbeing from a medical context for some time (Oleribe et al., 2018). The World Health Organisation's (WHO) (1948) definition of health extended this definition to physical, mental and social wellbeing. According to the WHO (1948), "health is a state of complete physical, mental and social wellbeing and not merely the absence of disease or infirmity" (https://www.who.int/about/who-we-are/constitution). It also suggests that it is the fundamental human right of every human being to attain the highest standard of health irrespective of their race, religion, political belief, economic or social condition. However, the definition is limited, as it does not cover the spiritual wellbeing of human beings, which is an integral part of their complete wellbeing. Therefore, different views of health that are currently represented in discussions on health are discussed next.

The biomedical model of health and wellbeing

In Western societies, the current approach to health and wellbeing stems predominantly from a *biomedical model of health* (Kurtz et al., 2018). This model became popular in the formative years of the 19th century and is still the dominant perspective today (Marks, Murray, & Estacio, 2018). Through the lens of this model, health is conceptualised as the absence of disease or illness (Deacon & McKay, 2015; WHO, 2003). Marks, Murray, and Estacio (2018) note the biomedical model maintains that illnesses will usually have a biological cause. Furthermore, this model surmises that disease occurs due to the invasion of pathogens such as a virus, bacterium or microorganism into the body. Despite this model evolving to adopt more holistic views of health, it still does not account for non-biological factors. Examples of such factors include relationships with family, social relationships with friends and community, and interactions within environments. Consequently, the predominant weakness of this model is its minimal consideration and adoption of psychological, sociological, environmental or behavioural variances associated with illness (Deacon & McKay, 2015).

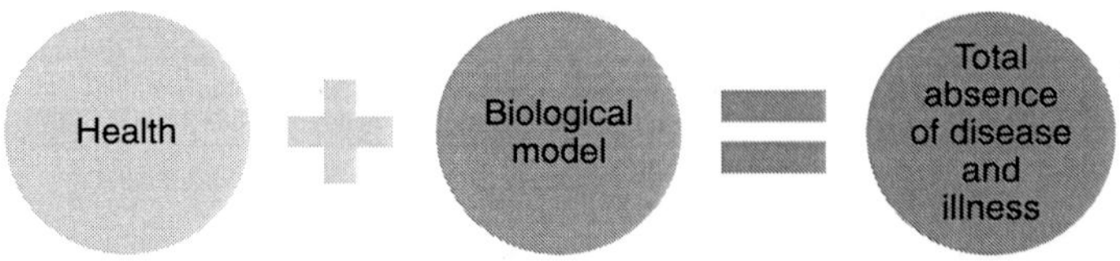

Figure 3.1 The biomedical model of health

For example, if you take a person out of their house that has mould (a type of fungi), they become hospitalised, and they receive treatment for the illness caused by the mould. They get better and return to their place of residence, and then eventually they come back into hospital because the mould (which has not been treated) has made them sick again. Unless you address the issue of the mould, the person will continue to be sick. As the example denotes, factors related to the environment were not considered during the treatment of the illness. The biomedical model does not take these factors into account when investigating and responding to a person's health and wellbeing. The biomedical model focuses on the disease and takes the approach of cure rather than prevention. It focuses attention primarily on the disease and specific part of the body or the organ, often ignoring the social origins of the disease (Germov, 2019). Dubbin, Chang, and Shim (2013) note this approach is growing to incorporate a more patient-/client-centred care approach, with the overarching goal of placing the person's cultural values, needs and preferences at the forefront of their ongoing health care (Figure 3.1).

Box 3.3 Reflection—Putting the biomedical model into practice

Australia continues to be an increasingly diverse country. With a growing population of people moving to Australia each year, the population is forecasted to grow from 21.0 million people in 2007 and increase to between 30.9 and 42.5 million by 2056 (Australian Bureau of Statistics, 2008). A third of the Australian population is overseas born (Australian Bureau of Statistics, 2020). More than one-fifth (21%) of Australians speak another language other than the English language at home (Australian Bureau of Statistics, 2016). Based on Australia's current demographic composition of the population and reliance on the traditional biomedical approach, do you feel it can sustain the health needs of the ever-increasing population? Open a new webpage, locate the most current form of population data and consider the racial and ethnic statistics that make up Australia. After reflecting on this diverse population, consider, based on the definitions given earlier (biomedical, primary health care and non-Western models of health), the following questions:

1. Based on the statistics provided, both born in Australia and overseas, compare the differences in health care that may exist in the immigrants' country of origin and the host country.
2. Pick an ethnic group and search for the diverse ways their country of origin's definition of health and wellbeing may be expressed.
3. Can the biomedical model accurately assist in these issues?

Australian Bureau of Statistics (2016). *2016 Census: Multicultural.* https://www.abs.gov.au/ausstats/abs@.nsf/lookup/media%20release3

Critiques of the biomedical model

As previously noted, the biomedical model considers health to be defined by an absence of disease and illness. In a way, this model is simplistic in nature; it does not account for the complexities of lived health. As Straub (2017) suggests, human life is messy, wonderful, challenging and rewarding, amongst other things. Therefore, our perceptions of health should accommodate these "messes" as health. Health is not simply the absence of illness; it encompasses a person's environment, mental and spiritual health, emotional state, connections to friends and family, the experiences individuals have growing up and a lot more. The biomedical model does not recognise that health is multifaceted. The problem with this approach is its dominance in Western nation-states. However, most Western nation-states are deeply diverse with many groups of people coming from non-Western nation-states and by extension these nations' First Peoples. Therefore, approaches to health and wellbeing must be reflective of this diversity.

Ethnocentrism, Eurocentrism and health

Ethnocentrism centres itself around the importance of one's own cultural beliefs and values as superior; therefore, every other culture is scaled in comparison, rated in reference to the individual's own culture (Baer, Singer, Long, & Erickson, 2016). Ethnocentrism differs slightly to *Eurocentrism* in that respect (Capell, Dean, & Veenstra, 2008; Liamputtong & Suwankhong, 2019). In this connection, Capell, Dean, and Veenstra (2008) and Liamputtong and Suwankhong (2019) note that ethnocentrism can impact an individual's engagement with health practices, which may not complement their own cultural health beliefs. For example, there may be a cultural clash with Eurocentric biomedical approaches if the consumer is from a background that places greater emphasis on traditional medicines such as Traditional Chinese Medicine or Indigenous Bush Medicine. People who perceive their cultural understanding of health to be marginalised would likely not engage with biomedical health services for more serious health concerns such as cardiovascular disease, cancer, diabetes or kidney disease or mental health issues (Capell, Dean, & Veenstra, 2008; Logan, Steel, & Hunt, 2016). It is important to see the value for the diversity of cultural beliefs concerning health practices are gaining greater recognition whereby many culturally diverse individuals domiciled in Western nations would engage with these alternative health practices (Pérez & Luquis, 2008).

Eurocentrism is a cultural phenomenon that views the histories and cultures of non-Western societies from a European or Western perspective (Joseph, 2015). Europe, more specifically Western Europe or *the West*, functions as a universal signifier in that it assumes the superiority of European cultural values over those of non-European societies. Countries that form *the West* are countries with colonial ties, such as Canada, America, New Zealand, Alaska and Australia. Although Eurocentrism is anti-diversity in nature, it presents itself as a universalist phenomenon and advocates for the imitation of a Western model of health based on *Western values*. This model focuses on individuality, human rights, equality, democracy, free markets, secularism, and social justice as a cure to all kinds of problems, no matter how different various societies are socially, culturally, and historically constructed (Bhopal, 2007; Dixey, 2014; Joseph, 2015).

Box 3.4 Reflection—Eurocentrism and ethnocentrism in practice

- Explain how Eurocentrism and health intersect and create inequalities.
- Do they exacerbate unhealthy outcomes due to the one-dimensional approach of the biomedical approach?

- When you are feeling sick, have you ever visited a qualified Traditional Chinese Medicine clinic?
- Do you engage with other alternative remedies that may not be considered "Western"? What kind of practices are they?

The biopsychosocial model of health and wellbeing

Considered in its infancy by some (Hatala, 2012; Pilgrim, 2015; Sarafino & Smith, 2014; Straub, 2017), the *biopsychosocial model of health and wellbeing* (BPS model) has been around for at least four decades since its proposition by Engel (1977). It emerged from a realisation that the biomedical model was inadequate for comprehensive health care. While there has been an epidemiological shift to noncommunicable diseases, such as cardiovascular diseases, drug and alcohol abuse disorders and lung cancer from communicable diseases, such as tuberculosis, influenza and measles (Hatala, 2012), the biomedical model lacked in versatility across the disease continuum, calling for models that tie in the socio-environmental conditions that influence population health.

George Engel originally conceptualised the BPS model in 1977 to form a new medical model, as diseases are multi-determined and may result from a combination of biological, psychological or social processes within the various forms of human interaction (Pilgrim, 2015). Therefore, BPS model attempts to answer the multifarious impacts of health contrasts to the traditional biomedical model, which does not consider the social factors that underlie health conditions (Lehman, David, & Gruber, 2017; Matsui, Adamson, & Peng, 2019; Pilgrim, 2015; Suls & Rothman, 2004). For example, the biomedical model of health views one's genetic predisposition to disease and illness, and psychological and/or behavioural concerns may consider a person's lifestyle choices or health beliefs, whereas the BPS model considers social factors such as a person's relationships, socioeconomic status, religion, and access to social support as a direct influencer of their health outcomes (Hatala 2012; Lehman, David, & Gruber, 2017; Matsui, Adamson, & Peng, 2019). These different perceptions of health treated separately fail to recognise the nuances of what influences human beings, and thus, the term and approach of the BPS model of health and wellbeing emerged to address the intersections of identity and health.

Pilgrim (2015) posits the BPS model began as an idea to answer these intersecting issues and as such address issues concerning health to be more complex than one simply being sick with a disease or illness. This model takes into consideration that when you are in an environment that may be unhealthy, you take a person out of it to make them feel better but then do not change the conditions in which they live and place them back, how does one expect a person to get better (Lehman, David, & Gruber, 2017; Matsui, Adamson, & Peng, 2019)? Conversely, this is more so the case for many people from all diverse backgrounds. However, Straub (2017) argues it is becoming increasingly common to overlook the reasons that perpetuate illness and disease (Figure 3.2).

Critiques of the biopsychosocial model

A person's biology, their psychological functions and their social environment underpin the BPS model. Going further than the biomedical model to consider that health is multidimensional, is a strength of this approach. However, this model is under-researched and not as popular as the biomedical model, despite this model encompassing more parts of human life (Deacon & McKay, 2015; Straub, 2017). While the model indeed explains that health is not simply not being burdened with disease or illnesses, it is not as universal in Western nation-states.

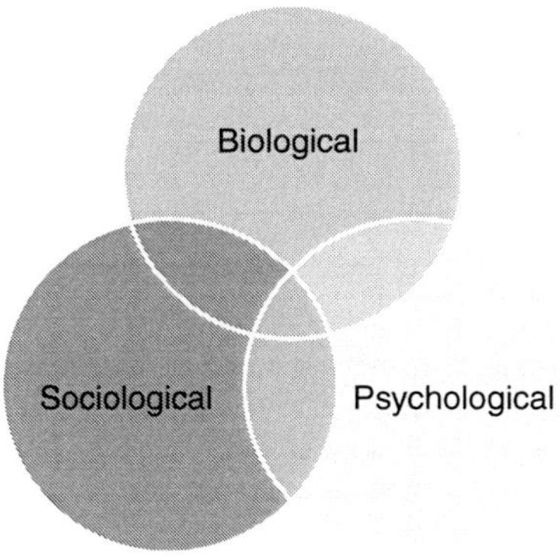

Figure 3.2 The biopsychosocial model of health

Primary health care models and cultural safety

Primary health care encompasses a philosophy that "is a whole-of-society approach to health and wellbeing centred on the needs and preferences of individuals, families and communities ... addresses the broader determinants of health and focuses on the comprehensive and inter-related aspects of physical, mental and social health and wellbeing" (WHO, 2019). This model is centred on principles of social justice, equity and self-determination, where individuals and communities are encouraged to actively participate in decisions and actions regarding their health and wellbeing (WHO, 2019). Furthermore, primary health care models look to address various determinants, including social, economic, cultural and environmental that may impact health and wellbeing (Talbot & Verrinder, 2017).

In the Australian context, primary health care models have been identified as best practice for addressing health inequities experienced across culturally diverse groups (Campbell, Hunt, Scrimgeour, Davey, & Jones, 2018; Campinha-Bacote, 2002; Weightman, 2013). For example, in Aboriginal and Torres Strait Islander communities, good health is more than just the absence of disease or illness, but one that addresses health from the lens of a holistic and communal approach (Davy, Harfield, McArthur, Munn, & Brown, 2016; Taylor & Guerin, 2014). For this population, the concept of health and wellbeing encompasses physical, social, emotional, cultural, spiritual and ecological wellbeing, for both the individual and the community (see Figure 3.3) (Australian Institute of Health and Welfare, 2018). In contrast to the biomedical model and, expanding on the BPS model, primary health care models include more than the absence of being sick physically, psychologically or the sociological reasons for why one may be sick (Australian Institute of Health and Welfare, 2018). Conversely, this may allow conflict to manifest between these competing perspectives of health, where the alternative ways of health and wellbeing are culturally significant; however within the contemporary Australian health environment Indigenous ways of understanding health are often disregarded (Davy et al., 2016). Community-controlled models of primary health care such as Aboriginal Community Controlled Health Organisations (ACCHOs) adopt the philosophy of primary health care and advocate for the provision of culturally safe care (Campbell et al., 2018). These models of primary health care address health inequities directly related to specific cultural groups and effectively address specific aspects of health by embracing principles shared in primary health care. For a more holistic approach and to aid in the development of culturally safe health environments, health practitioners should aim to have a total sense of how health and wellbeing are conceptualised and experienced across culturally diverse groups (Figure 3.3).

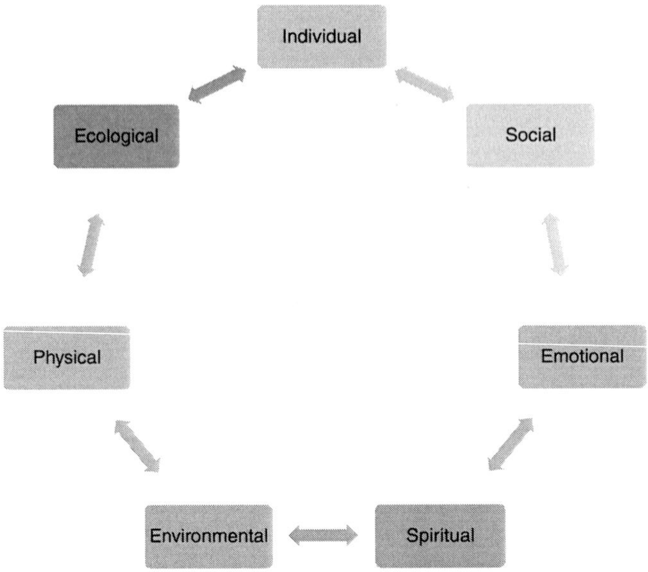

Figure 3.3 Concept of health and wellbeing for Indigenous communities

Box 3.5 Case study—The five constructs into practice

The biomedical model proposes that to be healthy, we as individuals must have two pieces of fruit and three vegetables a day, we must drink at least two litres a water a day, wash daily and practice good personal hygiene. The goal of these directives is to prevent the spread of disease and illnesses. For many citizens in societies that are considered Westernised, educated, industrialised, rich and democratic (WEIRD), this is easily achievable, and they may exercise these activities daily without any conscious thought. Arguably, some people take having access to these things for granted. Now, imagine those who live and work in an impoverished community in far-remote Australia or a community of low socioeconomic status somewhere outside their home city's suburban area. The local supermarket is a few hours' drive away or around the corner, but the cost of fruits and vegetables may not be in the budget. For those individuals who live rurally, there has been no rain for months (which is what you rely upon for drinking water and bathing water), and you see that for the people living in this community, not only do they not have access to fresh fruits and vegetables, but they also do not have access to other sources of pre-packaged non-perishable food. As a health practitioner, you are stunned to find that local people take offence to a poster you put up saying to be healthy you must:

1. Drink 2 litres of water a day
2. Eat two pieces of fruit and three vegetables a day
3. Must wash yourself daily and practice good personal hygiene

The town is resistant to your poster because the things we take for granted are luxury items for some, and having access or the capacity to purchase these items is hard to achieve. But they can provide certain items for their loved ones that may not meet the requirements as outlined by the WHO.

Considering cultural perspectives on health and wellbeing

Understanding cultural perspectives on health and wellbeing, such as in Indigenous health, can be challenging due to the generational and intergenerational impacts of colonisation, issues regarding culturally safe practices and government policy within broader health care systems (Smith, 2016; Taylor & Guerin, 2014, 2019). There have been attempts to publicly address these challenges and impacts for certain populations in Australia. In 2008, former Prime Minister Kevin Rudd offered a national apology into the historical and contemporary treatment of Indigenous people (Askew, Brady, Mukandi, Singh, Sinh, Brough, & Bond, 2020; Commonwealth of Australia, 2020; Prime Minister of Australia, 2020). After this, there was a pledge to combat the ever-growing gap of health outcomes between Indigenous and non-Indigenous Australians from life expectancy outcomes (10 years lower), health-related issues such as cardiovascular disease, diabetes and mental health-related issues, to name a few. (Commonwealth of Australia, 2020; Joseph, 2015). For many Indigenous people this apology was to begin a new page in the book of their proud and long history. Thus, the *Closing the Gap* campaign arose to combat the issues of health within this community; however, there are many critiques of this campaign, which currently have not been addressed (Australian Institute of Health and Welfare, 2018; Gannon, 2018). While health was one of the primary focuses, there are many other social determinants of health (SDH), which were also highlighted, such as poor educational outcomes (both in early childhood and educational achievements), child mortality, and employment outcomes (Bond & Singh, 2020; Commonwealth of Australia, 2020).

A review of the campaign found that current models of health such as the biomedical model ignore the nuances of life for many cultural groups including Indigenous people and may not consider the philosophical principles that underpin primary health care models (Askew et al., 2020; Commonwealth of Australia, 2020). Supporting this perception is the concept of Eurocentrism previously defined in this chapter. The Closing the Gap campaign on health took the stance of a Western view of health and by extension other social determinants of health as well. The view of being healthy requires meeting certain criteria such as actuarial risk assessment. This process is often used in criminal justice proceedings to determine the likelihood of a person receding back into criminality. A person's life is compiled into a list, and boxes are ticked such as the likelihood of criminality determined by various outcomes such as marital/relationship status, socioeconomic conditions, education, ethnic status, gender, sexuality and many more (Findlay, Odgers, & Yeo, 2014). The Closing the Gap campaign acted much the same as a risk assessment tool; to be healthy a person must achieve this level of education, this level of health and, these levels of healthier choices. The campaign and the money pledged did achieve some positive outcomes; however, it failed to take into consideration Indigenous ways of living, knowing and being (Askew et al., 2020). As represented in the diagram in Figure 3.3, Indigenous life is not a singular thing; it is heavily influenced by many aspects of everyday life. Askew et al. (2020) argued that these health outcomes, while positive in theory, failed in many other aspects, including practice.

Box 3.6 Reflection—Closing the gap, and happiness

For example, a Ted Talk from Sheree Cairney in a study on Indigenous wellbeing and happiness found that for Indigenous children to be more successful in education, they should first experience traditional knowledge education and then Westernised education. If this occurs the outcomes are more positive. On the contrary if they receive education from a Westernised view of education first, they are more *unsuccessful* by the Closing the Gap standards.

- What do you think is missing from the Closing the Gap campaign?
- Which group's knowledge and way of life is being prioritised here?

Check out the following video:
What Aboriginal knowledge can teach us about happiness | Sheree Cairney | TEDxStKilda https://youtu.be/Cf-dK8HFP2c

Reflections on the primary health care models and cultural perspectives of health and wellbeing

Health is more than the individual—health is part of the community and those deep connections of kin, to land and country (Oppong, Brune, & Mpofu, in press). Primary health care models such as community-controlled health organisations in Indigenous health demonstrate a more inclusive approach by exploring the various aspects of a person's life compared to the biomedical or BPS models of health. Some health practices of groups such as Aboriginal and/or Torres Strait Islander peoples, adopt unique perspectives on health and wellbeing that apply to all facets of life (Waterworth, Pescud, Braham, Dimmock, & Rosenberg, 2015; Westerman, 2010). Primary health care is universal in accordance with Western definitions (i.e., applicable to all), in the sense that it does not discriminate against any part of a person's identity and therefore is the most inclusive approach to health. Primary health care models such as ACCHOs (Campbell et al., 2018) embrace the variety of perspectives on health and combine principles of accessibility, acceptability, community participation, equity, social justice and community empowerment, to achieve great cultural safety in health care. As a result, health services that adopt primary health care models can be described as "by the people, for the people, according to their needs, and in harmony with their holistic view of health … the decision-making base is shifted from the medical professions to community elected boards of directors" (Eckermann et al., 2010, p. 199).

Box 3.7 Reflection—Holistic review to Indigenous health and wellbeing

The Indigenous health and wellbeing approaches to health in perspective:
Wurrimiyanga's (Nguiu) Holistic approach to mental health. Located in Bathurst Island, this community centre has taken an alternative approach to health and wellbeing that focuses primarily on the Indigenous way of health and wellbeing. Please review the following YouTube link:
https://www.youtube.com/embed/jQWqBWy8HRE?feature=oembed
Discuss with your peers:

1. How does this approach support Indigenous health?
2. How is this approach relevant or not relevant to non-Indigenous people in Bathurst?
3. Does the approach need to be inclusive to all groups? Why might you say yes? Why might you say no?

Non-Western models of health and wellbeing

The models of health and wellbeing for people traditionally from the *East* differs from the biomedical model but has similar approaches to the Aboriginal and Torres Strait Islander concept of health embraced in primary health care models, in the sense that their approaches are multifaceted and encompass more than the absence of disease or illness (Mpofu, 2006; Oppong et al., in press). The *Eastern model of health and wellbeing* embraces much more than just the disease or illness an individual may experience, but this model has a deep connection to the region's philosophical and spiritual values (Chan, Ho, & Chow, 2002; Newcombe, 2012; Sulman, Savage, & Way, 2002). Tsuei (1978) notes that at the individual level, health comes from the teachings of Taoism, Buddhism, Confucianism, Shintoism, and Traditional Chinese Medicine, which advocate for a holistic understanding and practice of health. Health comes from yin and yang in that health is in an equilibrium, playing out between these two forces. There are extra layers that influence the outcome of one's health, such as the five elements (fire, water, earth, wood and air), six environmental conditions (dry, wet, hot, cold, wind and flame), other external sources of harm (physical injury, insect bites, poison, overheat and overwork) and the seven emotions (joy, sorry, anger, worry, panic, anxiety and fear) (Chan, Ying Ho, & Chow, 2002) (Figure 3.4).

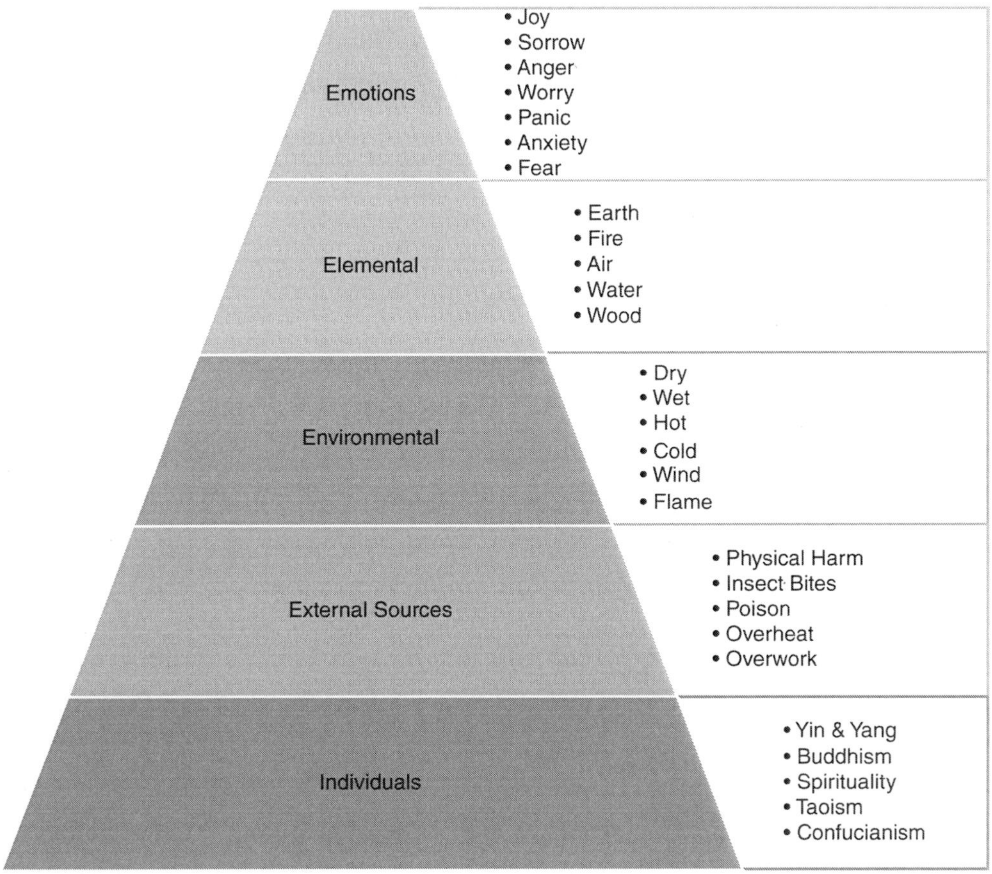

Figure 3.4 The Eastern model of health and wellbeing

Eastern ways of health and wellbeing in practice

Life operates in balance where individuals live in harmony with their environment. For people who view and practice health from an Eastern perspective, health is simply a way of being. Religious, philosophical, ethical and spiritual practices are at the forefront of being healthy. For example, Confucianism is an ethical perspective as well as a way of life, and yet is deeply rooted into the fabric of the Eastern way of life.

Box 3.8 Reflection—Eastern model of health and wellbeing

The Eastern model of health and wellbeing in perspective:
It is important to understand the clear distinction between the Western (biomedical) model and the Eastern model of health. For instance, while the Western model uses a deductive approach where it divides health from the disease, in contrast, the Eastern model uses an inductive approach, meaning it considers health as a balanced state versus disease as an unbalanced state (Tsuei, 1978). Further, the Eastern model tends to adopt the environment; in contrast the Western approach (biomedical approach) prefers to change the environment (Tsuei, 1978)

1. How does Eastern medicine differ from Western medicine?
2. Does the approach need to be inclusive to all groups? Why might you say yes? Why might you say no?

Critiques of non-Western models of health

With the increase in chronic conditions, people are more likely to seek help from alternatives. Western medicine (within the biomedical model), with the introduction of the new medication and medical technology, has contributed to reduced death rates for stroke, heart disease and cancer. For example, the death rate from heart disease has decreased by 60% since 1970 and the death rate for HIV/AIDS has dropped more than 75% since 1995 (Sullivan, 2018). However, the Eastern medicines, in particular Traditional Chinese medicine, herbal medicine and other alternative medicine, are growing in use but are limited to an acute and emergency health crisis (Sullivan, 2018). For example, acupuncture practice is recognised and has been rapidly increasing for the past two decades since the 1990s. There are nearly 4000 acupuncturists registered with the Chinese Medicine Board of Australia (Zheng, 2014).

Conclusion

In singularity the approaches to health and wellbeing presented in this chapter surmise a similar outcome, the absence of disease and illness to create good health and by extension good wellbeing. However, as you have read in this chapter and will continue to read throughout this entire book, health is a far more nuanced and complex issue than simply being absent of disease and illness. Some cultural models draw on various aspects of life including multifarious cultural approaches, emigrational experiences, geographical location, socioeconomic status, gender, gendered identity, sexuality, age or generation, education, religious status, to connect and shape understandings of health.

At the start of this chapter, you were asked to reflect on what health means to you. After reading throughout this chapter, has your answer changed, did it stay the same, or was your perspective of health aligned more so with one of the models put forth? When considering what it means to be healthy, people are divided into a few categories, and this is completely okay to have our own perceptions of what health means. Conversely, as a health practitioner, being receptive to the notion that other people's views may be quite different from yours is challenging (Horwitz et al., 2011). The same can be said about the life choices someone makes. How they chose to live their life, the type of work they do, whom they chose to love and the capacity they have to cope with issues they may have is what makes us as human beings unique.

Based on the information gathered throughout this chapter, let's now place what we have learned into practice. So far, throughout this chapter and by extension this book, you have begun to challenge the dominant narratives associated with health critically. Understanding that the one-dimensional biomedical approach currently held in Westernised nation-states traditionally upholds the values and teachings from the biomedical model does not account for other ways of being "healthy". Conversely, the non-Western and primary health care models of health and wellbeing encompass multiple ways of life to highlight how health is not one singular aspect that makes a person a person.

References

Askew, D. A., Brady, K., Mukandi, B., Singh, D., Sinha, T., Brough, M., & Bond, C. J. (2020). Closing the gap between rhetoric and practice in strengths-based approaches to Indigenous public health: A qualitative study. *Australian and New Zealand Journal of Public Health, 44*(2), 102–105. https://doi.org/10.1111/1753-6405.12953.

Australian Bureau of Statistics. (2008). *Population projections, Australia* (no. 3222.0). https://www.ausstats.abs.gov.au/ausstats/subscriber.nsf/0/0E09CCC14E4C94F6CA2574B9001626FE/$File/32220_2006 to 2101.pdf.

Australian Bureau of Statistics. (2016). *Census of population and housing: Reflecting Australia: Stories from the census, 2016* (no. 2071.0). https://www.abs.gov.au/ausstats/abs@.nsf/Lookup/by Subject/2071.0~2016~Main Features~Cultural Diversity Data Summary~30.

Australian Bureau of Statistics. (2020). *Migration Australia, 2018–19* (no. 3412.0). https://www.abs.gov.au/ausstats/abs@.nsf/Latestproducts/3412.0Main Features32018-19?opendocument&tabname=Summary&prodno=3412.0&issue=2018-19&num=&view=

Australian Institute of Health and Welfare. (2018). *Australia's health 2018*. https://www.aihw.gov.au/get-media/f3ba8e92-afb3-46d6-b64c-ebfc9c1f945d/aihw-aus-221-chapter-5-3.pdf.aspx.

Baer, H. A., Singer, M., Long, D., & Erickson, P. (2016). Rebranding our field? Toward an articulation of health anthropology. *Current Anthropology, 57*(4), 494–510. https://doi.org/10.1086/687509.

Bhopal, R. S. (2007). *Ethnicity, race, and health in multicultural societies: Foundations for better epidemiology, public health and health care*. Oxford University Press.

Bond, C. J., & Singh, D. (2020). More than a refresh required for closing the gap of Indigenous health inequality. *Medical Journal of Australia, 212*(5), 198–200. https://doi.org/10.5694/mja2.50498.

Campbell, M. A., Hunt, J., Scrimgeour, D. J., Davey, M., & Jones, V. (2018). Contreibution of aboriginal community-controlled health services to improving Aboriginal health: An evidence review. *Australian Health Review, 42*(2), 218–226. https://doi.org/10.1071/AH16149.

Campinha-Bacote, J. (2002). The process of cultural competence in the delivery of healthcare services: A model of care. *Journal of Transcultural Nursing, 13*(3), 181–184. https://doi.org/10.1177/10459602013003003.

Capell, J., Dean, E., & Veenstra, G. (2008). The relationship between cultural competence and ethnocentrism of health care professionals. *Journal of Transcultural Nursing, 19*(2), 121–125. https://doi.org/10.1177/1043659607312970.

Chan, C., Ho, P. S.Y., & Chow, E. (2002). A body–mind–spirit model in health: An Eastern approach. *Social Work in Health Care, 34*(3–4), 261–282. https://doi.org/10.1300/J010v34n03_02.

Commonwealth of Australia. (2020). Closing the gap report 2020. https://ctgreport.niaa.gov.au/sites/default/files/pdf/closing-the-gap-report-2020.pdf.

Cora-Bramble, D., Tielman, F., & Wright, J. (2004). Traditional practices folk remedies, and the Western biomedical model: Bridging the divide. *Clinical Pediatric Emergency Medicine*, *5*(2), 102–108. https://doi.org/10.1016/j.cpem.2004.01.006.

Davy, C., Harfield, S., McArthur, A., Munn, Z., & Brown, A. (2016). Access to primary health care services for Indigenous peoples: A framework synthesis. *International Journal for Equity in Health*, *15*(1), 1–9. https://doi.org/10.1186/s12939-016-0450-5.

Deacon, B., & McKay, D. (2015). The biomedical model of psychological problems: A call for critical dialogue. *The Behavior Therapist*, *38*(7), 231–235.

Dixey, R. (2014). After Nairobi: Can the international community help to develop health promotion in Africa? *Health Promotion International*, *29*(1), 185–194. https://doi.org/10.1093/heapro/dat052.

Dubbin, L. A., Chang, J. S., & Shim, J. K. (2013). Cultural health capital and the interactional dynamics of patient-centered care. *Social Science and Medicine*, *93*(1), 113–120. https://doi.org/10.1016/j.socscimed.2013.06.014.

Dune, T., & Liamputtong, P. (2019). Gender and sexuality and social determinants of health. In P. Liamputtong (Ed.), *Perspectives on social determinants of health* (pp. 215–242). Oxford University Press.

Eckermann, A. K., Dowd, T., Chong, E., Gray, R., & Nixon, L. (2010). *Binan Goonj: Bridging cultures in Aboriginal health*. Elsevier.

Engel, G. L. (1977). The need for a new medical model: A challenge for biomedicine. *Science*, *196*(4286), 129–136. https://doi.org/10.1126/science.847460.

Findlay, M., Odgers, S., & Yeo, S. (2014). *Australian criminal justice* (5th ed.). Oxford University Press.

Gannon, M. (2018). *Closing the gap: 10 year review*. Australian Medical Association. https://ama.com.au/ausmed/closing-gap-10-year-review.

Germov, J. (2019). Imagining health problems as social issues. In J. Germov (Ed.), *Second opinion: An introduction to health sociology* (6th ed. pp. 5–22). Oxford University Press.

Hatala, A. R. (2012). The Status of the biopsychosocial model in health psychology: Towards an integrated approach and a critique of cultural conceptions. *Open Journal of Medical Psychology*, *1*(4), 51–62. https://doi.org/10.4236/ojmp.2012.14009.

Horwitz, I., Sonilal, M., & Horwitz, S. (2011). Improving health care quality through culturally competent physicians: Leadership and organisational diversity training. *Journal of Healthcare Leadership*, *3*(1), 29. https://doi.org/10.2147/jhl.s15620.

Ike, R. O. C. L., & King, M. L. (2008). Educating clinicians about cultural competence and disparities in health and health care. *Journal of Continuing Education in the Health Professions*, *28*(3), 157–164. https://doi.org/10.1002/chp.20127.

Joseph, A. J. (2015). The necessity of an attention to Eurocentrism and colonial technologies: An addition to critical mental health literature. *Disability and Society*, *30*(7), 1021–1041. https://doi.org/10.1080/09687599.2015.1067187.

Kurtz, D. L. M., Janke, R., Vinek, J., Wells, T., Hutchinson, P., & Froste, A. (2018). Health sciences cultural safety education in Australia, Canada, New Zealand, and the United States: A literature review. *International Journal of Medical Education*, *9*(1), 271–285. https://doi.org/10.5116/ijme.5bc7.21e2.

Lehman, B. J., David, D. M., & Gruber, J. A. (2017). Rethinking the biopsychosocial model of health: Understanding health as a dynamic system. *Social and Personality Psychology Compass*, *11*(8), 1–17. https://doi.org/10.1111/spc3.12328.

Liamputtong, P. (2019). Social determinants of health: An introduction. In P. Liamputtong. (Ed.), *Perspectives on social determinants of health* (pp. 1–27). Oxford University Press.

Liamputtong, P., & Suwankhong, D. (2019). Culture as social determinant of health. In P. Liamputtong (Ed.), *Perspectives on social determinants of health* (pp. 51–82). Oxford University Press.

Logan, S., Steel, Z., & Hunt, C. (2016). Intercultural willingness to communicate within health services: Investigating anxiety, uncertainty, ethnocentrism and help seeking behaviour. *International Journal of Intercultural Relations*, *54*, 77–86. https://doi.org/10.1016/j.ijintrel.2016.07.007.

Marks, D. F., Murray, M., & Estacio, E.V. (2018). *Health psychology: Theory, research and practice* (5th ed.). Sage.

Matsui, E. C., Adamson, A. S., & Peng, R. D. (2019). Time's up to adopt a biopsychosocial model to address racial and ethnic disparities in asthma outcomes. *Journal of Allergy and Clinical Immunology*, *143*(6), 2024–2025. https://doi.org/10.1016/j.jaci.2019.03.015.

Mortensen, A. (2010). Cultural safety: Does the theory work in practice for culturally and linguistically diverse groups? *Nursing Praxis in New Zealand Inc*, *26*(3), 6–16.

Mpofu, E. (2006). Majority world health care traditions intersect indigenous and complementary and alternative medicine. *International Journal of Disability, Development and Education*, *53*, 375–379. https://doi.org/10.1080/10349120601008340.

Newcombe, S. (2012). Global hybrids? Eastern traditions of health and wellness in the West. In S. Nair-Venugopal (Ed.), *The gaze of the West and framings of the East* (pp. 202–217). Palgrave Macmillan.

Oleribe, O. O., Ukwedeh, O., Burstow, N. J., Gomaa, A. I., Sonderup, M. W., Cook, N., Waked, I., Spearman, W., & Taylor-Robinson, S. D. (2018). Health: redefined. *The Pan African Medical Journal*, *30*, 292. https://doi.org/10.11604/pamj.2018.30.292.15436.

Oppong, S., Brune, K., & Mpofu, E. (in press). Indigenous communities health. In E. Mpofu (Ed.), *Sustainable community health: Systems and practices in diverse settings*. Palgrave Macmillan.

Pérez, M. A., & Luquis, R. R. (2008). *Cultural competence in health education and health promotion*. Jossey-Bass.

Pilgrim, D. (2015). The biopsychosocial model in health research: Its strengths and limitations for critical realists. *Journal of Critical Realism*, *14*(2), 164–180. https://doi.org/10.1179/1572513814Y.0000000007.

Prime Minister of Australia. (2020). *Address, Closing the Gap statement to Parliament*. https://www.pm.gov.au/media/address-closing-gap-statement-parliament.

Rose, P. R. (2018). *Health disparities, diversity, and inclusion context, controversies, and solutions*. Jones and Bartlett.

Sarafino, E. P., & Smith, T. W. (2014). *Health psychology: Biopsychosocial interactions*. John Wiley & Sons.

Smith, J. D. (2016). *Australia's rural, remote and Indigenous health*. Elsevier.

Straub, R. O. (2017). *Health psychology: A biopsychosocial approach* (5th ed.). Worth Publishers.

Sullivan, T. (2018). *Modern medicine vs alternative medicine: Different levels of evidence*. https://www.policymed.com/2011/08/modern-medicine-vs-alternative-medicine-different-levels-of-evidence.htm.

Sulman, J., Savage, D., & Way, S. (2002). A body-mind-spirit model in health cecilia. *Social Work in Health Care*, *34*(3–4), 315–332. https://doi.org/10.1300/J010v34n03.

Suls, J., & Rothman, A. (2004). Evolution of the biopsychosocial model: Prospects and challenges for health psychology. *Health Psychology*, *23*(2), 119–125. https://doi.org/10.1037/0278-6133.23.2.119.

Talbot, L., & Verrinder, G. (2017). *Promoting health: The primary health care approach* (6th ed.). Elsevier.

Taylor, K., & Guerin, P. (2014). *Health care and Indigenous Australians, cultural safety in practice* (2nd ed.). Palgrave Macmillan.

Taylor, K., & Guerin, P. (2019). *Health care and Indigenous Australians, cultural safety in practice* (3rd ed.). Red Globe Press.

Tsuei, J. J. (1978). Eastern and Western approaches to medicine. *Western Journal of Medicine*, *1*(128), 551–557.

Tucker, C. M., Arthur, T. M., Roncoroni, J., Wall, W., & Sanchez, J. (2015). Patient-centered, culturally sensitive health care. *American Journal of Lifestyle Medicine*, *9*(1), 63–77. https://doi.org/10.1177/1559827613498065.

Waterworth, P., Pescud, M., Braham, R., Dimmock, J., & Rosenberg, M. (2015). Factors influencing the health behaviour of Indigenous Australians: Perspectives from support people. *PLoS ONE 10*(11), e0142323. https://doi.org/10.1371/journal.pone.0142323.

Weightman, M. (2013). The role of Aboriginal community controlled health services in indigenous health. *Australian Medical Student Journal*, *4*(1), 49–52.

Westerman, T. G. (2010). Engaging Australian Aboriginal youth in mental health services. *Australian Psychologist*, *45*, 212–222.

Wilkerson, J. M., Rybicki, S., Barber, C. A., & Smolenski, D. J. (2011). Creating a culturally competent clinical environment for LGBT patients. *Journal of Gay and Lesbian Social Services*, *23*(3), 376–394. https://doi.org/10.1080/10538720.2011.589254.

World Health Organisation (WHO). (1948). *Constitution of the World Health Organization*. https://apps.who.int/gb/bd/PDF/bd47/EN/constitution-en.pdf?ua=1.

World Health Organisation (WHO). (2003). *Behavioural mechanisms explaining adherence: What every health professional should know*. https://www.who.int/chp/knowledge/publications/adherence_annexes.pdf?ua=1.

World Health Organisation (WHO). (2019). *Primary health care*. https://www.who.int/news-room/fact-sheets/detail/primary-health-care-:text=Primary health care is a, and social health and wellbeing.

Zheng, Z. (2014). Acupuncture in Australia: Regulation, education, practice, and research. *Integrative Medicine Research*, *3*(3), 103–110. https://doi.org/10.1016/j.imr.2014.06.002

Part II

Culturally safe health care practice

4 Principles of cultural safety

Robyn Williams, Tinashe Dune and Kim McLeod

Learning outcomes

After working through this chapter, students should be able to:

1. Demonstrate an understanding of the history, rationale, and principles of cultural safety as a theorised model of health care.
2. Reflect on power, racism, Whiteness, intersectionality, and the related impact on health professionals, clients and health services.
3. Consider the definition of cultural safety and the related conceptual confusion with other terms, including cultural competence.
4. Examine the principles of cultural safety in relation to the impact of cultural values, attitudes and beliefs, shared decision making, power and responsibility, respect, and trust and relationship building.
5. Explore what cultural safety means for personal and professional identity.

Key terms

Cultural safety: An environment that is spiritually, socially and emotionally safe, as well as physically safe for people; where there is no assault challenge or denial of their identity, of who they are and what they need.

Racism: Any cognition, affective state or behaviour that advances the differential treatment of individuals or groups due to their racial, ethnic, cultural or religious background.

Respect: An essential component of a high-performance organization. It helps to create a healthy environment in which clients feel cared for as individuals, and members of health care teams are engaged, collaborative and committed to service. Within a culture of respect, people perform better, are more innovative and display greater resilience. On the contrary, a lack of respect stifles teamwork and undermines individual performance. It can also lead to poor interactions with clients. Cultivating a culture of respect can truly transform an organization and leaders set the stage for how respect is manifested (James, 2018).

Self-awareness: The capacity to become the object of one's own attention. In this state one actively identifies, processes and stores information about the self.

Self-reflection: A genuine curiosity about the self, where the person is intrigued and interested in learning more about his or her emotions, values, thought processes and attitudes.

Social justice: A political and philosophical theory that broadens the concept of justice beyond those embodied in the principles of civil or criminal law, economic supply and demand or traditional moral frameworks. Social justice tends to focus more on just relations between groups within society as opposed to the justice of individual conduct or justice for individuals.

Trust: Refers to people's expectations, typically for goodwill, advocacy, and competence (and/or good outcome). As such, it is future-directed; although past experiences and other forms of knowledge influence the degree of current trust in another; measuring trust itself requires measuring the beliefs of the person who trusts about the trustee's behaviour (Goold, 2002). Patient or client trust in their health care professional is central to clinical practice. Clients must be able to trust health professionals with their health and to work in their best interest and outcome. Trust in the health care professional is a central factor in effective treatments and fundamental for patient-centered care (Australian Commission Safety Quality Health Care, 2011; Birkhäuer et al., 2017).

Whiteness: Whiteness and White privilege are ways of conceptualising racial inequalities that focuses as much on the advantages that Whites accrue as on the disadvantages that people of colour experience. Unlike theories of overt racism or prejudice, which suggest that people actively seek to oppress or demean other racial groups, theories of White privilege assert that the experience of Whites is viewed by Whites as normal rather than advantaged. Whites as a group hold social advantages rather than experiencing a "normal" state of existence.

Chapter summary

This chapter will formally introduce students to the theory of cultural safety as an interdisciplinary and interprofessional model of health care. The history, contention, criticisms of, and necessity for cultural safety will also be discussed, along with related topics of racism, White privilege, discrimination and power. The principles of cultural safety, including social justice, trust, respect, self-awareness, and self-reflection, will be discussed in relation to forming the basis of culturally safe practice. The need for robust partnerships negotiated with diverse groups of people and their respective health needs will also be highlighted as a key component of cultural safety. Furthermore, this chapter will include a focus on the availability, accessibility and acceptability of health care for diverse populations as a health equity issue. Mind maps and other resources will also be used to explore ways in which the cultural values, attitudes and beliefs of individuals, health care organisations and health systems can impact and shape health care relationships.

Introduction

Cultural safety is defined as:

> The effective nursing practice of a person or family from another culture and is determined by that person or family. Culture includes, but is not restricted to, age or generation; gender; sexual orientation; occupation and socioeconomic status; ethnic origin or migrant experience; religious or spiritual belief; and disability. The nurse delivering the nursing service will have undertaken a process of reflection on their own cultural identity and will recognise the impact their personal culture has on their professional practice. Unsafe cultural practice comprises any action which diminishes, demeans or disempowers the cultural identity and wellbeing of an individual.
>
> (Nursing Council of New Zealand, 2012)

Principles of cultural safety

The cultural safety model has its roots in the field of nursing education and health care in Aotearoa, New Zealand, and is based on the work of Doctor Irihapeti Ramsden (2002) and others. Cultural safety is premised on working towards *social justice* and better health outcomes for those experiencing health inequity. It is a philosophy of practice that is concerned with *how* a health professional does something, not what they do, in order to engage in and support culturally safe practice (Nursing Council of New Zealand, 2011, p. 7).

Cultural safety provides a means to examine how people are treated in society and how they are affected by the systemic and structural issues and social determinants of health (Williams, 2016). It represents a key philosophical shift from providing care regardless of who an individual is, to acknowledging that each person's identity is central to the provision of health care (Eckermann et al., 2010; Kurtz et al., 2018; Taylor & Guerin, 2019). Cultural safety takes into account peoples' unique needs and requires an ongoing process of practitioner *self-reflection*, cultural *self-awareness* and an acknowledgement of how these factors impact on care (De Souza, 2008; Ramsden, 2002). Importantly, cultural safety uses a broad definition of culture that does not reduce it to ethnicity only. Instead, it includes a range of variables, such as age/generation, sexual orientation, socio-economic status, religious or spiritual beliefs, gender and ability (Cox, 2016).

Cultural safety works on the premise that professions and workplaces also have cultures (not only the clients). Cultural safety is therefore as applicable to working with colleagues as it is to actual health care (Furlong & Wight, 2011; Johnstone & Kanitsaki, 2008). Originally based on a Māori knowledge construct, cultural safety has a crucial role to play in Australian health care as it provides a decolonising model of practice based on dialogue, communication, power sharing and negotiation and acknowledgement of Whiteness and privilege (Mkandawire-Valhmu, 2018; Richardson, 2015; Taylor & Guerin, 2019; Wepa, 2015). These actions are a means to challenge *racism* at personal and institutional levels and to establish trust in health care encounters.

Unlike other models of health care between self and different "others", cultural safety is not about progress through certain levels of awareness and practice along a staged or linear continuum. The process is a lifelong one and does not require the study of any culture other than one's own—so as to be aware of the impacts and implication of our own cultures, open-minded and flexible in our attitudes towards others (Cox, 2016). Identifying what makes others different is simple—understanding our own culture and its influence on how we think, feel and behave is much more complex. This is particularly the case when one is a member of the dominant culture in a society, as the features of dominant cultures become social norms, and the standard by which others are judged. The features of the more dominant cultures become normalised and therefore invisible.

A cornerstone of cultural safety is that ultimately it is the receiver of health services who determines if their care was culturally safe or not (McEldowney & Connor, 2011; Richardson, 2012; Universities Australia, 2011; Woods, 2010). This can then be linked with the philosophical framework of primary health care and that of Indigenous community-controlled organisations for example.

Why cultural safety?

Some prominent writers in social science disciplines support the notion that people living and working within a culture other than their own need to at least comprehend certain factors about working cross-culturally[1] (Betancourt et al., 2003; De Souza, 2015; Tseng & Streltzer, 2010; Wepa, 2015). One of the main reasons for health professionals needing to develop cross-cultural understandings is that their own beliefs and actions will have an impact upon their behaviour and care of, or service provision to, their clientele. Acknowledgement of the impact of values and beliefs on behaviour in general and health interactions specifically reinforces the idea that cultural safety is a process contingent on effective communication, self-reflection, cultural self-awareness and changing practice accordingly.

Much of the literature on cultural safety relates to the nursing profession, although other disciplines have also adopted the concept and are adapting it to suit their own purposes. The social work profession (Bennett et al., 2013; Bennett, 2015), psychologists (McGough, 2016; McGough, Wynaden, & Wright, 2018) and other allied health professions (Gerlach, 2015) provide some exemplars. In addition, many government program areas, community-controlled health organisations and national advocacy organisations each have their own particular interpretation of cultural safety. Instances include the Australian Indigenous Doctors Association (AIDA), Royal Australian College of General Practitioners (RACGP), Indigenous Allied Health Australia (IAHA), Congress of Aboriginal and Torres Strait Islander Nurses and Midwives (CATSINaM), National Rural Health Alliance of Australia (NRHA), Nursing and Midwifery Board of Australia (NMBA), Australian Health Practitioner Regulation Agency (Ahpra) and Universities Australia. Nonetheless, cultural safety is still a contested area, particularly regarding terminology and interpretations. This conceptual confusion will be addressed in the next section.

Box 4.1 Reflection—Conceptual confusion

There is limited literature referring to the inconsistent use of and confusion about cultural safety terminology. Many terms including cultural awareness, cultural appropriateness, cultural sensitivity, cultural competency and cultural safety are often used interchangeably, even though they do not share the same meaning. This conceptual confusion and inconsistent use of terminology is reflected in much of the literature on Indigenous health, cultures and health care.

Consider the definition of cultural competence, for example: a set of congruent behaviours, attitudes and policies that come together in a system, agency or among professionals and enable that system, agency or those professionals to work effectively in cross-cultural situations (National Health and Medical Research Council, 2005, p. 6).

How is this definition different from cultural safety?

Who is the focus of cultural competence, and why might that be problematic? The health professional or the health consumer?

Understanding cultural safety in health care

The Nursing and Midwifery Board of Australia (NMBA), Australian College of Midwives (ACM), Australian College of Nurses (CAN), Australian Nursing and Midwifery Federation (ANMF), and Congress of Aboriginal and Torres Strait Islander Nurses and Midwives CATSINaM),[2] released a joint statement on culturally safe health care in February 2018. The joint statement affirmed "that regulations and codes establishing health professional standards must clearly communicate the requirement for cultural safety" (Nursing and Midwifery Board of Australia, 2019). Cultural safety was not redefined as part of this process as the definition was already based on Ramsden's (2002) work and that of the Nursing Council of New Zealand (2011).

Conversely, the Australian Health Practitioner Regulation Agency (Ahpra) undertook a consultation process April 3rd to May 15th, 2019,[3] to ascertain feedback on a proposed definition of cultural safety to be applied in the context of the National Registration and Accreditation Scheme (NRAS), and by National Health Leadership Forum (NHLF) member organisations, as a foundation for embedding cultural safety across the NRAS for all registered professions. It was intended that the final definition would be used to inform documents such as future codes of conduct for the professions regulated in the National Scheme and/or registration standards and guidelines (Australian Health Practitioner Regulation Agency, 2019). The definition proposed for discussion was

> Cultural safety is the individual and institutional knowledge, skills, attitudes and competencies needed to deliver optimal health care for Aboriginal and Torres Strait Islander Peoples as determined by Aboriginal and Torres Strait Islander individuals, families and communities.
>
> (Australian Health Practitioner Regulation Agency, 2019, p. 2)

In February 2020, Ahpra released a statement about the launch of a strategy for embedding cultural safety into the Australian health system. *The National Scheme's Aboriginal and Torres Strait Islander Health and Cultural Safety Strategy 2020–2025* is focused on "achieving patient safety for Aboriginal and Torres Strait Islander Peoples as the norm and the inextricably linked elements of clinical and cultural safety" (https://www.ahpra.gov.au/News/2020-02-26-strategy-for-embedding-cultural-safety.aspx). Cultural safety for the National Scheme is now defined as such:

> Cultural safety is determined by Aboriginal and Torres Strait Islander individuals, families and communities. Culturally safe practise [sic] is the ongoing critical reflection of health practitioner knowledge, skills, attitudes, practising behaviours and power differentials in delivering safe, accessible and responsive health care free of racism.
>
> (https://www.ahpra.gov.au/About-AHPRA/Aboriginal-and-Torres-Strait-Islander-Health-Strategy.aspx)

In terms of informing codes of conduct, registration standards and guidelines, and thereby shaping health professionals' practice, this definition still highlights several ongoing concerns regarding true understanding and appropriate use of cultural safety. The draft Ahpra definition was loose and very general and was at best about delivery of health services for Indigenous peoples, and it did not fully capture the principles of cultural safety. However, the Strategy's definition now refers specifically to some cultural safety principles such as social justice; an emphasis on health inequities rather than cultural differences; and the potential to challenge power imbalances, racism and White dominance in educational, research and clinical practices. It must be noted that the primary focus is still on Indigenous peoples and therefore does not address other key aspects of cultural safety including age, gender, generation, ability, or sexuality.

Unintended consequences of using the Ahpra definition might include perpetuation of confusion over the terminology and concept of cultural safety and the misconception that cultural safety is only about ethnicity and in this case about Indigenous peoples. In an article addressing concerns raised initially by Ahpra's proposal, Cox and Best (2019) questioned why cultural safety would need further definition as it already has the capacity for wide application in any context plus the potential to address systemic racisms and intersectionality concerns.

In summary, cultural safety is a process that means working in partnership and negotiating an environment that is spiritually, socially and emotionally safe, as well as physically safe for people. By contrast, unsafe cultural practice is any action that diminishes, demeans or disempowers the cultural identity and wellbeing of an individual or group (Williams, 1999). The transformative potential of cultural safety in the way it grapples with racism, power, and inequity in health care is in danger of being diluted or weakened by current efforts to redefine it or at least not being clearly defined. Additionally, official definitions of cultural safety that are used to refer to only one particular group (that is, Indigenous peoples) are problematic. This is primarily because those that are unaffected (that is, White people) do not have to take responsibility for their role in transforming these circumstances.

Cultural safety is NOT:

1. Cultural awareness. This is a beginning step on a continuum toward understanding that there is difference. Cultural awareness courses are usually designed to sensitise participants to formal cultural aspects, for example, "ritual and practice", rather than the emotional, social, economic and political context in which people exist. It comprises selected information and "facts" about specific group and often is a "recipe" or "cookbook" approach. Cultural awareness definitely has a place though, but only if generated and managed or facilitated by local or regional people with the right to tell those stories.
2. Cultural competence. This is also problematic, as it assumes an endpoint and presumes acceptance of particular perspectives with a specific focus on the health professional and their individual "cultural standpoint". A key feature of this approach is the focus on understanding the "other" who has "culture"; therefore, it shifts focus away from understanding the self. In addition, cultural competence locates "difference" in others, thus maintaining the invisible privilege/s of dominant groups/positions. What we need to aim for is the concept of self-reflexive and culturally safe practice.
3. Cultural responsiveness. This has its origins in North America and is a relative of the earlier work of transcultural nursing and the later work of cultural competency. Indigenous Allied Health Australia (IAHA) defines cultural responsiveness as an action of cultural safety—a negotiated process of what constitutes culturally safe health care as decided by the recipient of that care. It is also clearly about the centrality of culture and how that shapes each individual; their worldviews, values, beliefs and attitudes; and their interactions with others. This is a more useful consideration of cultural safety as defined by the recipient (in this case IAHA).

Access to health care

This section briefly refers to factors that impact on whether people from different cultures physically access a health service and feel comfortable, culturally safe, happy and confident as service users. Relevant issues will be addressed further on in the text and include

- Key attributes of culturally safe health care.
- Addressing racism in the health system is vital for improving health outcomes for any cultural or ethnic minority.
- Whiteness and White privilege refer to systems that privilege some people while disadvantaging others. In health care, sections of the population will experience institutional racism and discrimination if they do not hold the social advantages of Whiteness
- Our current health care system is designed for the dominant group.
- Health systems that are culturally safe are more likely to be used by people in the greatest need.

Effects of power and authority on health care

The question of the misuse of, or lack of awareness about, the power relationship between health professionals and their clients lies at the heart of culturally unsafe practices. It is this issue that cultural safety is attempting to address. Cultural safety is unashamedly about health professionals' power to support healing. At one level, it is about the care a health professional gives to the concerns expressed by their particular clients. For example, in the context of Indigenous health, it is about non-Indigenous health professionals recognising the reality and the lived experiences of the people who come before them (Milne et al., 2016). Similarly, contextualisation and recognition of the reality and lived experiences of refugees will impact on the health encounter and challenge health professionals to be reflective and critical thinkers. At another level, it is about the primacy of health professionals needing to recognise the limitations their cultural beliefs impose on their practice with clients of other cultures (Katsikitis et al., 2013).

According to Willis and Elmer (2011) certain discussions (or discourses) about health and illness will be dominant at particular points in time, and the ideas and practices that constitute these discourses will carry more weight or legitimacy. These dominant discourses are the ideas and practices that are most socially accepted as the "right" way to think about issues, categories of people, social factors and behaviours. The power or "might" of discourse lies in the authority and power that can be exercised when one's ideas, values and beliefs are accepted as the "right" way of understanding an issue or situation. 'There are many different discourses about health and illness, and they vary in their degrees of influence and "authority" (Willis & Elmer, 2011, p. 23). The discourses of science and medicine are very influential and are considered authoritative in most Western societies, and the scientific knowledge that underpins contemporary medicine is primarily a product of its history and social context.

The institution of medicine is a useful arena in which to begin to explore the notion of power and authority. Most people can immediately recognise the authority that medicine has, particularly doctors who hold the highest level of specialist skills and knowledge when viewed within the biomedical model that dominates the Australian health care system.

Historically, ideologically and contextually, the external systems of mainstream health care have not allowed other cultural systems to operate effectively if at all. The external systems have not developed the practices to support and validate these cultural systems, and so the mainstream systems continue to dominate. The effect of this dominance is a constant "grinding away" at cultures and spirit. That is, the health system is predominantly "culturally unsafe", not just individuals.

The cultural "unsafety" of the health system stems from people's inability to acknowledge and legitimise difference, the centrality of culture and the integrity of identity. The language of the dominant group often makes it hard to accept the differences that exist between the members of the dominant group and others. The way notions of difference are constructed and maintained brings with it a number of implicit and explicit expectations.

Paradies, Harris, and Anderson (2008) state that

> ... it is well established that Indigenous Australians and Māoris have higher levels of ill health and mortality than non-Indigenous people. It is also clear that the disadvantage suffered by Indigenous peoples is associated with both historical and contemporary racism, colonisation and oppression. Both an "adequate state of health" and "freedom from racism" are rights enshrined in legislation in Australia and Aotearoa (New Zealand).
>
> (2008, p. 1)

It would appear that there is still a long way to go regarding the cultural unsafety of the Australian health system, as Indigenous peoples have also been subject to non-Indigenous medical treatment and health services, which have largely failed to recognise the cultural bases of their traditional health care, or the ongoing impacts of colonisation. Indigenous health inequities are evident in terms of how racism has influenced service delivery to Indigenous Australians (Paradies, Harris, & Anderson, 2008), the quality and suitability of health services provided

(Henry, Houston, & Mooney, 2004) and the continued failure of the health system to provide culturally safe care (Brown, Middleton, Fereday, & Pincombe, 2016).

For example, Naomi Williams, a 27-year-old Wiradjuri (Aboriginal) woman from New South Wales was six months pregnant when she died at a rural hospital in Tumut in January 2016. As recently reported in the media, an autopsy showed the cause of death was sepsis associated with a serious infection that is treatable with antibiotics. In other words, her condition was treatable and her death avoidable. Williams had attended the hospital 18 times in the seven months before her death complaining of pain, vomiting and nausea. She had been discharged for the last time just 15 hours before her death (Jackson, 2019). Seven of the recommendations handed down by the coroner in July 2019 related to employing more Indigenous health professionals, addressing implicit racial bias, increasing representation of Indigenous people on the local health advisory committee and the Local Health District Board, and improving access to culturally safe and appropriate health care. To date, Tumut Hospital has implemented further cultural awareness programs in partnership with the local Indigenous community to build connections and develop relationships. Meetings between Indigenous community representatives and Tumut Hospital managers and involvement of Indigenous community representatives in the Local Health Advisory Committee have been introduced (Hayter & King, 2019).

Naomi Williams' experience, as an Aboriginal woman, of being repeatedly ignored and not treated appropriately, is an example of implicit bias and racism existing within the health system. What happened to Naomi Williams is by no means an isolated incident and is an indicator of the major systemic failures in the Australian health system (Robinson, 2019).

As you have seen in Chapters 1, 2 and 3, there are strong connections between culture, identity and health, although these may not at first seem obvious, particularly to some health professionals. However, there needs to be consideration of the extent to which identity and health are linked, particularly given the different kinds of definitions of health that exist. However, in Australia one particular sociocultural framework dominates over others resulting in varying levels of disadvantage and health inequities—Whiteness.

Whiteness, White privilege, White fragility

What is "Whiteness[4]", and why do we have to talk about it? Sentance describes Whiteness as:

> In conversations about diversity, we should also talk about whiteness. Let me add by whiteness I'm not referring to racial categorisation or skin colour, I am referring to a system of exclusion ... that makes Western thought and white people the invisible but highly visible default or "normal". Or as George Yancy more elegantly puts it "The power of whiteness is we don't see white bodies as white bodies; we see them as just bodies.

Many have noted that it is its invisibility is how Whiteness maintains its power because it is removed from scrutiny, so we need to continue to identify it and talk about it, [as] if it is named and seen, if we can point a finger at it, Whiteness can be challenged ... (Nathan mudyi Sentance on Twitter March 2020).

So what is "Whiteness"? King and Springwood (2001, p. 160) indicate that:

> Whiteness is simultaneously a practice, a social space, a subjectivity, a spectacle, an erasure, an epistemology, a strategy, an historical formation, a technology, and a tactic. Of course, it is not monolithic, but in all of its manifestations, it is unified through privilege and the power to name, to represent, and to create opportunity and deny access.

Implicit in this definition of Whiteness is a delineation of those who reap benefits from Whiteness and those who do not—those who are White and those who are non-White (Du Bois, 1917). As noted by Moreton-Robinson (2004, p. 137) "Whiteness as a racial identity… confers dominance and privilege (that) remains unmarked and unnamed".

Dune et al. (2018) explain that non-White refers to individuals who are excluded from being beneficiaries of Whiteness as a result of their racial, ethnic, cultural, religious, linguistic or national identities (Sue, 2006). Describing those who are White is, however, a more challenging task (Anderson, 2003; Feagin, 2013; Lewis, 2004; Sue, 2006). This is because Whiteness is more concerned with analysing, describing, characterising and excluding those who do not belong within it, but provides little clarification about what defines or characterises Whites (Lewis, 2004). This ambiguity results from a colloquial, quotidian and unquestioned sociocultural framework in which Whiteness is the invisible benchmark, normative, ideal and default standard from which non-Whites are evaluated (Moreton-Robinson, 2004; Sue, 2006).

Notably, a particular "luxury of belonging to the advantaged racial group is that one's own racialness often is invisible to oneself" (Lewis, 2004, p. 641) and seemingly requires no explanation (Sue, 2006). As explained by Lewis (2004, pp. 624–625), this phenomenon leads individuals to perceive those in non-White groups as "social problems" resulting in "failure to situate one's self in one's whiteness, and within the larger racial discourse". Importantly Whites are in no way a homogenous group (as with non-Whites)—nor are their group/collective identities under examination in this inquiry. Whiteness, however, and its consequences for how non-Whites are perceived and engaged, is an important piece of this research. As noted by Sue (2006, p. 15) "…Whiteness, White supremacy, and White privilege are three interlocking forces that disguise racism so it may allow White people to oppress and harm persons of color while maintaining their individual and collective advantage and innocence". Of course, this is not to say that all Whites experience the same advantages and to the same degrees or that Whiteness has always looked the same or that it lacks impermeable and flexible boundaries. It is acknowledged that Whiteness (and the delineators for those who benefit, or are excluded, from it) is constantly under negotiation (Lewis, 2004). Even within this constant state of flux, the role of Whiteness and its consequences endure (Guess, 2006). It is therefore important to consider and identify the impact of this construct on the whole of Australian society, and especially non-Whites. Given the invisible and pervasive nature of Whiteness, the power tactics required to sustain it as well as its construction of non-Whites as social problems, the consequences for non-Whites are profound. Notably, the negative health outcomes and experiences of non-Whites within health care settings are well documented and related to systems and practitioners that harbor constructions of health and wellbeing based on frameworks of Whiteness (Dune, Caputi, & Walker, 2018). In this way people who are identified as White experience more privileges that improve their social determinants and therefore health outcomes.

Box 4.2 Reflection—Whiteness, White privilege and White fragility

The topics of Whiteness, White privilege and White fragility can be confronting and can create conflicting thoughts and feelings intra-personally (within yourself) and inter-personally (between you and others). Importantly, people from a range of backgrounds find this concept very confronting and difficult to understand in the context of their own as well as others' health outcomes. In order to investigate our perspectives on this construct, it is important to have discussions about what it means, whether or not it exists, and how it might affect the health outcomes of all Australians.

To practice thinking about the diverse perspectives on these topics, prepare points to support or challenge the following statements. When you are done, have a debate with your classmates to explore these perspectives further.

Importantly, please respect the views of your classmates even if they differ to your own. It is important to debate these topics as future health professionals who will carry their perspectives into client interactions that affects health outcomes.

1. White privilege is a concept created by people in minority groups who blame others because they have chosen not to take the initiative to work hard and overcome the restrictions that everyone faces.
2. White privilege is not about people who are Caucasian at all. It is a social construct that demonstrates the impact of the dominant culture in Australia on the health, wellbeing and outcomes for Australians who are not Caucasian.
3. White privilege does not exist because race does not exist. Being Caucasian does not provide people with an immediate set of advantages. Such a perception is a myth.
4. The purpose of discussing White privilege is simply to make people who are Caucasian feel guilty about things they did not do and were not a part of. Such discussions and constructs are actually a form of racism towards Caucasian people and do nothing to create equity or equality.
5. White privilege, as a result of colonisation, is the basis for the disadvantage and difficulties that many minority populations in Australia experience. If minority groups were offered the same privileges on a daily basis they would not suffer poor social determinants and therefore poor health outcomes.

White privilege

In critical race theory, White privilege is a way of conceptualising racial inequalities that focuses as much on the advantages that White people accrue as on the disadvantages that people of colour experience. Unlike theories of overt racism or prejudice, which suggest that people actively seek to oppress or demean other racial groups, theories of White privilege assert that the experiences of White people are viewed by themselves as normal rather than advantaged. This normative assumption causes all discussion of racial inequality to focus on the disadvantages of other racial groups and on what can be done to bring them up to White (i.e., "normal") standards, effectively making racial inequality an issue that does not involve White people. Researchers suggest that more equitable attitudes can be achieved by refocusing such discussions to include White people as a group that holds social advantages rather than experiencing a "normal" state of existence (National Academies of Sciences, Engineering, and Medicine, 2017).

White privilege is where a person is not assumed to speak as a representative of one's group. The concept of Whiteness has been helpful in moving discussions of racism away from prejudice by exposing the unearned benefits and advantages that accrue to dominant group members solely by virtue of occupying a dominant social position and often regardless of one's attitude, volition, or belief.

White privilege is not experienced similarly by all people ascribed Whiteness, so what privilege looks like for a "broke White person" is different from what privilege looks like for someone like the prime minister of Australia or the chief executive officer of Qantas or another national company.

In her seminal work on racism, Eddo-Lodge (2018) stated, "*white privilege is the fact that if you're white, your race will almost certainly positively impact your life's trajectory in some way. And you probably won't even notice it*" (Eddo-Lodge, 2018, p. 87).

Therefore, even if experienced differently, all White people in some way benefit from Whiteness. Those who do not experience racism will more likely profess its non-existence or diminish its effects and, consequently, also relieve themselves of having to consider how they might be complicit in perpetuating a system that to them does not exist. What does this mean for us as health professionals? Rather than resting assured that one is fighting racism, we must all continually be open to reflection and interrogating the consequences of one's ethical and political practice on both the self and the world.

Box 4.3 Article—Explaining White Privilege to a Broke White Person by Gina Crosley-Corcoran

Key points:

- "Impossible to deny that being born with White skin in America affords people certain unearned privileges in life that people of other skin colors simply are not afforded".
- "Poverty colours nearly everything about your perspective on opportunities for advancement in life. Middle-class, educated people assume that anyone can achieve their goals if they work hard enough".
- More nuanced concept of privilege: the term "intersectionality".

(https://www.huffingtonpost.com/gina-crosleycorcoran/explaining-white-privilege-to-a-broke-white-person_b_5269255.html)

White fragility

Robin DiAngelo, a White American academic, created the term *White fragility* to describe the common reactions of "disbelieving defensiveness" that White people exhibit when their ideas about race and racism are challenged. In her most recent book DiAngelo examines the phenomenon of White people's sensitivity and resistance to being challenged. She argues that the way most societies are structured, in fact insulates White people from racial discomfort and inculcates a sense of entitlement to peace and deference, leading to an inability to engage in difficult conversations and challenge assumptions. Discussions in this space then often lead to responses of "emotions such as anger, fear and guilt, and behaviours such as argumentation, silence, and withdrawal from the stress-inducing situation" (DiAngelo, 2011, p. 54).

White fragility gives a name to the ubiquitous practice in which White people react with a range of defensive moves that compensate for even the slightest distress caused by challenges to their racial worldviews and/or to their racial innocence. White fragility is the "state in which even a minimum amount of racial stress becomes intolerable, triggering a range of defensive moves" (DiAngelo, 2011, p. 54).

As a way forward, DiAngelo maintains that White people need to cultivate "psychosocial stamina" (DiAngelo, 2011, p. 56) or the resilience required to acknowledge the violence Whites themselves enact. In addition, DiAngelo counsels White people to take the first step and to "let go of your racial certitude and reach for humility" (DiAngelo, 2015).

Box 4.4 Reflection—Understanding White fragility

1. Why don't White people see themselves in racial terms or Whiteness as a position of status?
2. Why does the term *White fragility* generate such strong reactions?

Reverse racism?

Is there such a concept as reverse racism? DiAngelo disagrees, and notes that:

"Reverse is an interesting term … Why not just say racism is racism? Reverse suggests it is going in the wrong direction. People who complain about reverse racism never seem to complain about racism otherwise. These are not racial justice advocates" (Iqbal, 2019). (https://www.theguardian.com/world/2019/feb/16/white-fragility-racism-interview-robin-diangelo).

Racism is not directional

Racism is not the same thing as prejudice, bigotry or discrimination.

Prejudice, bigotry and discrimination are wrong. They are wrong no matter what person or group is enacting them. Yes, people of colour can sometimes be prejudiced about White people. They can hold negative views about White people as a group. They can act on these negative views. This can and does happen.

Racism is a system rather than just a slur; it is prejudice plus power. And is designed to benefit and privilege Whiteness by every economic and social measure. People of colour can show prejudice against White people …. but this form of discrimination does not come with systemic privilege and so is not racism as per the modern definition.

DiAngelo cautions us against complacency and reminds us,

> Interrupting the forces of racism is ongoing, lifelong work because the forces conditioning us into racist frameworks are always at play; our learning will never be finished.
>
> (DiAngelo, 2018, p. 9)

Box 4.5 Case study—Codes of conduct and White privilege

Background

The Nursing and Midwifery Board of Australia (NMBA) officially launched the Codes of Conduct in March 2018. The new codes are for all nurses and midwives in Australia and set out the legal requirements, professional behaviour and conduct expectations for all nurses and midwives in all practice settings.

To support cultural safety in nursing and midwifery, the NMBA worked closely with CATSINaM to develop the principle in the new codes. This principle is for nurses and midwives to "provide care that is holistic, free of bias and racism, challenges belief based upon assumption and is culturally safe and respectful for Aboriginal and Torres Strait Islander peoples" (NMBA, 2018).

"Cultural safety is about acknowledging how our own culture and assumptions can have an impact on the care we give. It's about ensuring we are self-aware and work in a genuine partnership with people, both the people we care for and our colleagues," NMBA Chair, Associate Professor Lynette Cusack RN said.

"Systemic racism contributes to poor health outcomes experienced by Aboriginal and Torres Strait Islander Australians. By providing health care in a culturally safe and respectful way, and contributing to culturally safe and respectful health systems, nurses and midwives can make a real contribution to health equity for all Australians," Janine Mohamed, the former Chief Executive Officer of CATSINaM, said (NMBA, 2018).

Reactions to the launch of the codes

In this case study you will be asked to reflect on reactions when the Codes of Conduct were launched.

In the popular media, headlines like "White privilege outrage" were released, with claims the new nursing code will force White nurses to declare "White privilege".

The code for nurses and midwives, which came into effect in March 2018, does talk about Indigenous patients, and the glossary does say this about White privilege (NMBA, 2019, p. 16). The glossary is not the code that nurses must adhere to, and nurses are not required, forced or even encouraged to announce their White privilege to patients before treating them, or indeed at all.

Yet that unsubstantiated claim gathered momentum for weeks. According to that new code from the Nursing and Midwifery Board of Australia:

Rather than saying "I provide the same care to everyone regardless of difference," cultural safety means providing care that takes into account Aboriginal and/or Torres Strait Islander peoples' needs.—Nursing & Midwifery Board of Australia code of conduct for nurses and code of conduct for midwives, March, 2018.

Box 4.6 Reflection—Nursing and Midwifery Board of Australia

Read a statement from the Nursing and Midwifery Board of Australia (NMBA). Read a response to Media Watch from the Nursing and Midwifery Board of Australia. Consider what might be behind the claims that "people will have to apologise for being white" and that nurses and midwives "must announce their "white privilege" before treating Aboriginal and Torres Strait Islander patients).

(NMBA, 2018)

The question asked earlier this section as to what Whiteness or White Privilege means, is succinctly and powerfully answered in the following quote:

… it's not just strangers but people you know and care for who have suffered and are suffering because we are excluded from the privilege you have to not be judged, questioned, or assaulted in any way because of your race. As to you "being part of the problem," trust me, nobody is mad at you for being white. Nobody. Just like nobody should be mad at me for being black. Or female. Or whatever. But what is being asked of you is to acknowledge that white privilege does exist, and to not only to treat people of races that differ from yours "with respect and humor," but also to stand up for fair treatment and justice, to not let "jokes" or "off-color" comments by friends, co-workers, or family slide by without challenge, and to continually make an effort to put yourself in someone else's shoes, so we may all cherish and respect our unique and special contributions to society as much as we do our common ground. (https://onbeing.org/blog/what-i-said-when-my-white-friend-asked-for-my-black-opinion-on-white-privilege/)

Conclusion

Cultural safety does have a crucial role to play not only in regard to Indigenous health (Browne & Varcoe, 2006; Purdie et al., 2010) in Australia but also for other sections of the population, for example, refugees, migrants, LGBTIQA+, elderly, disability, and so on, primarily as it provides a model of practice based on:

- Dialogue
- Communication
- Power sharing and negotiation
- Acknowledgement of Whiteness and privilege.

These actions are a means to challenge racism at personal and institutional levels and to establish trust in health care encounters. Therefore, it is not about progress through certain levels of awareness and practice along a staged or linear continuum, as the process is a lifelong one, and does not require the study of any culture other than one's own—so as to be open-minded and flexible in attitudes towards others. Identifying what makes others different is simple—understanding our own culture and its influence on how we think, feel and behave is much more complex. Ultimately, it is the receiver of services who determine if their care was culturally safe or not (Cox & Simpson, 2015).

The bottom line is whatever the context or specific group, that health professionals looking at cultural safety ask themselves What does cultural safety mean to me, and how can these "good practices" be embedded in my own work practice?

Finally, being an effective and culturally safe health professional, no matter what the context, means obtaining skill sets that include effective communication, developing relationships, and building trust.

Box 4.7 Reflection—Chapter review questions

1. How would the theory of cultural safety be described as an interdisciplinary and interprofessional model of health care?
2. Why is the model of cultural safety contested along with related topics of racism, White privilege, discrimination and power?
3. The principles of cultural safety, including social justice, trust, respect, self-awareness, and self-reflection form the basis of culturally safe practice. How does cultural safety differ from other terms used, often interchangeably?
4. Why is the need for robust partnerships negotiated with diverse groups of people and their respective health needs considered to be a key component of cultural safety?

Box 4.8 Reflection—Chapter discussion

1. What might be some of the challenges in relation to culturally safe and effective health care?
2. How might use of cultural safety strategies contribute to improvement of health outcomes?

Box 4.9 Reflection—Questions for personal reflection

1. The availability, accessibility and acceptability of health care for diverse populations is a health equity issue. What are some of your cultural values, attitudes and beliefs of that might impact and shape health care relationships?
2. What might be some of the personal and professional actions you can take in preparation for being a culturally safe and effective practitioner?

Notes

1 The term *working cross-culturally* is used in this context as broadly concerning any form of interactivity between members of distinct cultural groups. It is not to be conflated with cultural safety or culture-centred approaches (Dutta, 2008).
2 They are five of the peak Australian nursing and midwifery organisations.
3 The consultation period was extended until May 24th as more interested parties found out about the Ahpra proposal and wanted to submit feedback.
4 The capitalisation of the "W" in White and non-White is one of contentious scholarly debate. A capital W is used in this chapter in line with *The Diversity Style Guide* (2019) to acknowledge the racialisation and concomitant characterisation of ethnic, religious, cultural and linguistic affiliation in terms of proper nouns used to construct identities and not simply to inaccurately describe phenotypical traits.

References

Australian Commission Safety Quality Health Care. (2011). *Patient centred care: Improving quality and safety through partnerships with patients and consumers*. https://www.safetyandquality.gov.au/sites/default/files/migrated/PCC_Paper_August.pdf.

Australian Health Practitioner Regulation Agency. (2019). *Public consultations on the definition of cultural safety*. https://www.ahpra.gov.au/News/Consultations/Past-Consultations.aspx.

Bennett, B. (2015). Stop deploying your white privilege on me! Aboriginal and Torres Strait Islander engagement with the Australian Association of Social Workers. *Australian Social Work*, *68*(1), 19–31. https://doi.org/10.1080/0312407X.2013.840325.

Bennett, B., Green, S., Gilbert, S., & Bessarab, D. (2013). *Our voices: Aboriginal and Torres Strait Islander social work*. Palgrave Macmillan.

Birkhäuer, J., Gaab, J., Kossowsky, J., Hasler, S., Krummenacher, P., Werner, C., & Gerger, H. (2017). Trust in the health care professional and health outcome: A meta-analysis. *PLoS One*, *12*(2), 1–17. https://doi.org/10.1371/journal.pone.0170988.

Brown, A. E., Middleton, P. F., Fereday, J. A., & Pincombe, J. I. (2016). Cultural safety and midwifery care for Aboriginal women—A phenomenological study. *Women and Birth*, *29*(2), 196–202. https://doi.org/10.1016/j.wombi.2015.10.013.

Browne, A., & Varcoe, C. (2006). Critical cultural perspectives and health care involving Aboriginal peoples. *Contemporary Nurse*, *22*(2), 155–167. http://search.informit.com.au/documentSummary;dn=641204474741333;res=IELHEA

Cox, L. (2016, October 31–November 2). *Social change and social justice: Cultural safety as a vehicle for nurse activism [Paper presentation]. 2nd International Critical Perspectives in Nursing and Healthcare*, Sydney, Australia. http://sydney.edu.au/nursing/pdfs/critical-perspectives/cox-social-change.pdf.

Cox, L., & Best, O. (2019). *Cultural safety history repeats: Why are we taking the redefinition road?* Croakey. https://croakey.org/cultural-safety-history-repeats-why-are-we-taking-the-redefinition-road/.

Cox, L., & Simpson, A. (2015). Cultural safety, diversity and the servicer user and carer movement in mental health research. *Nursing Inquiry*, *22*(4), 306–316. https://doi.org/10.1111/nin.12096.

De Souza, R. (2008). Wellness for all: The possibilities of cultural safety and cultural competence in New Zealand. *Journal of Research in Nursing*, *13*(2), 125–135. https://doi.org/10.1177/1744987108088637.

De Souza, R. (2015). Culturally safe care for ethnically and religiously diverse communities. In D. Wepa (Ed.), *Cultural safety in Aotearoa New Zealand* (2nd ed., pp. 189–203). Cambridge University Press.

DiAngelo, R. (2011). White fragility. *International Journal of Critical Pedagogy*, *3*(3), 54–70.

DiAngelo, R. (2015). *White fragility: Why it's so hard to talk to white people about racism. Dr. Robin DiAngelo explains why white people implode when talking about race.* The Good Men Project. https://goodmenproject.com/featured-content/white-fragility-why-its-so-hard-to-talk-to-white-people-about-racism-twlm/.

DiAngelo, R. (2018). *White fragility: Why it's so hard for white people to talk about racism.* Beacon Press.

Du Bois, W. E. B. (1917). Of the culture of white folk. *The Journal of Race Development*, 7(4), 434–447.

Dune, T., Caputi, P., & Walker, B. (2018). A systematic review of mental health care workers' constructions about culturally and linguistically diverse people. *PLoS ONE*, *13*(7), e0200662. https://doi.org/10.1371/journal.pone.0200662.

Dutta, M. J. (2008). *Communicating health: A cultured-centered approach.* Polity Press.

Eckermann, A. K., Dowd, T., Chong, E., Nixon, L., Gray, R., & Johnson, S. (2010). *Binan Goonj: Bridging cultures in Aboriginal health* (3rd ed.). Elsevier.

Eddo-Lodge, R. (2018). *Why I'm no longer talking about race.* Bloomsbury Publishing.

Furlong, M., & Wight, J. (2011). Promoting critical awareness and critiquing cultural competence: Towards disrupting received professional knowledges. *Australian Social Work*, *64*(1), 38–54. https://doi.org/10.1080/0312407X.2010.537352.

Gerlach, A. (2015). Sharpening our critical edge: Occupational therapy in the context of marginalized populations. *Canadian Journal of Occupational Therapy*, *82*(4), 245–253. https://doi.org/10.1177/0008417415571730.

Goold, S. D. (2002). Trust, distrust and trustworthiness: Lessons from the field. *Journal of General Internal Medicine*, *17*(1), 79–81. https://doi.org/10.1046/j.1525-1497.2002.11132.x.

Guess, T. J. (2006). The social construction of whiteness: Racism by intent, racism by consequence. *Critical Sociology*, *32*(4), 649–673. https://doi.org/10.1163/156916306779155199.

Hayter, M., & King, R. (2019). Naomi Williams inquest concludes with coroner calling for change at NSW hospital. *ABC News.* https://www.abc.net.au/news/2019-07-29/naomi-williams-tumut-sepsis-death-inquest-findings/11355244.

Henry, B. R., Houston, S., & Mooney, G. H. (2004). Institutional racism in Australian healthcare: A plea for decency. *Medical Journal of Australia*, *180*(10), 517–520. https://doi.org/10.5694/j.1326-5377.2004.tb06056.x.

Iqbal, N. (2019). Academic Robin DiAngelo: We have to stop thinking about racism as someone who says the N-word. *The Guardian.* https://www.theguardian.com/world/2019/feb/16/white-fragility-racism-interview-robin-diangelo.

James, T. A. (2018). *Setting the stage: Why health care needs a culture of respect.* Harvard Medical School Lean Forward. https://leanforward.hms.harvard.edu/2018/07/31/setting-the-stage-why-health-care-needs-a-culture-of-respect/.

Jackson, G. (2019). *Naomi Williams inquest: Coroner finds bias in way hospital treated Aboriginal woman.* The Guardian. https://www.theguardian.com/australia-news/2019/jul/29/naomi-williams-inquest-coroner-finds-bias-in-way-hospital-treated-aboriginal-woman.

Johnstone, M. J., & Kanitsaki, O. (2008). The politics of resistance to workplace cultural diversity education for health service providers: An Australian study. *Race Ethnicity and Education*, *11*(2), 133–154. https://doi.org/10.1080/13613320802110258.

Katsikitis, M., McAllister, M., Sharman, R., Raith, L., Faithfull-Byrne, A., & Priaulx, R. (2013). Continuing professional development in nursing in Australia: Current awareness, practice and future directions. *Contemporary Nurse*, *45*(1), 33–45. https://doi.org/10.5172/conu.2013.45.1.33.

King, C. R., & Springwood, C. F. (2001). *Beyond the cheers: Race as spectacle in college sport*. State University of New York Press.

Kurtz, D. L. M., Janke, R., Vinek, J., Wells, T., Hutchinson, P., & Froste, A. (2018). Health sciences cultural safety education in Australia, Canada, New Zealand, and the United States: A literature review. *International Journal of Medical Education*, *9*, 271–285. https://doi.org/10.5116/ijme.5bc7.21e2.

Lewis, A. E. (2004). What group? Studying whites and whiteness in the era of color-blindness. *Sociological Theory*, *22*(4), 623–646.

McEldowney, R., & Connor, M. J. (2011). Cultural safety as an ethic of care: A praxiological process. *Journal of Transcultural Nursing*, *22*(4), 342–349. https://doi.org/10.1177/1043659611414139.

McGough, S. (2016). Tackling cultural safety and disparities in mental health: Striving or surviving? *International Journal of Mental Health Nursing*, *25*(S1), 32–33.

McGough, S., Wynaden, D., & Wright, M. (2018). Experience of providing cultural safety in mental health to Aboriginal patients: A grounded theory study. *International Journal of Mental Health Nursing*, *27*(1), 204–213. https://doi.org/10.1111/inm.12310.

Milne, T., Creedy, D. K., & West, R. (2016). Development of the awareness of cultural safety Scale: A pilot study with midwifery and nursing academics. *Nurse Education Today*, *44*, 20–25. https://doi.org/10.1016/j.nedt.2016.05.012.

Mkandawire-Valhmu, L. (2018). *Cultural safety, healthcare and vulnerable populations: A critical theoretical perspective*. Routledge.

Moreton-Robinson, A. (2004). Whiteness, epistemology and Indigenous representation. In A. Moreton-Robinson (Ed.), Whitening race: Essays in social and cultural criticism (pp. 75–88). *Aboriginal Studies Press*.

National Academies of Sciences, Engineering and Medicine. (2017). The root causes of health inequity. In *National Academies of Sciences, Engineering, and Medicine, Health and Medicine Division, Board on Population Health and Public Health Practice, Committee on Community-Based Solutions to Promote Health Equity in the United States*, A. Baciu, Y. Negussie, A. Geller, & J. N. Weinstein (Eds.), Communities in action: Pathway to health equity (pp. 99–184). National Academies Press. https://doi.org/10.17226/24624.

National Health and Medical Research Council. (2005). *Cultural competency in health: A guide for policy, partnerships and participation*. Commonwealth of Australia. https://www.nhmrc.gov.au/about-us/publications/cultural-competency-health#block-views-block-file-attachments-content-block-1.

Nursing and Midwifery Board of Australia. (2018). *NMBA and CATSINaM joint statement on culturally safe care*. Ahpra. https://www.nursingmidwiferyboard.gov.au/news/2018-02-01-nmba-catsinam.aspx.

Nursing and Midwifery Board of Australia. (2019). *Nursing and midwifery board of Australia codes of conduct*. https://www.nursingmidwiferyboard.gov.au/Codes-Guidelines-Statements/Position-Statements/leading-the-way.aspx.

Nursing Council of New Zealand. (2011). *Guidelines for cultural safety, the Treaty of Waitangi and Maori health in nursing education and practice*. https://ngamanukura.nz/sites/default/files/basic_page_pdfs/Guidelines%20for%20cultural%20safety%2C%20the%20Treaty%20of%20Waitangi%2C%20and%20Maori%20health%20in%20nursing%20education%20and%20practice%282%29_0.pdf.

Nursing Council of New Zealand. (2012). Code of conduct for nurses. https://www.nursingcouncil.org.nz/Public/Nursing/Standards_and_guidelines/NCNZ/nursing-section/Standards_and_guidelines_for_nurses.aspx.

Paradies, Y., Harris, R., & Anderson, I. (2008). *The impact of racism on Indigenous health in Australia and Aotearoa: Towards a research agenda*. Cooperative Research Centre for Aboriginal Health. http://dro.deakin.edu.au/eserv/DU:30058493/paradies-impactofracism-2008.pdf.

Purdie, N., Dudgeon, P., & Walker, R. (2010). *Working together: Aboriginal and Torres Strait Islander mental health and wellbeing principles and practice*. Australian Government Department of Health and Ageing.

http://web.archive.org/web/20160314115103/http://aboriginal.telethonkids.org.au/media/54847/working_together_full_book.pdf.

Ramsden, I. (2002). Cultural safety and nursing education in Aotearoa and Te Waipounamu. [Doctoral Dissertation, Victoria University of Wellington]. https://croakey.org/wp-content/uploads/2017/08/RAMSDEN-I-Cultural-Safety_Full.pdf.

Richardson, F. (2012). Editorial: Cultural safety 20 years on time to celebrate or commiserate? *Whitireia Nursing Journal, 19*, 5–8.

Richardson, F. (2015). Building inclusive frameworks for practice. In J. Davis, Y. Birks, & Y. Chapman (Eds.), *Inclusive practice for health professionals* (pp. 39–67). Oxford University Press.

Robinson, M. (2019). *Calls to address the public health threat of racism in healthcare – #JusticeForNaomi.* Croakey. https://www.croakey.org/calls-to-address-the-public-health-threat-of-racism-in-health-care-justicefornaomi/.

Sue, D. W. (2006). The invisible whiteness of being: Whiteness, white supremacy, white privilege, and racism. In M. G. Constantine & D. W. Sue (Eds.), *Addressing racism: Facilitating cultural competence in mental health and educational settings* (pp. 15–30). Wiley.

Taylor, K., & Guerin, P. T. (2019). *Health care and Indigenous Australians: Cultural safety in practice* (3rd ed.). Red Globe Press.

Tseng, W. S., & Streltzer, J. (2010). *Cultural competence in health care.* Springer.

Universities Australia. (2011). *National best practice framework for Indigenous cultural competency in Australian universities.* https://www.universitiesaustralia.edu.au/uni-participation-quality/Indigenous-Higher-Education/Indigenous-Cultural-Compet - .XPin7NMzbSw.

Wepa, D. (2015). *Cultural safety in Aotearoa New Zealand* (2nd ed.). Cambridge University Press.

Williams, R. (1999). Cultural safety—what does it mean for our work practice? *Australian and New Zealand Journal of Public Health, 23*(2), 213–214. https://onlinelibrary.wiley.com/doi/pdf/10.1111/j.1467-842X.1999.tb01240.x.

Williams, R. (2016). Culture and health. In J. D. Smith (Ed.), *Australia's rural, remote and Indigenous health* (3rd ed., pp. 45–75). Elsevier.

Willis, K., & Elmer, S. (2011). *Society, culture and health: An introduction to sociology for nurses.* Oxford University Press.

Woods, M. (2010). Cultural safety and the socio-ethical nurse. *Nursing Ethics, 17*(6), 715–725. https://doi.org/10.1177/0969733010379296

5 Policy and advocacy in culturally diverse health care

Keera Laccos-Barrett and Angela Brown

Learning outcomes

After working through this chapter, students should be able to:

1. Review health policy in relation to culturally diverse health care.
2. Explore the role of the health care professional in health advocacy.
3. Critique the inclusiveness of Australian health policy.
4. Identify the barriers and enablers of cultural safety in the context of organisational policies and structures.
5. Explore systemic racism and discrimination embedded in health care policy.
6. Apply cultural safety principles in advocacy at individual and organisational levels.

Key terms

Aboriginal and Torres Strait Islander peoples: The first peoples of this land now called Australia are the Aboriginal peoples; however, they also have other names that they use to refer to themselves: Goori, Koori, Arrernte, Kamilaroi, Yungl, Yaegl and so on. Torres Strait Islanders are a seafaring peoples, whose traditional countries are in the Torres Strait, off the Australian mainland's northernmost point. The region has over 270 islands in the strait of ocean between the northern tip of Queensland, Cape York, and the south-east coast of Papua New Guinea.
Cultural diversity: The presence of many different cultural or ethnic groups within a society.
Cultural safety: An environment that is spiritually, socially and emotionally safe, as well as physically safe for people; where there is no assault challenge or denial of their identity, of who they are and what they need.
Culture: The evolved human capacity to classify and represent experiences with symbols, and to act imaginatively and creatively. Cultures are differentiated by the distinct ways that people, who live differently, classify and represent their experiences.
Health advocacy: Means providing care to health care consumers that includes the promotion of health and access to services.
Institutional discrimination: A form of racism expressed in the practice of social and political institutions. It affects racial minorities but is also a term used to describe the discrimination experienced by people of minority such as, but not limited to, ethnic, cultural, sexual orientation, gender identity and religious groups. It is reflected in disparities regarding wealth, income, criminal justice, employment, housing, health care, political power and education, among other factors.
Institutional racism: A form of racism expressed in social and political institutions that devalue and ignore people of a racial minority

Chapter summary

This chapter will focus on policy and advocacy aspects of culturally diverse health care. Students will explore the various roles that health professionals across a range of disciplines can play in terms of advocacy, community development and capacity building to address the social determinants of health. Students will review relevant documents, including national guidelines, professional codes of conduct and policies. Using cases from contemporary research, students will review a number of scenarios that can challenge health practitioners and their engagement with culturally safe practice. In doing so, students will critique policies and their application—whether inclusive and/or exclusive. The enablers and limitations to cultural safety will be discussed in the context of organisational policies and structures. Students will be provided with examples and encouraged to develop their own ideas about how to work within (or advocate for changes of) policy and practice relating to cultural safety. Students will be encouraged to reflect on these perspectives on cultural safety and its application in groups or online portfolios that can support peer feedback and exposure to perceptual variation.

Introduction

In thinking about *cultural diversity* within this chapter, it is important to explore its meaning. First, what is culture? *Culture* is sometimes considered as the traditions and practices within groups of people. However, culture is much more than that, it is everything about a person or group of people, it's their history, traditions, worldview, practice, protocols and beliefs and the way they relate to others within the world. Culture evolves and is experienced differently by individuals. When considering cultural diversity in society, our understandings are often framed from the perspective of dominant White culture. White culture represents the societal norm and is framed on a background of invasion, White dominance and an historical context of policies that privileged White peoples. White culture defines what is considered 'normal' and values White perspectives and ways of knowing. Think about some of the icons used to portray Australian identity. Often they are based on White culture, and this fails to acknowledge the cultural diversity in Australia. For example, the Australian flag clearly shows British dominance of this country and its "White" identity. White culture manifests itself much deeper than simple icons. White culture can define the way Australian people should dress, think, act, speak and behave and is silently reinforced as the norm. This chapter will highlight the depth of the embodiment of White culture within Australian policy. We will then explore how we may advocate for our patients and clients when our practice is shaped by those policies.

How we view health care differs depending on our own cultural background. Consider your own culture, what is your worldview of health and wellness? How does this differ from the health care that you have access to? How might your gender, age or disability change the way that you consider this? What potential issues or challenges can you think of if you were not from the dominant culture and you needed health care? Perhaps you do not speak English or have religious considerations that are important to you and that are not the norm where you live and work.

Health policy in Australian health care

Responsibility for Australia's health policy is shared between the Commonwealth Government and eight state and territory governments (Fisher et al., 2016). Individual states and territories have developed their own strategic health plans that encompass the core values of the Commonwealth government. For example, New South Wales (NSW) has enacted its NSW

State Health Plan (NSW Government, 2014) that outlines the core values and attributes within the health system. Cultural diversity and the concepts that underpin it do not feature in any depth within the plan and more specifically the key priorities.

The nature of the governance of health systems and policy make it difficult to determine the shared values within individual state and territory policies. It is difficult again when you consider the different worldviews and cultural backgrounds that make up the Australian population and the complexity of attempting to embed those views within a system that is already deeply aligned with White societal beliefs and norms and a biomedical view of health as identified in Chapter 3.

Social determinants of health and policy

We are now going to consider the role of the social determinants of health and how they can impact on health policy. Consider the health inequality between *Aboriginal and Torres Strait Islander peoples* and non-Indigenous Australians that is explored in Chapters 1 and 7. Currently the gap in life expectancy is approximately 10 years (Australian Institute of Health and Welfare, 2018). What do you think about this? How can health policy reduce the inequality? There is no doubt that health inequity exists, that it is unfair and that it is avoidable (Marmot et al., 2008). Health policy must address the inequities in the health system because of the cultural diversity that exists within Australian society. Policymakers also have an ethical responsibility to ensure cultural diversity is considered and addressed within health policy.

Let us review the social determinants of heath that were covered in Chapter 2. The World Health Organisation (2019) defines these as the conditions in which we live, work and age and include the forces and systems that shape our lives. They also include economic policies and systems, social policies and norms and the political systems.

Review the health needs of a recent migrant from a non-English-speaking country whose religious affiliation is often problematised (Muslim) and is accessing health care. What policies are in place at the health services that would support cultural diversity, equity and responsive systems? Responsive health systems support all Australians in policy, service delivery and access to care rather than only those from White Australia. For example, Muslim patients can experience racial discrimination, stigmatisation and stereotyping in Australian society that is also experienced in health care and impacts on health-seeking behaviours for this community (Al Abed, Davidson, & Hickman, 2014; Rassool, 2015). This creates barriers to health equity when the health professionals and health services should, in fact, be advocating for the health of the people seeking care. Systems are governed by policies, the policies written by administrators and health care professionals, and for the most part this is through the lens of the dominant White culture. The Australian population is dominated by people of Anglo-Celtic backgrounds (Biddle, Khoo, & Taylor, 2015). Consider a hospital in Australia that may be accessed by a person who had been born in China. This person's view of health and wellbeing may be different from the health care culture of mainstream Australia. For example, they may use traditional Chinese medicine for health and healing. Accessing health care within the Australian system would mean that they would not have access to treatment from Chinese medicine practitioners within a hospital. This is because the hospital systems, treatments and policies all stem from the dominant White culture. Practitioners working within these institutions are for the most part also from the dominant White culture, where perhaps Chinese traditional medicine is not valued as a "valid" treatment option for sickness and health. It is also important to remember when thinking about these issues that cultural differences are not the same for every person from non-White backgrounds. Two people born in China may have very different worldviews and beliefs, whilst one person may prefer traditional Chinese medicine, and the other may prefer Western-style medicine, for example. Other factors such as country of origin, language, education, socioeconomic status and length of time within Australia can also impact on the health-seeking behaviours, understanding and needs within a health service (Vedio et al., 2017).

Consider your own definition of health. Health can mean different things for different people. For instance, many Aboriginal and/or Torres Strait Islander peoples view health very differently from the biomedical view of health. For many Aboriginal and/or Torres Strait Islander peoples, health encompasses the social, emotional and cultural wellbeing of the whole community (Gee et al., 2014). Conversely within the biomedical model, health is often viewed from the standpoint of the absence of disease as highlighted in Chapter 3. Health care is provided in this way to manage disease. Consider a person who has a view of health and wellbeing that differs from the dominant White culture. For instance, the person who wishes to access traditional Chinese medicine within a South Australian health hospital or health service may encounter barriers. According to the policy requirements in their *Guideline Complementary and Alternative Medicines* (SA Health Policy Committee, 2017), SA Health does not support, supply or administer "complementary alternative medicines" that are not listed on the Australian register of therapeutic goods. Consider those who access homeopathy or naturopathy; these forms of treatment do not align with mainstream health treatments. Do you think people who wish to access "alternative medicines" are placed at a disadvantage when trying to access health care that is not aligned to their worldview? If you agree, then what structures are in place that reinforce this? These structures may not always be related to cultural aspects of a person's worldview but can be related to choices that do not align to mainstream treatments.

Policy and standards in Australian health care

What sort of policies govern health care in Australia? Can you think of any? Perhaps review some of the governing documents for your profession, and look for the inclusion of cultural diversity. We will now examine the Australian Health Practitioners Agency, Medical Board of Australia's policies and codes that govern the profession. The Code of Conduct for Doctors in Australia (2017) states that good practice involves "genuine" efforts to understand the cultural needs of patients. The code asks doctors to respect the needs of the community that they serve; acknowledge the social, economic and cultural factors that impact on health; and to understand their own culture (Medical Board of Australia, 2017). What do genuine efforts look like, and how are they governed? Cultural needs are often the least-considered aspect of health care, with many health care providers only focusing on the physical needs of their patients. Consider some of the Australian state coroners' court findings. Rarely is culture considered a factor in people seeking or accessing care or even contributing to negative outcomes. However, culture can be used to "blame" people for not accessing health care. Rarely are care providers subjected to blame for not offering acceptable services to the community that they serve. Some well-known cases include Tanya Day (Victorian Coroner's Court Findings) and Julieka Dhu (West Australian Coroner's Court findings). You might like to review them but also to search some of the other findings on these sites.

Box 5.1 Reflection—Cultural diversity

In groups review the Tanya Day or Julieka Dhu case, and look for the inclusion of cultural diversity and the potential impact on health outcomes.

https://www.coronerscourt.vic.gov.au/
https://www.coronerscourt.wa.gov.au/
Some prompts can include

- Was the cultural diversity of the person an important factor in the delivery of health care?

Can you identify areas in the coroner's report where culturally safe care was restricted and/or hindered or supported by policy? Explain how this was done.

Consider a pregnant woman who attends for antenatal care at a service that is designed for White Australian women. Perhaps the woman is a lesbian. Structures, policies and the system are geared towards men and women having a baby together, and the woman may not feel safe attending for care where she may be questioned and feel her relationship is not acknowledged or respected by the system. Think about the paperwork at the hospital where the father's name is asked and recorded. The visual representations within a maternity hospital are often representations of White Australia with a mother and a father. For some people this could make them not wish to attend the service. What are the implications of this? Let's say, for example, that the woman decides not to attend for antenatal care—the flow on effect for her baby could be devastating. Every structure within the system is telling us what "normal" looks like, and these forms of institutional discrimination are rarely noticed by members of the dominant culture.

Hospital policies can also act to disempower the people they are created to serve, particularly in relation to cultural difference (Brown et al., 2016). Consider a policy that restricts visitors to a health service. If we review an Aboriginal and/or Torres Strait Islander view of health that can encompass the whole community, policies that restrict those interactions are inherently racist and place the health and wellbeing of the person seeking care at a significant disadvantage. Placing restrictions on visitors can have significant consequences in connection to culture that may not be an issue for White Australia in the same way. For example, there are many cultures after birth where the woman's mother or partner play a significant role in helping the woman care for her new baby. Hospital structures do not allow this connection to culture, and the distress these policies cause can go unnoticed.

Consider the case of Julieka Dhu in Western Australia. Julieka was an Aboriginal woman who died in 2014 whilst in Police custody. She had been arrested for unpaid fines (Coroner's Court of Western Australia, 2016). The coroner described Julieka's family's belief that she had experienced institutional racism and assumptions about her were made that impacted on her receiving the care that she needed (Coroner's Court of Western Australia, 2016). Ultimately Julieka died of septicaemia despite being transported to a health service twice within the time she was in custody.

Health national standards

In July 2010 the Health Practitioner Regulation National Law came into effect in each state and territory (Ahpra, 2017a). The development of this law meant that 16 health professions in Australia were to be consistently regulated under the National Registration and Accreditation Scheme. Table 5.1 shows the 15 boards that are supported by the Australian Health Practitioner Regulation Agency, also known as Ahpra (2017a). The roles and responsibilities of Ahpra include, but are not limited to, registering 700,000+ Australian health professionals, auditing, compliance

Table 5.1 The 15 National Boards regulated by the Ahpra (2017b)

Aboriginal and Torres Strait Islander Health Practice Board of Australia
Chinese Medicine Board of Australia
Chiropractic Board of Australia
Dental Board of Australia
Medical Board of Australia
Medical Radiation Practice Board of Australia
Nursing and Midwifery Board of Australia
Occupational Therapy Board of Australia
Optometry Board of Australia
Osteopathy Board of Australia
Paramedicine Board of Australia
Pharmacy Board of Australia
Physiotherapy Board of Australia
Podiatry Board of Australia
Psychology Board of Australia

and publication of the online register (Ahpra, 2017a, 2018). Those allied health professionals that are not governed by Ahpra are self-regulated within their profession by associations that function similarly to Ahpra. The accreditation provided by the professional associations is required for the allied health professionals to access some essential services such as Medicare, private health insurers and other services (Ahpra, 2019).

Currently, the Medical Board of Australia (2017), in *Good Medical Practice: A Code of Conduct for Doctors in Australia,* focuses on culturally safe care and partnerships with patients in Section 3.7.

Box 5.2 Reflection—Good medical practice: A code of conduct for doctors in Australia (Medical Board of Australia, 2017)

Section 3.7 in *Good Medical Practice: A Code of Conduct for Doctors in Australia* provides guidelines for culturally safe and sensitive practice.

Good medical practice involves genuine efforts to understand the cultural needs and contexts of different patients to obtain good health outcomes. This includes

1. Having knowledge of, respect for, and sensitivity towards, the cultural needs of the community you serve, including Aboriginal and Torres Strait Islander Australians and those from culturally and linguistically diverse backgrounds.
2. Acknowledging the social, economic, cultural and behavioural factors influencing health, both at individual and population levels.
3. Understanding that your own culture and beliefs influence your interactions with patients and ensuring that this does not unduly influence your decision making.
4. Adapting your practice to improve patient engagement and health care outcomes.

Source: Medical Board of Australia (2017). *Good medical practice: A code of conduct for doctors in Australia.* https://www.medicalboard.gov.au/codes-guidelines-policies/code-of-conduct.aspx

Ahpra (2019) has proposed a singular definition of *cultural safety* which is

> Cultural safety is the individual and institutional knowledge, skills, attitudes and competencies needed to deliver optimal health care for Aboriginal and Torres Strait Islander Peoples as determined by Aboriginal and Torres Strait Islander individuals, families and communities.

This proposed definition is to be used as a "foundation for embedding cultural safety across the National Scheme". The idea is that the one definition will be used by all professions in future codes of conduct/standards or guidelines (Ahpra, 2019).

Box 5.3 Reflection—Australian Health Practitioner Regulation Agency (Ahpra) and cultural safety

Reflecting on what you have learnt about culturally safe care in previous chapters, compare the proposed Ahpra (2019) definition of cultural safety with the current culturally safe and sensitive practice guidelines in *Good Medical Practice: A Code of Conduct for Doctors in Australia* (Medical Board of Australia, 2017). Knowing that the proposed Ahpra definition will be embedded in all future codes of conduct/standards or guidelines, consider the following points:

- Will this enable policy to be more culturally safe for Aboriginal and/or Torres Strait Islander peoples?
- What about those people from culturally diverse backgrounds who are not Aboriginal and/or Torres Strait Islander peoples?
- What will this cultural safety definition, which will be embedded in our professional codes and standards, mean for them?

Consider both the recipient of care and the health professional in your responses.

McDermott (2012) believes there to be a false dichotomy between clinical competence and self-reflection within the Australian health professions, where the capacity for reflection converting into practice varies greatly between health professionals. Understanding your own culture and its impact on your relationship with the people you care for is important. Self-refection is the ability to review and improve your practice with deep exploration of all aspects of care provision and the impact on patients/clients and other health staff. A practitioner can be clinically excellent but lack those reflection skills. Likewise, reflective practitioners can explore their practice, understand the barriers some policies create for patients/clients and act in an advocacy role to ensure equitable access to health care. For example, consider a White diabetes nurse caring for a recent Indian migrant. The nurse could have the highest clinical knowledge yet still provide care that is unsafe for the patient. The nurse may not have explored his/her own bias towards migrants or consider some of the cultural factors around diet (including fasting) and food for Indian cultures.

Cultural safety and policy considerations

The Nursing Council of New Zealand (2011) has defined cultural safety as shown in Table 5.2.

Table 5.2 Nursing Council of New Zealand cultural safety definition (2011)

The effective nursing practice of a person or family from another culture, and is determined by that person or family. Culture includes, but is not restricted to, age or generation; gender; sexual orientation; occupation and socioeconomic status; ethnic origin or migrant experience; religious or spiritual belief; and disability. The nurse delivering the nursing service will have undertaken a process of reflection on his or her own cultural identity and will recognise the impact that his or her personal culture has on his or her professional practice. Unsafe cultural practice comprises any action which diminishes, demeans or disempowers the cultural identity and well being of an individual.

Box 5.4 Reflection—Considering cultural safety

Consider the cultural safety definition just given, and think about the last time you were in a health care centre, perhaps a doctor's surgery or a hospital.

- How have you seen cultural safety principles embedded in the system?
- Was there recognition of cultural diversity and the capacity to meet the needs of people who are not of the dominant culture?

If you have worked in a health care institution (or plan to), you might like to consider how these features might translate into policy.

Mandatory cultural safety training is not present in all institutions or institutional policy. The lack of education in this area could reflect the value, or lack thereof, that is inherent within the dominant culture's psyche and reflected within policy. The value of holding these sessions could be increased by making it mandatory prior to applying for a job and more advanced training required for promotion as a means of encouraging staff to progress on their cultural safety journey. Policymakers could embed these requirements into their institutions. The very setup of a hospital, for example, is geared towards the dominant White culture. The Western view of health is presented, and the structures and systems are not oriented towards the cultural diversity present in Australian society.

Critiques in policies

Let us consider cultural safety and policy for Aboriginal and/or Torres Strait Islander peoples. It has been over a decade since the rollout of the Closing the Gap strategy and campaign (Department of the Prime Minister and Cabinet, 2018), although with changes to funding, administration and shifting policies, progress to reaching the targets outlined have been suspended (Holland, 2018). The strategy has failed with inequality persisting at unacceptable levels. In fact, the Australian Medical Association Chair has described a lack of resourcing and investment in Aboriginal and/or Torres Strait Islander peoples' health and wellbeing that is contributing to unacceptable gaps across a range of outcomes (Bartone, 2019). Not only is this a failure of the Australian government in advocating for Aboriginal and/or Torres Strait Islander peoples but it is also a failure to adhere to the United Nations Declaration on The Human Rights of Indigenous People (United Nations, 2007). When the declaration was passed in 2007, Australia was one of four countries that voted against it but has since reversed its position. The declaration provides policymakers a minimum standard that works towards supporting Indigenous peoples around the world and protects their basic human rights (United Nations, 2019). These include rights for Indigenous people to be involved in decision making directly affecting them, the right to use their own medicines and "informed consent by Indigenous people before adopting and implementing legislative or administrative measures affecting them" (United Nations, 2019). These standards emulate very basic human rights that Aboriginal and/or Torres Strait Islander peoples are still denied. An example of how the breaching of these basic rights, culturally unsafe care and deeply entrenched racism, particularly *institutional racism,* is impacting Aboriginal and/or Torres Strait Islander peoples is the staggering life expectancy gap between Aboriginal and/or Torres Strait Islander peoples and non-Indigenous people in Australia (Holland, 2018).

Review of the Closing the Gap (CTG) Strategy in 2018 demonstrated many failures on behalf of the government (Holland, 2018). These failures included poor engagement with Aboriginal leaders and communities, a lack of clarity and the promotion of the government's agenda that did not include Aboriginal and/or Torres Strait Islander peoples (Holland, 2018). Aboriginal and/or Torres Strait Islander peoples were not involved in the "refreshed" CTG strategy, again breaching a basic human right outlined by the United Nations (2019; Holland, 2018). This is a very strong stance on where the Australian government currently stands regarding cultural safety considerations in health policy development and review.

Policy and cultural safety for health professionals

Having a deeper understanding of the key features of cultural safety will enable you to identify when a scenario has the *potential* to be culturally unsafe for the person that you are caring for (Fleming et al., 2018; Laverty et al., 2017). The Nursing Council of New Zealand (2011) defines unsafe cultural practices as those that diminish, demean or disempower a person's identity and wellbeing. How do we then ensure these professional standards transpire into competent and culturally safe practice within a strictly White biomedical setting?

A study by Brown (2016) that involved interviews with birthing Aboriginal women about their care in a large tertiary South Australian hospital clearly demonstrated culturally unsafe practices. These practices included stereotyping, judgements and even hospital policies that restricted visitors or prevented fast return to community or the use of traditional medicine (Brown, 2016). In the following quote, the woman identifies a divide between her health beliefs and practices and the policies at the hospital from which she was seeking care (Brown, 2016):

> Well, in our law, like, when we have a baby we go back to community and we go back to bush medicine, that's what we do at home, it makes them grow strong … bush medicine for flu and all that, for diarrhoea, for everything.

Institutional discrimination occurs when an organisation, like a hospital, has policies and procedures that disempower and do not represent the cultural values of the people who are seeking care. Consider the preceding quote and the woman's requirements around her own culture and how they differ from the Western biomedical model. This is an example of systemic or institutional racism where you can clearly see the contrasts between the cultural values, meanings and protocols. When health care delivery is culturally unsafe, it can then proceed to have a significant impact on the physical health of the person seeking care. Review Box 5.5 where you can see an example of how feeling safe can impact on a person's health-seeking activity.

Box 5.5 Reflection—Feeling safe at a health service

Alex is a 25-year-old non-binary person. Alex has been experiencing abdominal pain and attends a hospital emergency department. At check-in, Alex is asked to fill out the paperwork for registration including identification as male or female. Alex does not identify as either sex although was born female. Alex prefers the pronoun "they" when referring to identity as opposed to male or female. There is no box for non-binary on the registration form so Alex writes "non-binary". The nurse at the desk asks Alex what sex they were born as. Alex says, "I am non-binary" and would prefer not to say. The nurse tells Alex that in order to proceed he would need Alex to provide the information as it was required in the organisation. The nurse does this quite loudly at the desk and the conversation is overheard by others.

Once Alex has provided the information to the nurse, Alex feels uncomfortable and shamed. They decide to use the toilet and must decide between the male/female or disabled toilets. This makes Alex feel unsafe. Alex decides to go home and maybe wait for longer and see if the pain gets better. Alex's identity is not supported in the structural processes and facilities within the institution. The nurse has not considered Alex's needs or placed any value on a respectful partnership with Alex. Alex's health is compromised as they have decided to leave the institution.

1. What policy changes could be implemented to make Alex feel safe when accessing health care?
2. What behaviours could the nurse have implemented to ensure a safe experience for Alex?
3. What institutional changes can be made to support Alex and other non-binary people?

Cultural safety is often poorly understood in clinical settings. It can sometimes be aligned with physical safety or there can be a tick box mentality where some health professionals feel it is something that they can get "signed off" with no further development or self-reflection. Some health professionals who have undergone basic cultural competency training will not continue to develop their understanding of cultural safety and begin their personal journey towards cultural safety development.

There is evidence that cultural safety or cultural care is not valued or prioritised by some health care professionals (Brown et al., 2016; Wilson et al., 2015). Attitudes of disregard of culture and cultural safety prevail, and the forcing of their own individualised cultural beliefs upon the people they care for follows. This can result in *institutional discrimination* whereby the organisational policies act to devalue, ignore and impose the dominant culture's worldview. We will explore institutional discrimination in more detail later in this chapter.

Consider the needs of an asylum-seeking person who has very different needs from a White middle-class person seeking health care. Health systems and structures must adapt to meet these needs and must be supported by inclusive policies. Frequently people entering into the health care system when seeking asylum experience misunderstanding and receive care that does not recognise the trauma that they have experienced.

Trauma that can be associated with Australian policies include fear of uncertainty about one's future, years of detention, bridging visa that may restrict a person's ability to work and access legal assistance with the visa application, only then to be granted a three-year temporary visa (Procter et al., 2018). Between 2014 and 2016 there were 11 asylum seeker suicides. One man, Amini, left a suicide note:

> A statement [written] with my blood for those who call themselves human beings, I ask that you stand up for the rights of refugees and stop people being killed just because they have become refugees. Humanity is not a slogan; every human being has a right to live. Living shouldn't be a crime anymore.
>
> (Procter et al., 2018)

Box 5.6 Reflection—Australian policies regarding people seeking asylum

- Review the Universal Declaration of Human Rights (UDHR), and identify how many articles within the declaration are in breach by the policies Australia has in place in regards to people seeking asylum.
- Consider how years in detention and an uncertain future may impact on your mental health.
- Consider a child born into detention and knowing no other life—what are the potential ramifications for that person's health?

Review the latest media coverage regarding Australian policy and people seeking asylum, think of the barriers to basic health care these people may face physically, mentally and culturally.

Medical professionals have taken a stance on detention and human rights with vocal advocacy groups working to support removing people from detention. The #doctorsforasylumseekers campaign saw medical professionals and some of the country's peak medical bodies work together to campaign for the removal of children from detention in Nauru. The Royal Australasian College of Physicians (RACP) developed social media kits to assist medical officers to advocate for the children of Nauru.

Policies, enablers and limitations towards culturally safe care

Person-centred care allows a person's individuality and unique needs to be determined by health care providers as it places them at the centre of their own care (Eklund et al., 2018). Person-centred approaches to health care provision are supported by many Australian organisations and in policies, reports and initiatives including the Australian Charter of Health care rights, Australian Safety and Quality Framework for Health Care and the National Safety and Quality Health Service Standards (Australian Commission on Safety and Quality in Health Care, 2011. A person-centred approach to care provision can offer a way to provide care that may be experienced as culturally safe in health care.

If we consider the features of cultural safety (Table 5.2), it is clear that institutions must design health policy that aims to educate, evaluate and ensure that people from culturally and linguistically diverse (CALD) backgrounds are consulted meaningfully to develop policies that reflect their different worldviews. Cultural safety must also be valued as critical to care provision and culturally unsafe practices seen as reportable breeches to patient safety.

Institutional discrimination

Institutional discrimination is deeply embedded within institutional norms. It takes the form of racial, cultural and social discrimination based on a person's race, culture, choices, lifestyle, age or religion. Health care settings and our society normalise this form of discrimination to the point that it is being generally unnoticed with the effects from the top of the institutional hierarchy flowing down to manifest and engrain itself throughout the entire setting (Brennan, 2016). Institutional discrimination includes the control of information, materials and resources that disadvantage a sector of the population and advantage another; examples of these include access to quality health care, housing and education (Jones, 2000; Paradies, 2005). It is evident in the differential access to goods and services that members of the disadvantaged sector receive (Jones, 2000).

Within policy, discrimination can operate under several guises including, but not limited to, anti-racism policy, the "colour-blind" and monoculturalistic ideology. A monoculturalistic ideology occurs when only one culture is considered. In the Australian health system that is the dominant White culture. Often this view adopts an "everyone is the same" mantra, for example, when considering race, the differences that come with race are ignored, White is "normal" and anything that does not fit within this monoculturalistic view is "other". Colour-blind ideology is framed in meritocracy and equality (Flintoff 2018), where systems aim to treat all people the same and are framed within dominant cultural view. Consider why traditional Chinese medicine is classified as "alternative" within the biomedical model of health and the impact this broad umbrella term can have on the perception of these medicines and medical practices from both the health professional, patient and wider community's point of view. Failure to embed "difference" in policy can be related to ignorance or the magnitude of trying to capture the needs of a multi-cultural population becomes too overwhelming, and it is easier to provide a generic service that caters to the majority. Services operating under these generic "White default" policies become void of the difference and diversity within Australian society.

Institutional racism is often experienced by Aboriginal and/or Torres Strait Islander peoples in many institutions including health (Paradies, 2018). Anti-racism policy is initially viewed as inclusive in an effort to reduce racism, although it can result in paternalistic and disempowering actions undertaken by the health provider towards the patient (Paradies, 2005), actions that thereby manifest themselves as racist, stripping the minority of their voice and autonomy. When you consider racism and health policy, think about who was included in the development of the policy. Were the people whom the policy impacts on the people who developed the policy, or were they consulted in the development and to what extent were they consulted? Reflect on where you stand ethically writing or enforcing a policy for someone with a cultural background different to yours, particularly if you have minimal knowledge of these people, their beliefs and their practices. Consider further your knowledge or lack thereof of who was involved in the development of the policies. Box 5.7 contains an example of the misapplication of policy undertaken from a Western perspective that was thought to be culturally safe—work through the scenario and questions.

Institutions that have policy that is intended for all end users as one collective group have policies that can be labelled as "colour blind", and they are good examples of institutional racism. Colour-blindness is often used by health professionals in supporting an "equality" stance and used to deny that colour is noticed at all. This discourse disempowers people of colour and their experiences of race and racism. Colour-blind policies are disadvantageous to the non-dominant

Box 5.7 Reflection—Cultural safety and policy

Several years ago, whilst working in a tertiary hospital in the city, it was a standard hospital policy to refer all Aboriginal patients to the Aboriginal Liaison Officer (ALO), as the ALO had requested that all Aboriginal peoples were made aware of their role and given the option to access this service. The ALO was not involved in the development of the policy and the resulting policy became:

All ATSI [sic] people must be referred to the ALO.

The result this had on the ward was quite profound. Any issue or concern that the patient had, be it cultural or personal, was "fixed" by contacting the singular ALO, who at times attended people who were not aware a referral had been made and did not wish to access the service. So, whilst the ALO was inundated with an array of problems, the majority of the nurses believed that they had emulated cultural safety principles in their practice by passing on "Aboriginal problems" to "Aboriginal People" whilst they focused on physical care.

- What do you think about this?
- How might this be different when thinking about the principles of cultural safety?
- What responsibility do the health care providers have in relation to cultural safety?
- Can the responsibility be "handed over" to an Aboriginal person to manage?

cultural groups; they enforce poor attitudes and maintain covert racism through a monoculturalistic viewpoint (Jones, 2000). This monoculturalistic view has the ability to affect the level of care given by health professionals. Health professionals will tend to blame the patient for personal shortcomings such as "non-compliance" or "poor lifestyle choices" as opposed to the structural barriers faced by people from minority groups. This belief is generally accompanied by the view that racial discrimination was in the past and no longer occurs (Malat et al., 2010). Monoculturalistic and "colour-blind" majority decision making in health generally derives itself from a dominant Western set of values that verifies the Western views as the default "norm" that everything relating to the policy is then measured against (Came, 2014). Consider the following reflection activity (Box 5.8) on institutional racism. After reading the story try to identify how this relates to institutional racism and how this could have been managed or, even better, avoided altogether.

At this point you may begin to see the connections between the world of Western medicine, the monoculturalistic view, colour-blind ideology, victim blaming and the impact that it can have on culturally diverse people. Are you capable of reviewing your own specific standards and policies and identifying the wording and structures within them that may not be wholly inclusive of all cultures? How can we then redress institutional racism in policy? It is important to remember

Box 5.8 Reflection—Institutional racism

As a registered nurse working in the country I had the privilege of working in health alongside many people whom I knew as I was growing up. At the hospital I was working I was one of two Aboriginal staff at the entire facility. As an Aboriginal nurse I was very often allocated to care for patients whom were Aboriginal. I was allocated to care for a man who was a close friend of my father and was my cultural uncle. He had a wound on his pelvis that required dressing. Given the location of the dressing and the relationship I had with this man I requested the enrolled nurse I was working with to do the dressing as this was culturally inappropriate for me to do so. I was promptly reported to the senior nurse for not attending to my allocated workload and being "lazy", as this was not the first time this had happened while she was working with me. Following this report I was required to speak with my supervisor about the expectations of myself as an employee of the hospital having to "just get on with it, because this is your job now". The hospital was clear in its expectations of me but offered no flexibility where cultural differences were concerned, nor was the senior nurse culturally competent or reflective enough to understand these differences. As a result of this incident I felt ostracised from my co-workers, hurt and frequently questioned my choice in career. The next time a similar incident occurred, in a desperate attempt to try to "fit in", "do my job", "keep my job" and be accepted by peers I went against my cultural norms, and the result was a long-lasting fractured relationship with that patient and guilt that I did something that I knew was not acceptable—an incident that has haunted me ever since.

- How can you create a culturally safe workplace for both patients and colleagues?
- Are you, as a health professional, being culturally safe by assigning an Aboriginal staff member to care of an Aboriginal patient or are you simply avoiding your own cultural safety accountability?

Reflect on how policy can be culturally unsafe in its manoeuvrability from Western ideals. In some Aboriginal Community Controlled Health Organisations (ACCHOs), the facilities are divided in half with one side being for men's health and the other side women's health. Discuss how different care is in a tertiary hospital facility.

that not all Aboriginal and/or Torres Strait Islander people in Australia are from one large homogenous group, not all people who practice religion practice the same religion, not all people who do not look like you are the same. In order to redress institutional racism within health care policy, we must focus on the multi-layered standpoint of institutionalised, internalised and personally mediated racism (Jones, 2000). Consider your registration standards, codes of conduct and future workplace. Do they have an emphasis on cultural safety, cultural diversity or racism? As a health care professional learning about institutional racism in policy, consider the statement by Jones (2000, p. 1212) that "institutionalised racism is often evident as inaction in the face of need".

The role of health professionals in health advocacy

Health professionals have a responsibility to identify where policy may impede on a person's rights. Being able to critically appraise policy enables health professionals to advocate for systemic changes and to ensure marginalised people's unique health needs are reflected in organisational policies.

There are two important goals to consider when thinking about *health advocacy*: protection of the vulnerable and empowerment of the disadvantaged (Carlisle, 2011). These are referred to as representational advocacy that supports protection of the vulnerable and facilitational advocacy that supports empowerment of the disadvantaged (Carlisle, 2011). Scholars have argued that despite the measures put in place to reduce health inequality, advocacy is required to engage public support for health policy that will address the inequality (Garthwaite et al., 2016).

We define health advocacy as providing care to health care consumers that includes the promotion of health and access to services. This involves some levels of activism to ensure that access to services is fair and equitable. It is not simply around individual advocacy, but health care professionals have a larger role in public health advocacy and to ensure the voices of the marginalised are embedded in our institutions. For example, consider if a registered nurse found a policy of placing all women in the same ward yet was caring for a patient who did not identify as female. What levels of advocacy could the nurse take? He or she could first attempt to find an acceptable solution for the patient. This may be to locate a single room or consider offering to place the patient in the male ward. The nurse could then advocate for changes within the system and for changes to the policy that would avoid placing the patient in the situation in the first place. The nurse could take this further and advocate at a higher level again, outside of the institution, for changes to the health system as a whole. Advocacy can be achieved through many levels and can operate away from individual patients/clients to the entire health system and the development of inclusive policies.

Health professionals from the dominant culture may have to look harder to find discrimination in health policy when it comes to the inclusion of cultural diversity. It is often hidden from the dominant culture. If we take a step back and examine our practice, one way to discover if policy is negatively impacting on our clients/patients is to start a dialogue with them. We should ask them what they need and if they feel safe receiving care. For health professionals involved in writing policy it would be beneficial to ensure that members of the non-dominant culture are included in the development of policy.

The Medical Board of Australia's Code of Conduct (2017) acknowledges the role that doctors should play in health advocacy. Specifically, it acknowledges the health inequities present in different groups that occurs because of social, cultural and geographical factors (Medical Board of Australia, 2017). The code acknowledges the influence doctors have in society and encourages them to use this to further the health and wellbeing of patients and their communities (Medical Board of Australia, 2017). Now consider what you have learnt about institutional discrimination. Health care professionals must avoid seeing advocacy as speaking on behalf of people but actively creating spaces for their voices, opinions, wants and needs to be embedded in health policy. Now take a look at the standards, guidelines and policies that guide your profession and see what you can find around health advocacy.

Scenario 1

An Aboriginal woman and a small baby age 3 months old arrived at a small-country hospital one evening. The baby required treatment for a bronchial chest infection so was brought into hospital by the cultural mother, which resulted in a Royal Flying Doctor Service (RFDS) transfer to a tertiary hospital located within the nearest city. On arrival to the hospital, the cultural mother was questioned about the location of "the real mother", as staff noted contrasting skin colours between the baby and the cultural mother. The cultural mother explained that the baby was in her care, who in their culture is considered the equivalent of another mother, they were in a regional town for a family event over 1000 km from their home community.

Upon further questioning from the doctors, the cultural mother with the baby advised that she was there in place of the child's birth mother, who was currently at home caring for other children. The cultural mother was in contact with the birth mother and was concerned about the questioning and the attitudes towards her, which prompted the birth mother to write a letter. The letter was faxed from her local clinic on letterhead paper advising that this woman is the cultural mother and has full permission to give consent for the child. The cultural mother did not leave the child for the entire duration of the hospital stay. The doctor proceeded to submit a notification to the department of child protection as he was concerned about the birth mother being absent for the duration of the hospital stay. The baby was not under welfare up until this notification. Both the cultural mother and the birth mother were very distressed that the doctor was not interested in understanding their kin family dynamics and was quite open with his dissatisfaction about the birth mother not being with the child.

The letter written by the mother that she faxed from the clinic on their letterhead was not a legal document according to the Western law and policy, nor were the family dynamics of this family and their culture an "appropriate fit" into a Western ideal of what constitutes a family dynamic, nor was it acceptable by the doctor's ideals of "a family". The result was the notification to the department of child protection and subsequent involvement from a district of Families SA (South Australian child welfare), which became an ongoing involvement in the family's life for the next several years.

One-third of children in out-of-home care in South Australia are Aboriginal, and Aboriginal children are 10 times more likely to have involvement with child protection than non-Aboriginal children (Child Protection Systems Royal Commission, 2016).

Questions:

- When reviewing this scenario, consider Aboriginal peoples' family structures and how they fit within the strict policies and views of the Western medical systems.
- Who is suitable to provide consent?
- Who is considered family?
- How do you believe occurrences such as these can result in poor health outcomes for Aboriginal people?
- Do you think that the over-representation of Aboriginal children in state care may, in part, be contributed to by a lack of cultural understanding?
- Discuss how both health professionals and the health care system may create a standard of "norms" that can be damaging and culturally unsafe to people with differing societal and cultural views.

Scenario 2

A 28-year-old woman born in Afghanistan sought asylum in Australia two years ago. The woman and her husband have recently discovered that they are expecting their second child. Their first baby was born in Afghanistan. The family live in outer Melbourne in rented accommodation. The woman is a stay-at-home mum, and the man works in construction. He is developing his English skills, but they are basic. The woman has limited English, as she mainly associates with the Afghanistan community. Her primary language is Farsi. The family are Muslim and worship at their local mosque.

The woman attends a local public hospital for her antenatal care, although she doesn't understand much of what is happening in her pregnancy. She tells the staff that she does not want a male doctor via a translator. When it comes to the time of the birth the woman's sister-in-law is supporting her. The birth ends in an emergency caesarean. She felt confused about what happened in the birth, and the emergency caesarean happened so quickly that she did not understand what happened or give her informed consent. After the birth she asks the postnatal staff if her sister-in-law could stay and support her as she is feeling scared and her sister-in-law speaks English. They tell her they will not allow her to stay as they have a policy against relatives staying overnight at the hospital.

Questions:

- Consider the barriers she has experienced because of her culture—what are they?
- Would a White woman experience the same barriers? If no, why not?
- How does hospital policy influence this situation?
- How could you address these barriers considering what you have learnt about health advocacy? (Try to consider health advocacy at an individual level for the woman and at the policy level for other woman like her)

> **Box 5.9 Reflection—Cultural safety in future practice**
>
> We have discussed cultural diversity within this chapter, what does that mean for you now?
>
> How will understanding this impact on your future practice as a health professional?

Conclusion

In this chapter we have explored some of the government policies, health regulator policy, and the health care systems themselves to consider the inclusion of cultural diversity. We reviewed the social determinants of health and how these impact on policymakers and the difficulty of meeting the cultural needs of a person accessing care through a Western biomedical, monoculturalistic model of care. The models of care and institutional racism were explored. We hope that going forward as health professionals that you consider the institutional policies through a new lens and look for evidence of cultural diversity, cultural difference and the lack of a monoculturalistic view of health. We have left you with some case studies that have come from our years of practicing within health, and we encourage you to critically appraise these scenarios and your clinical encounters. Appraising policy with cultural safety at the forefront will assist you to identify areas of systemic racism embedded within the multifaceted levels of policy that govern us. In being able to identify the barriers in policies, you, as a health professional, are able to advocate for change for a more culturally inclusive health force, real consultation in policy development and the ability to challenge monoculturalistic views on health care.

References

Al Abed, N. A., Davidson, P. M., & Hickman, L. D. (2014). Healthcare needs of older Arab migrants: A systematic review. *Journal of Clinical Nursing, 23*(13–14), 1770–1784. https://doi.org/10.1111/jocn.12476.

Australian Commission on Safety and Quality in Health Care. (2011). *Patient centred care: Improving quality and safety through partnerships with patients and consumers.* https://www.safetyandquality.gov.au/sites/default/files/migrated/PCC_Paper_August.pdf.

Australian Health Practitioner Regulation Agency (Ahpra). (2015). *Role.* https://www.nursingmidwiferyboard.gov.au/About.aspx.

Australian Health Practitioner Regulation Agency (Ahpra). (2017a). *Who are we.* https://www.ahpra.gov.au/About-AHPRA/Who-We-Are.aspx.

Australian Health Practitioner Regulation Agency (Ahpra). (2017b). *National Boards.* https://www.ahpra.gov.au/National-Boards.aspx.

Australian Health Practitioner Regulation Agency (Ahpra). (2018). *What we do.* https://www.ahpra.gov.au/About-AHPRA/What-We-Do.aspx.

Australian Health Practitioner Regulation Agency (Ahpra). (2019). *Consultations*. www.ahpra.gov.au/news/consultations.

Australian Institute of Health and Welfare. (2018). *Deaths in Australia* https://www.aihw.gov.au/reports/life-expectancy-death/deaths-in-australia/contents/summary.

Bartone, A. (2019). *Closing the gap report not good news*. Australian Medical Association. https://ama.com.au/ausmed/closing-gap-report-not-good-news.

Biddle N., Khoo S. E., & Taylor J. (2015). Indigenous Australia, white Australia, multicultural Australia: The demography of race and ethnicity in Australia. In R. Sáenz, D. Embrick, N. Rodríguez (Eds.), *The international handbook of the demography of race and ethnicity*. Springer.

Brennan, F. (2016). *Race rights reparations: Institutional racism and the law*. Routledge.

Brown, A. (2016). *Midwives and Aboriginal and Torres Strait Islander women's experiences with cultural care in the birth suite: An interpretative phenomenological investigation* [University of South Australia].

Brown, A., Middleton, P., Fereday, J., & Pincombe, J. (2016). Cultural safety and midwifery care for Aboriginal women: A phenomenological study. *Women and Birth, 29*(2), 196–202. https://doi.org/10.1016/j.wombi.2015.10.013.

Came, H. (2014). Sites of institutional racism in public health policy making in New Zealand. *Social Science and Medicine, 106*, 214–220.

Carlisle, S. (2011). Health promotion, advocacy and health inequalities: A conceptual framework. *Health Promotion International, 15*(4), 369–376.

Child Protection Systems Royal Commission. (2016). *The life they deserve: Child protection systems royal commission report, volume 1: Summary and report*. Government of South Australia. https://www.agd.sa.gov.au/sites/default/files/preface_summary_and_recommendations.pdf?acsf_files_redirect.

Coroner's Court of Western Australia. (2016). *Inquest into the death of Ms DHU*. https://www.coronerscourt.wa.gov.au/I/inquest_into_the_death_of_ms_dhu.aspx?uid=1644-2151-2753-9965.

Department of the Prime Minister and Cabinet. (2018). *Closing the gap Prime Minister's report 2018*. https://www.pmc.gov.au/sites/default/files/reports/closing-the-gap-2018/sites/default/files/ctg-report-20183872.pdf?a=1.

Eklund, J. H., Holmström, I. K., Kumlin, T., Kaminsky, E., Skoglund, K., Höglander, J., Sundler, A. J., Conden, E., & Meranius, M. S. (2018). "Same same or different?" A review of reviews of person-centered and patient-centered care. *Patient education and Counselling, 102*(1), 3–11. https://doi.org/10.1016/j.pec.2018.08.029.

Fazeli Dehkordy, S., Hall, K. S., Dalton, V. K., & Carlos, R. C. (2016). The link between everyday discrimination, healthcare utilization, and health status among a national sample of women. *Journal of Women's Health, 25*(10), 1044–1051. https://doi.org/10.1089/jwh.2015.5522.

Fisher, M., Baum, F., Macdougall, C., Newman, L., & Mcdermott, D. (2016). To what extent do Australian health policy documents address social determinants of health and health equity. *Journal of Social Policy, 45*(3), 545–564. https://doi.org/10.1017/S0047279415000756.

Fleming, T., Creedy, D., & West, R. (2018). Cultural Safety continuing professional development for midwifery academics: An integrative literature review. *Women and Birth, 32*(4), 318–326. https://doi.org/10.1016/j.wombi.2018.10.001.

Flintoff, A. (2018). Diversity, inclusion and anti racism in health and physical education: What can a critical whiteness perspective offer? *Curriculum Studies in Health and Physical Education, 9*(3), 207–219. https://doi.org/10.1080/25742981.2018.1488374.

Garthwaite, K., Smith, K., Bambra, C., & Pearce, J. (2016). Desperately seeking reductions in health inequalities: Perspectives of UK researchers on past, present and future directions in health inequalities research. *Sociology of Health and Illness, 38*(3), 459–478. https://doi.org/10.1111/1467-9566.12374.

Gee, G., Dudgeon, P., Schultz, C., Hart, A., & Kelly, K. (2014). Aboriginal and Torres Strait Islander social and emotional wellbeing. In P. Dudgeon, H. Milroy, & R. Walker (Eds.), *Working together: Aboriginal and Torres Strait Islander mental health and wellbeing principles and practice* (2nd ed., pp. 55–68). Department of The Prime Minister and Cabinet. https://www.telethonkids.org.au/globalassets/media/documents/aboriginal-health/working-together-second-edition/working-together-aboriginal-and-wellbeing-2014.pdf.

Holland, C. (2018). *Close the gap: 10 year review 2018*. Australian Human Rights Commission. https://humanrights.gov.au/our-work/aboriginal-and-torres-strait-islander-social-justice/publications/close-gap-10-year-review?_ga=2.21025403.1733906288.1597784161-41442067.1597784161.

Jones, C. (2000). Levels of racism: A theoretic framework and a gardener's tale. *American Journal of Public Health, 90*(8), 1212–1215. https://doi.org/10.2105%2Fajph.90.8.1212.

Laverty, M., McDermott, D., & Calma, T. (2017). Embedding cultural safety in Australia's main health care standards. *Medical Journal of Australia, 207*(1), 15–16. https://doi.org/10.5694/mja17.00328.

Malat, J., Clark-Hitt, R., Burgess, D., Friedemann-Sanchez, G., & Van Ryn, M. (2010). White doctors and nurses on racial inequality in health care in the USA: Whiteness and colour-blind racial ideology. *Ethnic and Racial Studies, 33*(8), 1431–1450. https://doi.org/10.1080/01419870903501970.

Marmot, M., Friel, S., Bell, R., Houweling, T., & Taylor, S. (2008). Closing the gap in a generation: Health equity through action on the social determinants of health. *The Lancet, 372*(9650), 1661–1669. https://doi.org/10.1016/S0140-6736(08)61690-6.

McDermott, D. (2012). Can we educate out of racism? *Medical Journal of Australia, 197*(1), 15. https://doi.org/10.5694/mja12.10936.

Medical Board of Australia. (2017). *Good medical practice: A code of conduct for doctors in Australia.* https://www.medicalboard.gov.au/documents/default.aspx?record=WD10%2F1277&dbid=AP&chksum=eNjZ0Z%2FajN7oxjvHXDRQnQ%3D%3D

NSW Government. (2014). *NSW state health plan towards 2021.* https://www.health.nsw.gov.au/statehealthplan/Documents/brochure-NSW-SHPT-2021.pdf.

Nursing Council of New Zealand. (2011). *Guidelines for cultural safety, and the Treaty of Waitangi and Maori health in nursing education and practice.* http://pro.healthmentoronline.com/assets/Uploads/refract/pdf/Nursing_Council_cultural-safety11.pdf.

Paradies, Y. (2005). Anti-racism and Indigenous Australians. *Analyses of Social Issues and Public Policy, 5*(1), 1–28. https://doi.org/10.1111/j.1530-2415.2005.00053.x.

Paradies, Y. (2018). Racism and Indigenous health. *Oxford research encyclopedia global public health* https://doi.org/10.1093/acrefore/9780190632366.013.86.

Procter, N. G., Kenny, M. A., Eaton, H., & Grech, C. (2018). Lethal hopelessness: Understanding and responding to asylum seeker distress and mental deterioration. *International Journal of Mental Health Nursing, 27*(1), 448–454. https://doi.org/10.1111/inm.12325.

Rassool, G. H. (2015). Cultural competence in counselling the Muslim patient: Implications for mental health. *Archives of Psychiatric Nursing, 29*(5), 321–325. https://doi.org/10.1016/j.apnu.2015.05.009.

SA Health Policy Committee. (2017). *Guideline complementary and alternative medicines.* https://www.sahealth.sa.gov.au/wps/wcm/connect/a5da9c0042d5e889910af78cd21c605e/Guideline_Complementary+and+Alternative+Medicines_v1.0_27092017.pdf.

United Nations. (2007). *United Nations declaration on the rights of Indigenous peoples.* https://www.un.org/development/desa/indigenouspeoples/wp-content/uploads/sites/19/2018/11/UNDRIP_E_web.pdf.

United Nations. (2019). *Department of economic and social affairs: Indigenous peoples.* https://www.un.org/development/desa/indigenouspeoples/news/2019/00/.

Vedio, A., Liu, E. Z. H., Lee, A. C., & Salway, S. (2017). Improving access to health care for chronic hepatitis B among migrant Chinese populations: A systematic mixed methods review of barriers and enablers. *Journal of Viral Hepatitis, 24*(7), 526–540. https://doi.org/10.1111%2Fjvh.12673.

Wilson, A. M., Magarey, A. M., Jones, M., O'Donnell, K., & Kelly, J. (2015). Attitudes and characteristics of health professionals working in Aboriginal health. *Rural and Remote Health, 15*(1), 1–15. https://doi.org/10.22605/RRH2739.

World Health Organisation. (2019). *Social determinants of health.* https://www.who.int/health-topics/social-determinants-of-health#tab=tab_1.

Diversity Australia. n.d. https://www.diversityaustralia.com.au/.

The Australian Health Practitioner Registration Agency: n.d. https://www.ahpra.gov.au/.

The Australian. n.d. https://www.catsinam.org.au/.

The Congress of Aboriginal and Torres Strait Islander Nurses and Midwives. n.d. https://www.catsinam.org.au/.

The World Health Organisation. n.d. https://www.who.int

6 Culturally safe health care practice

Kim McLeod, Robyn Williams and Tinashe Dune

Learning outcomes

After working through this chapter, students should be able to:

1. Explain how the principles of cultural safety can inform health care practice.
2. Identify key elements of effective strategies for embedding cultural safety in individual practices, organisational policy and health care systems.
3. Engage with strengths-based approaches to promote cultural safety in practice.
4. Foster working partnerships with culturally diverse health professionals, organisations and community members.
5. Develop a personal action plan for enacting cultural safety in professional health practice.

Key terms

Bias: Refers to "generally negative feelings and evaluations of individuals because of their group membership (prejudice), overgeneralised beliefs about the characteristics of group members (stereotypes) and inequitable treatment (discrimination)" (van Ryn et al., 2011, p. 201).
Client-centred care: Health care where a person's cultural values, needs and preferences are placed at the forefront of their ongoing medical care.
Collaboration: Working together to achieve greater impacts than can occur in isolation.
Cultural safety: An environment that is spiritually, socially and emotionally safe, as well as physically safe for people; where there is no assault challenge or denial of their identity, of who they are and what they need.
Intersectionality: The interconnected nature of social categorisations such as race, class, and gender as they apply to a given individual or group, regarded as creating overlapping and interdependent systems of discrimination or disadvantage.
Partnership: Two or more individuals or groups or coming together to achieve a common purpose.
Racism: Any cognition, affective state, or behaviour that advances the differential treatment of individuals or groups due to their racial, ethnic, cultural or religious background.
Self-awareness: The capacity to become the object of one's own attention. In this state one actively identifies, processes, and stores information about the self.
Self-reflection: A genuine curiosity about the self, where the person is intrigued and interested in learning more about his or her emotions, values, thought processes and attitudes.
Social construct: A perception of an individual, group, or idea that is "constructed" through cultural or social practice.

Social determinants of health: Conditions in which people are born, grow, work, live, and age, and the wider set of forces and systems shaping the conditions of daily life. These forces and systems include economic policies and systems, development agendas, social norms, social policies and political systems.
Social justice: Social justice is a concept of fair and just relations between the individual and society, as measured by the distribution of wealth, opportunities for personal activity and social privileges.
Stereotypes: An expectation that all people within the same racial, ethnic or cultural group act alike and share the same beliefs and attitudes.

Chapter summary

In this chapter students begin to link their previous understandings to practical outcomes and goals. The chapter highlights how an ongoing, lifelong process of self-reflection and critical thinking enables the principles of cultural safety (as described in Chapters 4 and 5) to be translated into health care practice. Students will be given the opportunity to explore what it means to embed the principles of cultural safety in individual health care practice, organisational policy and processes and health care systems. This chapter will therefore include practical and applied approaches to working with diverse populations that highlight the importance of client-centred and flexible approaches. Students will explore the relevance and place of partnerships and advocacy in their health profession and careers. Case studies will provide students with opportunities to assess cultural safety in themselves, health care environments and systems. Students will also engage with multimedia in order to enhance their understandings of the process of acquiring and developing cultural safety as a lifelong journey and undertake activities to assist them in identifying the areas where they require further work.

Introduction

A culturally safe health care environment is one where "people feel safe and secure in their identity" (Williams, 1999, p. 213) and "no action is taken which diminishes, demeans or disempowers the cultural identity and well-being of an individual" (Nursing Council of New Zealand, 2011, p. 7). This chapter addresses what kind of *practice* on the part of health professionals enables culturally safe health care. For health professionals, it means enacting health care that is: regardful of and responsive to a client's background, personal circumstance and cultural needs; holistic, free of *bias* and *racism*, and determined as culturally safe by the recipient (Paradies et al., 2015; Ramsden, 2002). At this point, students often ask, how can I meet the expectation of providing health care in a way that people from a range of diverse backgrounds define as useful? How will I actually go about this? How will I ensure culturally safe practice as well as meet all the other expectations of my health practitioner role?

Box 6.1 Reflection—Cultural safety in your professional practice

What are the feelings that arise when you consider culturally safety as an integral part of your health profession role?
What questions do you have about being culturally safe in *practice*?

It is useful to revisit why culturally safe health practice is an important dimension of health professionals' work. A compelling body of research (see, for example, Pallok, De Maio, & Ansell, 2019) points to the harm that happens within the health system as a result of biased and discriminatory care. The good news is that health professionals can be change agents, both in their individual practice, and as advocates for change in health organisations and systems. It is widely recognised that culturally safe practice reduces inequalities within health care interactions and across health systems and contributes to improved health outcomes for all Australians (Australian Government, 2013). The importance of creating culturally safe health environments is acknowledged in various health profession codes of conduct and in Australian, state and organisational policies.

Box 6.2 Reflection—What does your health profession's code of conduct say about cultural safety?

Find out if there is a Code of Conduct for your health profession. If there isn't one, then have a look at the NMBA Code of Conduct for Nursing and Midwifery.

- What does it say about cultural safety, or about working with diverse clients?
- Make a note of the key elements. Does the Code of Conduct identify any principles or strategies for practice?
- What do you think your health profession expects in relation to cultural safety?
- What questions do you have about culturally safe health practice after reading the Code of Conduct?

Students often have many questions about *how to?* as they contemplate working towards becoming a culturally safe heath practitioner. They also commonly report a range of feelings about the challenges of translating ideas about *cultural safety* into practice. This chapter is designed to facilitate students' learning in relation to culturally safe health care practice in practical and applied settings. The following four sections of the chapter explore how the key principles of cultural safety can be translated into culturally safe practice, by:

- Addressing the impact of health professionals' own cultural realities, values, attitudes and behaviours on others.
- Recognising the importance of health care that is driven by individual clients, their families and communities.
- Acknowledging the factors that impact individual and community health.
- Providing care that is regard*ful* of culture.

Throughout this chapter, students will be invited to undertake the self-reflection and critical thinking that underpins these broad domains of culturally safe health practice. Students will locate themselves in their own learning journey and identify what they need to progress further in the lifelong process of becoming a culturally safe heath professional. This is consolidated at the end of the chapter, where students review their learning across the chapter and outline a personal action plan for enacting cultural safety in professional health practice.

Culturally safe practice addresses the impact of health professionals' cultural realities, attitudes and behaviours on others

This section explores how to embed the cultural safety principle of consistent, ongoing self-awareness and self-reflection into culturally safe practice that addresses the impact of health professionals' cultural realities, attitudes and behaviours on others. The focus of this section is on growing skills in the *self-awareness*, *self-reflection*, and critical thinking that underpin this key aspect of cultural safety. You, as in the student, might be asking, why is this necessary? This is because a person's cultural values, attitudes and beliefs shape how they interact with others (Downing, Kowal, & Paradies, 2011). A significant body of evidence indicates how health professionals' behaviour acts as a barrier to service access and contributes to disparities in health care, via to the application of *stereotypes* and differential treatment based on aspects of a client's identity (Burgess et al., 2007; van Ryn et al., 2011). It is therefore important that health professionals identify the implications of their own behaviour and the behaviour of colleagues that may place people at cultural risk by examining their own cultural realities, attitudes and behaviours and the impact they may have on others (Ramsden, 1993). The focus is not on understanding the cultural differences of others; rather, it centres on unpacking the practitioner's cultural underpinnings. In other words, to become a health professional who can consider and articulate, "What do I bring to this encounter, what is going on for me?" (Laverty, McDermott, & Calma 2017, p. 15).

This section of the chapter goes on to detail a process to support students in developing an awareness about their own identity, qualities, cultures, and groups, and how this may impact the care provided to others who differ in any way from themselves. The first step involves growing students' awareness of their own intersectional identity. As established in Chapter 1, *intersectionality* refers to the interconnected nature of social categorisations such as race, class and gender as they apply to a given individual or group, regarded as creating overlapping and interdependent systems of discrimination or disadvantage. An important dimension of this step is acknowledging privilege. Privilege is defined as those conditions and circumstances enjoyed by a person because they belong to, or have the characteristics of, the majority group in a society at any given point in time. Privilege reflects the complex social structures that reproduce seemingly "natural" advantages that are conferred on people who fit within a particular, privileged identity. It is important for health professionals to explore the forms of privilege and discrimination associated with different aspects of their identity so they can engage in critical dialogue about the impact this has on their ability to practice professionally (Van Herk et al., 2011).

Box 6.3 Reflection—Of course I am privileged: The question actually is ... what should I do about it?

Here is an example of a health professional who develops self-awareness about her privilege and changes her health care practice:

https://croakey.org/of-course-i-am-privileged-the-question-actually-is-what-should-i-do-about-it/

The concept of *social construction* is a useful "tool" for thinking critically about how the different aspects of a person's identity are "socially constructed" through being responded to

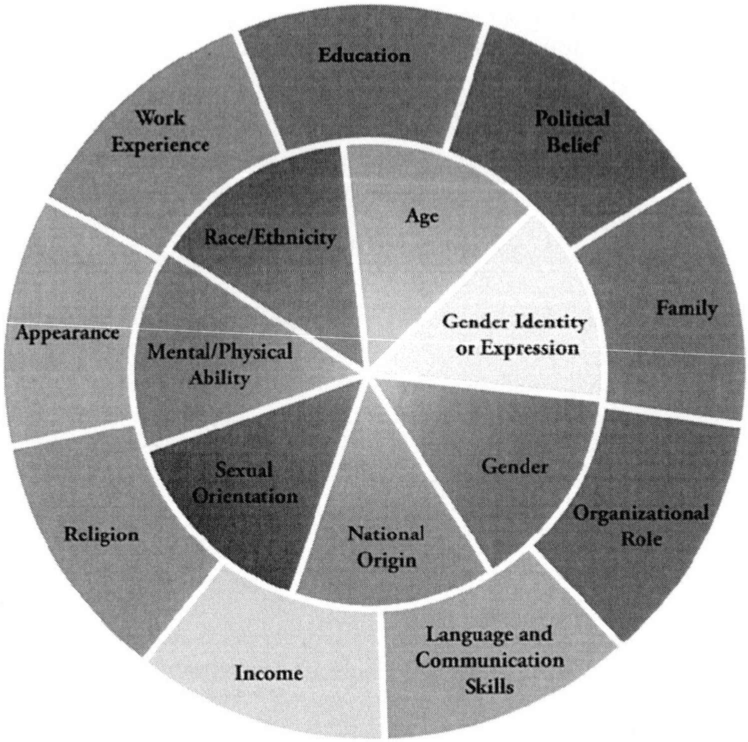

Figure 6.1 Diversity Wheel as used at Johns Hopkins University

in different ways by society. If a health professional can look at this squarely and acknowledge the benefits they receive, they can acknowledge the wealth of things they do not know and get better at listening to the experiences of others (Figure 6.1).

Box 6.4 Reflection—Exploring intersectional identity

- Make a list of your cultural groups and identities.
- Which cultural groups and identities affect your everyday life the most?
- Which cultural groups and identities affect your everyday life the least?
- Are some of your cultural groups and identities associated with privilege? Or discrimination and disadvantage?
- How are your cultural groups and identities viewed by others?
- Are positive or negative stereotypes applied to your cultural groups and identities?
- How do all your cultural groups and identities interact to shape your health and wellbeing?

Insight into their intersectional identity can assist health professionals to identify the areas that are the same, and those that are different between themselves and others. It provides a basis from which to understand the self and the other are multidimensional entities and enables critical reflection about health professionals' own identities, how the identity relates to others, and how they relate to people from different locations. In addition, a person's attitudes, values and beliefs are shaped by their cultural groups and identities. Explore this connection by thinking about these questions:

- How might my various cultural groups and identities influence my decisions and perceptions of others?
- How are my notions of positive regard, family involvement and perceptions of important and effective communication differently defined based upon my past and present cultural groups and identities?

The second step involves students investigating their values, attitudes and beliefs. It is widely recognised that a person's attitudes, beliefs and values affect the assumptions and practices they bring to the care of clients (Best, 2018; Mead & Bower, 2000; Taylor et al., 2010; Taylor & Guerin, 2019). Health professionals hold unconscious beliefs about people from different (usually) minority populations. These beliefs affect their treatment decisions, which ultimately affects client health and population-level health outcomes (Blair, Steiner, & Havranek, 2011; Chapman, Kaatz, & Carnes, 2013; Sahin & Akyol, 2010). Denial or disregard of difference affects how clients experience the encounter with a health professional. If a client feels discriminatory or prejudicial views about their difference, they worry they will only receive compromised care, or might not feel empowered to defend themselves (Ramsden, 2002). So, it is important that health professionals examine and identify their own biases, assumptions, stereotypes and prejudices. Bias refers to "generally negative feelings and evaluations of individuals because of their group membership (prejudice), overgeneralised beliefs about the characteristics of group members (stereotypes) and inequitable treatment (discrimination)" (van Ryn et al., 2011, p. 201). Generally, our values, attitudes and beliefs are unstated or assumed; we don't think about them until they are challenged. Interpretation of values is not easy and requires reflection.

Box 6.5 Reflection—Investigating values, attitudes and beliefs

Consider the five questions posed by Best (2018, p. 51). Best asked the questions in relation to Aboriginal and Torres Strait Islander peoples. However, this is applicable for other cultural groups or sections of the population. Ask yourself the questions in relation a range of diverse populations. What do the differences between your answers help you to learn about your beliefs, values and attitudes?

- What are your own beliefs, values and attitudes about?
- Where did you gain them from?
- How were they formed?
- Have you ever questioned whether they are valid or true?
- What are some of the commonly held views about?
- How are these views formed?

Exploration of a health professional's attitudes, values and beliefs can help them to avoid making assumptions based on generalisations about any aspect of a person's identity (Cioffi, 2013; Thorne, 2018). This insight can discourage or at least challenge stereotyping and open opportunities to instead establish connectedness, empathy and rapport with clients. Bias can be mitigated by developing empathy for others perceived as dissimilar and by direct "contact" with members of other groups (Burgess et al., 2007). This self-awareness will assist health professionals to not impose their own values on clients and supports an open-minded and flexible attitude towards others (Cox, 2016).

The skills in self-awareness and self-reflection developed through the activity in Box 6.5 can be extended to notice and respond to how bias might be operating at the level of the health care organisations and systems.

Box 6.6 Reflection—Responding to bias in the health care environments

Access the website for: Edith Cowan University, Creating Cultural Empathy and Challenging Attitudes through Indigenous Narratives:
https://altc.betterhealth.ecu.edu.au/scenarios/index.php
Register to use the website.
Go to Scenarios, and view the "Drunken Stereotypes" scenario.

- How can stereotypes and racist assumptions lead to limited treatment or a lack of services?
- How can health professionals discourage bias in their health care environments?

Vukic et al. (2012) report how Aboriginal nurses experience personal discrimination from co-workers and clients. Health professionals can ask how people from a diverse range of backgrounds are represented in the workplace and advocate for a more diverse workforce (Newman, Javanparast, Baum, & Hutchinson, 2015). In addition, does the workplace support the kind of learning process outlined in this chapter, is there paid leave to gain training in cultural safety? Is there a way to create a conversation amongst peers about how health professionals address privilege and bias across the organisation? An important element of creating a culturally safe work environment is to ensure staff are involved in the conversation and transformation (Butler-Henderson, Kemp, McLeod, & Harris, 2018).

This section has focussed on the first step of culturally safe practice: knowing yourself—who you are and the impact of this on interactions with others. This self-awareness provides the basis from which to develop the relationships to build trust.

Culturally safe practice recognises the importance of health care that is driven by the individual, family and community

This section focuses on what it means to embed the cultural safety principles of: trust and respect; collaboration, partnership and power sharing; and shared dialogue into the practice of relating with clients. These principles underpin the basis of culturally safe practice, which recognises the importance of health care that is driven by the individual, family and community.

Trust and respect

Clients are more likely to participate in a trusting and respectful relationship with their health professional if they feel they can rely on their health professional with confidence (Dinç &

Gastmans, 2012) and have a degree of control over their own situation (Shahid & Thompson, 2009; Taylor & Guerin, 2019). Ramsden (2002) argues that if the health professional is seen as respectful of the client's differences and can provide care that is enabling of a person, they will be regarded as trustworthy. Ramsden (2002) stresses that establishing trust and respect makes an inclusive and participatory relationship between health professional and client possible. If trust and respect is not present, a client will feel they need to protect their identity and "a divide is created between provider and client which results in the client receiving poor care that is unresponsive to who they are as human beings" (Van Herk et al., 2011, p. 29).

Trust is shaped by context and experienced in different ways (Ramsden, 2002). It is therefore important to take into account how different populations have particular historical legacies relating to their engagement with the health system. In the Australian context, personal and collective traumatic experiences of care by Indigenous Australians in mainstream health care has eroded trust (Shahid & Thompson, 2009). Therefore, health professionals need to "become very skilled at interpretation of the level of distrust experienced by Indigenous people when interacting with a health service which has its roots in the colonial administration" (Ramsden, 2002, p. 3). As Ramsden (2002) identifies, establishing trust and respect is crucial to culturally safe practice, as the client is then free to articulate their identity and be an active participant in the health care encounter.

Shared dialogue

Listening is a vital part of creating a shared dialogue with clients. Health professionals can cultivate some habits of engagement with clients: listen to the reason the client is there; elicit the client's perspective—what do they think the problem is or what do they think the solution might be (Taylor & Guerin, 2019)? Health professionals need to display empathy and compassion in their willingness to understand the point of view and the feelings of the client. Such approaches may help people feel more able to contribute to the communication dialogue.

A key to a shared dialogue is, don't assume, ask! Ask how someone wants to be addressed and respect how they choose to identify without questioning, assuming or stereotyping (Taylor & Guerin, 2019). For example, trans and gender diverse people embody a wide array of identities and practices; asking instead of assuming can help build trust while allowing clients to disclose relevant information about their sexual lives and sexual and romantic partners in the language of their choosing (McNair et al., 2012; Newman, Prankumar, Cover, Rasmussen, Marshall, & Aggleton, 2020; Persson et al., 2020).

A shared dialogue needs to be able to involve and encompass multiple worldviews (Durie, 2005; McKivett, Paul, & Hudson, 2018). If health professionals work only from the biomedical model, they will miss client priorities (Cass et al., 2002). Health professionals can think about respecting *both* evidence-based medical teaching and other paradigms during a clinical interview with a client. For example, a clinical interview with an Indigenous client can interweave information-giving steps with appropriate questions that target core concepts of Indigenous life. If the clinical interview includes respectful engagement and knowledge sharing, innovation results through Indigenous and Western knowledges coming together (Durie, 2005). Health professionals can also be flexible about the style of communication they use to achieve a shared understanding with a client. A question-and-answer interview, for example, may not be compatible with Indigenous frameworks for knowing (Cass et al., 2002). The use of storytelling, metaphors and visual representations of health concepts are effective ways to facilitate communication between health professionals and clients (Laholt, Guillemin, McLeod, Beddari, & Lorem, 2019; Taylor & Guerin, 2019). Shared dialogue is necessary to establish true engagement with a client to understand their unique needs, beliefs and preferred ways of doing things.

Collaboration, partnership and power sharing

Health care practice that is collaborative, builds partnerships and shares power enables individual clients, their families and communities to be active participants in health. This includes regarding clients as partners in health care, involved in the decision making and part of a team effort to maximise the effectiveness of the care (Hook et al., 2016; Laverty et al., 2017). Western health care has traditionally been hierarchical in nature. Health professionals may be in positions of power over their clients—wittingly or unwittingly—and need to actively consider how to shift this so power and responsibility is shared (Best, 2018; Mead & Bower, 2000; Nguyen, 2008).

Collaboration and *partnership* also underpin how health professionals can work with bi-lingual health workers, cultural liaison workers, and Aboriginal and Torres Strait Islander health workers—health professionals who clarify client-centred issues and enable more culturally congruent care for clients. Health professionals can actively build close, collaborative working relationships with these workers through a genuine sharing of personal and professional identities (Bennett et al., 2013). If it is possible to share knowledge, skills and experiences in these partnerships, new ways of knowing, being and doing emerge (Zubrzycki, Shipp, & Jones, 2017).

Box 6.7 Reflection—Collaboration and partnership between health workers

Watch this video made by The National Aboriginal and Torres Strait Islander Health Worker Association (NATSIHWA). It highlights the importance of collaboration and partnership with Aboriginal and Torres Strait Islander health workers:
https://www.natsihwa.org.au/good-gp-two-us-dr-rod-omond

- How do the heath workers relate to each other?
- How does the collaborative approach to health care positively impact the clients' health, and that of their families and communities?

The principles of collaboration, partnership and power sharing can also be used by health professionals to think critically about the extent to which their health care environments are informed by the different needs of individuals, families and communities. As outlined in Chapter 4, the (predominantly) biomedical Western health system in Australia is underpinned by frameworks of Whiteness (Dune, Caputi, & Walker, 2018). The dominance of this model of health and wellbeing has led to widely reported systemic harms being enacted on non-White clients. To think critically about their health environment, health professionals can ask:

- Does the health system, hospital or other health care environment actively share power by inviting collaboration and partnership with different organisations and communities?
- Are policies, processes and practices informed by a diversity of perspectives, worldviews and needs?
- To what extent does the health environment acknowledge and legitimise difference in processes and policies?
- To what extent are systems and practices defined by the groups of people who engage with the organisation?

Observations in response to these questions provide a basis for health professionals to advocate for enhanced collaboration and partnership between health organisations and the individual and communities who engage with them. Health professionals can actively work to build culturally safe approaches in their health care environments by advocating for ways of working that recognise, value and align more with other cultural perspectives.

Culturally safe practice acknowledges the factors that impact individual and community health

The capacity to take into account the factors that impact individual and community health is a key aspect of culturally safe practice. This is how health professionals can translate a key principle of cultural safety—understanding how social determinants, intersectionality and social construction shape health outcomes and access to culturally responsive health care—into practice. Students can think about the concepts of *social determinants of health*, social construction and intersectionality as "tools" for critical thinking about their clients' social worlds and their experiences of health and health inequity. For example, health professionals can consider clients in relation to what is known about their social determinants of health or, as discussed in Chapters 1 and 2, the conditions in which people are born, grow, work, live, and age, and the wider set of forces and systems shaping the conditions of daily life. This means developing an understanding of a client's social worlds and using the knowledge to inform health care. Building an understanding of the client in their context is a feature of *client-centred care* (Australian Institute of Health and Welfare, 2014; Mead & Bower, 2000). When growing this standpoint, it is important to bring a strengths-based rather than deficit-based perspective and acknowledge the strengths and abilities of clients and the people around them (Australian Human Rights Commission, 2010).

A health professional who seeks to take into account the factors that impact individual and community health aims for health care that recognises the whole person. Health care does become more complex when health professionals pursue health care "which involves all aspects of physical, social, emotional, spiritual and political concerns of the client" (Richardson & MacGibbon, 2010, p. 63). However, this approach enables health professionals to consider equity issues as part of their care of clients. As Kelly et al. (2015, p. 10) emphasise, clients do not all have the same resources available to them—which means some clients may need additional resources to ensure the same health outcomes. Health professionals can factor into their health care practice their understandings about the resources a client has access to:

> Many paramedics and ambulance clinicians may have already delivered a range of social interventions to address issues that impact clients' living conditions including simple interventions (such as changing a light bulb), active signposting to local services, and referral to the local authority social care team.
>
> (Tang, McBride, & Potts, 2019, p. 294)

Where possible, it is an important aspect of culturally safe practice to include interventions that respond to the wider determinants shaping a person's health. For example, this needs to be part of a health care encounter where a health professional is also using their clinical expertise to assist a client. How are health professionals to approach exploring factors that impact clients' health and wellbeing as part of a health care interaction with a client? The idea of "taking a social history" (Behforouz, Drain, & Rhatigan, 2014) is a useful resource here. A social history can be taken by asking questions such as:

- Where have people have come from?
- What are their social circumstances?
- Do they have social challenges?
- Do they have unmet social, physical, material needs?
- Does the client feel their social circumstances are impacting their health and wellbeing?
- Has discrimination impacted the client's health outcomes or their access to culturally sensitive care?

Kelly et al. (2015) developed tools to make visible, analyse and improve Aboriginal client journeys. They describe a comprehensive mapping process to capture the complexity of a client's journey through the health system. The mapping process includes prompts designed to help health professionals to recognise the whole person experiencing the client journey:

- Who is the person entering the journey?
- What is important for this person?
- What are this person's family and community commitments?
- How is the person's physical health?

These questions can help health professionals to identify these dimensions of health through conversation with clients. Kelly et al. (2015, p. 12) suggest the order the questions are asked is significant: "The physical/biological questions are purposefully positioned last so that the whole person is considered, not just their health condition or injury." They also suggest useful prompts for investigating the underlying factors that affect a client's access to, and quality of, care:

- What are the factors impacting access to health care?
- What is the preferred language, and are interpreters needed?
- How clear is communication between the client, family and staff?
- Is the client able to pay for health care, or is it difficult to pay?
- How does the client feel about accessing health services?
- Does the client or family/community have specific cultural or personal concerns or past experiences?
- Does the client have specific preferences for how his/her health care is delivered and how major decisions are made?

(Kelly et al., 2015, p. 13)

The questions are not prescriptive, but prompts to be drawn on to guide a dialogue that can be tailored for each health care encounter. Foronda, Baptiste, Reinholdt, and Ousman (2016) emphasise how health professionals can maintain on overall open stance to learning about the wider determinants shaping a client's health and wellbeing.

The concept of intersectionality can also assist health professionals to understand how different social determinants of health can intersect in ways that affect clients' wellbeing. Health professionals can understand how clients have multiple cultural groups and identities, which interact and intersect depending on the context and change with time. For example, socio-economic status may be more relevant than ethnicity in one context, and parental status may be more relevant than professional status in another context. As discussed in Chapter 1, and other chapters, a client's health is impacted by their intersecting identities. One crucial aspect of this is how the different aspects of a person's identity are "socially constructed" through being responded to in different ways by society. Some aspects of a person's identity may be associated with privilege, and others with disadvantage and discrimination. For example, racial discrimination works with and through gender, class and sexuality to predict barriers to health care (e.g., perceived difficulty accessing health services) (Bastos, Harnois, & Paradies, 2018; Paradies et al., 2015). Thus, intersectionality offers more precise identification of inequalities experienced by clients (Warner & Brown, 2011) and is a concept that can play a useful part in health professionals' critical thinking about how the wider determinants of health are at play in their clients' lives.

Acknowledging and responding to the factors that impact individual and community health is a significant dimension of culturally safe practice because it is a crucial component to embed the cultural safety principle of *social justice* into practice. For example, an important dimension of this work in the Australian context is acknowledging the ongoing impact of colonisation on Aboriginal and Torres Strait Islander peoples' contemporary health outcomes (Congress of Aboriginal and Torres Strait Islander Nurses and Midwives [CATSINaM], 2017). Mercer, Fitzpatrick, Gourlay, and Vojt (2007) found that engaging with clients about the wider determinants of their health for even a short time in a consultation can improve client empowerment, reduce health professionals' stress levels and improve care. There is increasing evidence that such interventions are effective in promoting health equity at the individual client level, and at broader community and structural levels (Andermann, 2018; Browne et al., 2012).

Health care professionals can also address the social determinants of health through health advocacy, or care that includes the promotion of health and access to services (see Chapter 5 for a detailed discussion). This requires assessing what is happening in the processes, policies and practices of the health professional's health care environment, as a basis for advocating for systemic change. Health professionals can also work to improve the wider determinants shaping health and wellbeing at a community level. This advocacy can happen in a range of ways, including: advocating for the needs of the community (Dobson, Voyer, Hubinette, & Regehr, 2015), forming partnerships with other public health organisations and community groups (Andermann, 2016) and working with community members and organisations to identify local solutions (Ingram et al., 2014). Opportunities for advocacy can arise through health care workplaces. Hospitals are increasingly recognising they need to become advocates for population health as they directly experience strain associated with broader failures to deal with the social determinants of health (Russell, Anstey, & Wells, 2015). "Health Promoting Hospitals" is an example of a program that health professionals might contribute to in an advocacy capacity. It can involve projects on multiple levels, including being a health-promoting setting, doing a health promotion project and promoting health in the wider community (Newman et al., 2015).

Culturally safe practice is regard*ful* of culture

This section outlines how the cultural safety principle of exploring diversity and difference in experiences and expectations of health and wellbeing can be translated into health care practice that recognises difference and acknowledges that everyone is cultured. In other words, for health care practice to be regard*ful* of culture. This means taking as a departure point that *everyone* is cultural and has worldviews, values and assumptions. It involves actively challenging the idea that culture resides in the exotic "other", or that everyone else is "diverse", and acknowledges diversity within and between cultures. Treating people the same (e.g., cultural blindness), regard*less* of culture, fails to acknowledge the unique needs and issues affecting those who are culturally different and will most likely result in inappropriate care. Users of health services should not have to discard their cultural values and preferred ways of doing things in order to receive health care in Australia (Cox & Taua, 2017; Taylor & Guerin, 2019). Instead, a person's cultural values, needs and preferences are placed at the forefront of their ongoing medical care, which Dubbin, Chang, and Shim (2013) describe as a more client centred care approach.

Being regardful of culture involves acknowledging that there are different models of health and experiences and understandings of health (see Chapter 3 for a detailed discussion). Health professionals can encompass a wide view of health—such as Indigenous health, which commonly involves cultural, physical, spiritual, psychological and social aspects for a person and community (Dudgeon, Milroy, & Walker, 2014). Cox and Taua (2013, p. 329) suggest health professionals can develop critical insight into working with multiple models of health by considering: what are their assumptions about health, illness and people; how does the client define health, and whose definitions of health are legitimised (by law and society)? What are the implications of these definitions for health care practice and the consequences of these definitions for health care practice? Critical reflection in this area will support health professionals to align to the needs of the person who is being cared for (Richardson & MacGibbon, 2010).

A key dimension of providing care that is regardful of culture is health professionals acknowledging the limitations of their own knowledge and perspectives (Best, 2018). This means understanding that our life experiences shape what we know, and there are limits to what we do know. Health professionals need to recognise the limitations their own cultural beliefs impose on their practice with clients of other cultures. This can be mediated by developing an accurate view of oneself culturally, including an awareness of the limitations of one's own cultural perspective and one's ability to understand another person's cultural background and experience (Hook et al., 2016). It is important to note this requires ongoing effort and reflection. Wilson et al., (2016) describe how health professionals with more than 15 years' experience working in Aboriginal health engaged in deep self-reflection about their work in Aboriginal health, giving serious consideration to their own position, stereotypes and biases. One of the key insights from such reflections was the awareness that, as one of the participants expressed "... firstly you have to admit that you don't know". This lends support to the importance of health professionals committing to ongoing learning, self-reflection

Box 6.8 Case study—Regard*ful* of culture

The following excerpt is from Peter Hartley's PhD: *Paramedic Practice and the Cultural and Religious Needs of Pre-Hospital Patients in Victoria*, p. 295 (Hartley, 2012). The PhD investigates how paramedics relate to the cultural and religious needs of African, Asian, Middle Eastern, Muslim, Jewish and Indigenous Australian communities in Victoria.

In the following quote, a Sikh research participant talks about his father's experiences with emergency paramedics during pre-hospital health care.

'We are a very traditional family, my father particularly. He was having some breathing problems from lung disease, he needs constant treatment. We have had many ambulances come, and almost always there is an issue with him. He is very spiritual, and also afraid when he is taken to hospital. His faith is very, very important to him. There have been times when the paramedics have just gone ahead to shave part of his arm and then they get angry when he pulls away. The removal of hair is forbidden, it is a sign of dedication to his spirituality. He always wears the Kirpan. It is purely a ceremonial sword a deeply religious symbol. It is not a weapon it has no sharp edges. Every time the paramedics take him to hospital they refuse to allow him to continue to wear the Kirpan. This is very distressing for him the fear of him dying without the Kirpan is overwhelming. One time the crew asked him to remove his Kara (steel bracelet worn as a symbol to remind the wearer of restraint in their actions and remembrance of God at all times). There was no reason for this. He now refuses to allow me to call for an ambulance; I must take him to hospital myself.'

If you were providing care for this client pre-hospital or in the hospital:

- How could you ensure health care with this client is regard*ful* of culture?
- What are the client's religious/cultural requirements? What are the client's religious values?
- Reflect on your own religious beliefs. How are they the same/different to the client? What would it mean to be aware of your own cultural values?
- What would make this situation culturally safe as defined by the client?

and a "willingness to learn one's strengths and limitations (knowing what you don't know)" (CATSINaM, 2017, p. 12).

Health care professionals can also assess their health care environment for practice that is regardful of culture. They can ask: are the practices, systems and policies of the health care environment regard*ful*, or regardless, of culture and cultural differences? To what extent is the health care environment open and accepting of difference? Newman et al. (2020) observe how this can happen to different extents in a health care environment. They discuss how inclusive health care environments for people of diverse sexual orientations and gender identities have predominantly focused on challenging the assumption that clients are heterosexual and cisgender until shown to be otherwise. However, this can be seen as a limited recognition of cultural difference. The authors suggest a health environment that is more comprehensively regardful of the cultural differences of people of diverse sexual orientations and gender identities would create a space whereby they feel "their difference is not erased by equal access, but is instead recognised in the way in which gender or sexual distinctiveness is seen as a significant and valued aspect of the contexts in which health care is sought out and provided" (p. 8). Health professionals can participate in interventions and health promotion programs that ensure the expression of cultural identities. As MacLean et al. (2017) identified, interventions that include opportunities for expression of cultural identities can have beneficial effects for Aboriginal and Torres Strait Islander peoples.

Health professionals can ask to what extent is the health service delivery I am part of regardful of culture? As described in Chapter 11, there is much to learn from Aboriginal Community Controlled Health Organisations: community controlled primary health care for Aboriginal and Torres Strait Islander peoples with an emphasis on provision of culturally safe care (Shannon, Carson, & Atkinson, 2006). ACCHOs have proven clinical effectiveness. The greater number of problems managed per consultation in ACCHOs, compared with Aboriginal and Torres Strait Islander clients in mainstream general practice, supports the assertion that ACCHOs fill an important role in the health system by providing care for their predominantly Indigenous clients with complex care needs (Larkins, Geia, & Panaretto, 2006). ACCHOs are supported by the National Aboriginal and Torre Strait Islander Health Plan 2013–2023, which emphasises strategies that integrate a focus on social and emotional wellbeing in all aspects of health care delivery and health promotion strategies.

Box 6.9 Reflection–Culturally safe practice

Many health programs focus on the delivery of health care, education and information to groups of people who have limited health access and/or literacy in a particular health area.

1. Make a list of some elements of programs that successfully support marginalised communities to increase their health and wellbeing.
   Watch the PHC Case Study —Culture and care in Australia video: https://www.youtube.com/watch?v=cC94MsIsje0
2. Does this program support some of the elements you noted down in Question 1?
3. How does this program put cultural safety into practice?

Conclusion

In this chapter students have been led through activities to facilitate the critical thinking and self-reflection that underpins culturally safe practice. It is important to recognise that by engaging with this textbook, and this chapter, students have already embarked on the lifelong process of becoming a culturally safe health professional. Ramsden (1993) identifies different dimensions to this process: health professionals need to understand their own self, history and attitudes; deconstruct any attitudes that delimit culturally safe practice; and grow skills to translate this learning and knowledge into health practice. Students can see this as an enduring, iterative learning process, involving ongoing feedback loops between thinking, learning, acting and reflecting. As students move into their health profession careers, they will have more opportunity in learn in and from their everyday professional practice. Becoming a culturally safe health practitioner involves learning new knowledge and contextualising the knowledge, which can be confronting (Best, 2018). Indeed, it necessarily involves unlearning and relearning in relation to dominant Western ways of doing and being (Walter & Baltra-Ulloa, 2016). A growing body of evidence indicates that collaborative reflection with peers supports unlearning processes in professional practice (McLeod et al., 2020). A community of practice (a small group of people) can be an effective way to support ongoing learning about cultural safety. As DeSouza and Higgins (2020) observe, a community of practice can be a space "where you can collectively draw on each other's skills and knowledge, brainstorm challenges and support each other's ongoing development" (pp. 86–87).

Health professionals need to be able to locate themselves in their own learning journey and identify what they need to do to progress further in the lifelong process of becoming a culturally safe heath professional. In this final part of the chapter, students are invited to review their learning across the chapter and use this process to articulate a personal action plan for enacting cultural safety in professional health practice.

Action plan for enacting cultural safety in professional health practice

1. Review your responses to Reflection Box 6.1. Have your feelings changed now that you have worked through the chapter?
2. Review your notes about Reflection Box 6.2. Do you feel better equipped to meet your health profession's expectations about cultural safety? Have additional questions arisen?
3. Review the material and the learning activities in each of the four domains that relate to culturally safe practice (Table 6.1).

4. Take a copy of the Action Plan Worksheet (Table 6.2). Fill in the first four columns, use this as a basis to define your "next steps" in relation to how you can further develop your critical thinking and self-reflection, and seek/build on opportunities for practice. Keep each worksheet, review and do again at different time points.

Table 6.1 Embedding cultural safety principles into practice through lifelong learning and critical reflection

Principles of cultural safety	*Culturally safe health care practice*
Consistent self-awareness and self-reflection	Addresses the impact of health professionals' own cultural realities, values, attitudes and behaviours on others
Trust and respect Collaboration, partnership and power sharing Shared dialogue	Recognises the importance of health care that is driven by the individual, family and community
Social Justice Understanding how social constructions, social determinants and intersectionality shape health outcomes, experiences and understandings of health, and access to culturally responsive health care	Acknowledges the factors that impact individual and community health
Exploring diversity and difference in experiences and expectations of health and wellbeing	Provides health care that is regard*ful* of culture

Table 6.2 Action Plan Worksheet

Domain of culturally safe practice	*What was particularly interesting?*	*What did you find challenging?*	*How does the domain intersect with your life, and/or health care practice if you are working?*	*What else do you feel you need to know about this domain of culturally safe practice?*	Next steps *To further develop critical thinking and self-reflection about this domain*	Next steps *To learn from practice or seek opportunities to learn from practice*
Addresses the impact of health professionals' own cultural realities, values, attitudes and behaviours on others						
Recognises the importance of health care that is driven by the individual, family and community						

(*continued*)

Table 6.2 (Continued)

Domain of culturally safe practice	*What was particularly interesting?*	*What did you find challenging?*	*How does the domain intersect with your life, and/ or health care practice if you are working?*	*What else do you feel you need to know about this domain of culturally safe practice?*	Next steps *To further develop critical thinking and self-reflection about this domain*	Next steps *To learn from practice or seek opportunities to learn from practice*
Acknowledges the factors that impact individual and community health						
Provides health care that is regard*ful* of culture						

References

Andermann, A. (2016). Taking action on the social determinants of health in clinical practice: A framework for health professionals. *Canadian Medical Association Journal, 188*(17–18), 474–483. https://doi.org/10.1503/cmaj.160177.

Andermann, A. (2018). Screening for social determinants of health in clinical care: Moving from the margins to the mainstream. *Public Health Reviews, 39*(1), 1–17. https://doi.org/10.1186/s40985-018-0094-7.

Australian Government. (2013). *National Aboriginal and Torres Strait Islander Health Plan 2013–2023.* https://www1.health.gov.au/internet/main/publishing.nsf/content/B92E980680486C3BCA257BF0001BAF01/$File/health-plan.pdf.

Australian Human Rights Commission. (2010). *Social justice and Aboriginal and Torres Strait Islander Peoples access to services [Speech]. QCOSS Regional Conference.* https://humanrights.gov.au/about/news/speeches/social-justice-and-aboriginal-and-torres-strait-islander-peoples-access.

Australian Institute of Health and Welfare. (2014). *The measurement of patient experience in non-GP primary health care settings.* https://www.aihw.gov.au/getmedia/88dc1aeb-17a0-49c0-a49c-da862eb-7cacf/17699.pdf.aspx?inline=true.

Bastos, J. L., Harnois, C. E., &Paradies, Y. C. (2018). Health care barriers, racism, and intersectionality in Australia. *Social Science and Medicine, 199*, 209–218. https://doi.org/10.1016/j.socscimed.2017.05.010.

Behforouz, H. L., Drain, P. K., & Rhatigan, J. J. (2014). Rethinking the social history. *The New England Journal of Medicine, 371*(14), 1277–1279. https://doi.org/10.1056/NEJMp1404846.

Bennett, B., Green, S., Gilbert, S., & Bessarab, D. (2013). *Our voices: Aboriginal and Torres Strait Islander social work.* Palgrave Macmillan.

Best, O. (2018). The cultural safety journey: Australian nursing context. In O. Best & B. Fredericks (Eds.), *Yatdjuligin: Aboriginal and Torres Strait Islander nursing and midwifery care.* Cambridge University Press.

Blair, I. V., Steiner, J. F., & Havranek, E. P. (2011). Unconscious implicit bias and health disparities: Where do we go from here? *The Permanente Journal, 15*(2), 71–78.

Browne, A., Varcoe, C., Wong, S., Smye, V., Lavoie, J., Littlejohn, D., Tu, D., Godwin, O., Krause, M., Khan, K. B., Fridkin, A., Rodney, P., O'Neil, J., & Lennox, S. (2012). Closing the health equity gap: Evidence-based strategies for primary health care organizations. *International Journal for Equity in Health, 11*(1), 59. https://doi.org/10.1186/1475-9276-11-59.

Burgess, D., van Ryn, M., Dovidio, J., & Saha, S. (2007). Reducing racial bias among health care providers: Lessons from social-cognitive psychology. *Journal of General Internal Medicine, 22*(6), 882–887. https://doi.org/10.1007/s11606-007-0160-1.

Butler-Henderson, K., Kemp, T., McLeod, K., & Harris, L. (2018). Diverse gender, sex and sexuality: Managing culturally safe workplaces. *HIM—Interchange*, *8*(3), 10–14.

Cass, A., Lowell, A., Christie, M., Snelling, P. L., Flack, M., Marrnganyin, B., & Brown, I. (2002). Sharing the true stories: Improving communication between Aboriginal patients and healthcare workers. *Medical Journal of Australia*, *176*(10), 466–470. https://doi.org/10.5694/j.1326-5377.2002.tb04517.x.

Chapman, E. N., Kaatz, A., & Carnes, M. (2013). Physicians and implicit bias: How doctors may unwittingly perpetuate health care disparities. *Journal of General Internal Medicine*, *28*(11), 1504–1510. https://doi.org/10.1007/s11606-013-2441-1.

Cioffi, J. (2013). Communicating with culturally and linguistically diverse patients in an acute care setting: Nurses' experiences. *International Journal of Nursing Studies*, *30*(3), 299–306. https://doi.org/10.1016/s0020-7489(02)00089-5.

Congress of Aboriginal and Torres Strait Islander Nurses and Midwives (CATSINaM). (2017). *The nursing and midwifery Aboriginal and Torres Strait Islander Health curriculum framework: An adaptation of and complementary document to the 2014 Aboriginal and Torres Strait Islander Health curriculum framework*. https://www.catsinam.org.au/static/uploads/files/nursing-midwifery-health-curriculum-framework-final-version-1-0-wfffegyedblq.pdf.

Cox, L. (2016). *Social change and social justice: Cultural safety as a vehicle for nurse activism*. In T. Rudge (Ed.), *Proceedings of the 2nd Critical Perspectives in Nursing and Health Care International Conference* (pp. 1–11). University of Sydney.

Cox, L., & Taua, C. (2013). Socio-cultural considerations and nursing practice. In J. Crisp, C. Taylor, C. Douglas, & G. Rebeiro (Eds.), *Potter and Perry's fundamentals of nursing* (4th ed., pp. 320–340). Elsevier.

Cox, L., & Taua, C. (2017). Understanding and applying cultural safety: Philosophy and practice of social determinants approach. In J. Crisp, C. Douglas, G. Rebeiro, & D. Waters (Eds.), *Potter and Perry's fundamentals of nursing* (5th ed., pp. 251–287). Elsevier.

DeSouza, R. & Higgins, R. (2020). Cultural safety: An overview. In J. Lillie, K. Larsen, C. Kirkwood, & J. J. Brown (Eds.), *The relationship is the project: Workimg with communities* (pp. 81–88). The Lifted Brow.

Dinç, L., & Gastmans, C. (2012). Trust and trustworthiness in nursing: An argument-based literature review. *Nursing Inquiry*, *19*(3), 223–237. https://doi:10.1111/j.1440-1800.2011.00582.x.

Dobson, S., Voyer, S., Hubinette, M., & Regehr, G. (2015). From the clinic to the community: The activities and abilities of effective health advocates. *Academic Medicine*, *90*(2), 214–220. https://doi.org/10.1097/ACM.0000000000000588.

Downing, R., Kowal, E., & Paradies, Y. (2011). Indigenous cultural training for health workers in Australia. *International Journal for Quality in Health Care*, *23*(3), 247–257. https://doi.org/10.1093/intqhc/mzr008.

Dubbin, L. A., Chang, J. S., & Shim, J. K. (2013). Cultural health capital and the interactional dynamics of patient-centered care. *Social Science and Medicine*, *93*, 113–120. https://doi.org/10.1016/j.socscimed.2013.06.014.

Dudgeon, P., Milroy, H., & Walker, R. (Eds.) (2014). *Working together: Aboriginal and Torres Strait Islander mental health and wellbeing principles and practice*. (2nd ed.). Commonwealth of Australia. http://aboriginal.telethonkids.org.au/kulunga-research-network/working-together-2nd-edition-%281%29/.

Dune, T., Caputi, P., & Walker, B. (2018). A systematic review of mental health care workers' constructions about culturally and linguistically diverse people. *PLoS One*, *13*(7), e0200662. https://doi.org/10.1371/journal.pone.0200662.

Durie, M. (2005). Indigenous knowledge within a global knowledge system. *Higher Education Policy*, *18*(3), 301–312. https://doi.org/10.1057/palgrave.hep.8300092.

Foronda, C., Baptiste, D. L., Reinholdt, M. M., & Ousman, K. (2016). Cultural humility: A concept analysis. *Journal of Transcultural Nursing*, *27*(3), 210–217. https://doi.org/10.1177/1043659615592677.

Hartley, P. (2012). Paramedic practice and the cultural and religious needs of pre-hospital patients in Victoria. [Doctoral dissertation, Victoria University]. Research Repository. http://vuir.vu.edu.au/21301/.

Hook, J. N., Boan, D., Davis, D. E., Aten, J. D., Ruiz, J. M., & Maryon, T. (2016). Cultural humility and hospital safety culture. *Journal of Clinical Psychology in Medical Settings*, *23*(4), 402–409. https://doi.org/10.1007/s10880-016-9471-x.

Kelly, J., Dwyer, J., Pekarsky, B., Mackean, T., Willis, E., de Crespigny, C., Perkins, S., O'Donnell, K., King, R., Mackean, L., Brown, A., Lawrence, M., & Dixon, K. (2015). Managing two worlds together. *Stage*

3: Improving Aboriginal patient journeys—Study report. The Lowitja Institute. https://www.lowitja.org.au/content/Document/Lowitja-Publishing/Project-Report-layout-WEB.pdf.

Ingram, M., Schachter, K. A., Sabo, S. J., Reinschmidt, K. M., Gomez, S., De Zapien, J. G., & Carvajal, S. C. (2014). A community health worker intervention to address the social determinants of health through policy change. *The Journal of Primary Prevention, 35*(2), 119–123. https://doi.org/10.1007/s10935-013-0335-y.

Laholt, H., Guillemin, M., McLeod, K., Beddari, E., & Lorem, G. (2019). How to use visual methods to promote health among adolescents: A qualitative study of school nursing. *Journal of Clinical Nursing, 28*(13–14), 2688–2695. https://doi.org/10.1111/jocn.14878.

Larkins, S. L., Geia, L. K., & Panaretto, K. S. (2006). Consultations in general practice and at an Aboriginal community controlled health service: Do they differ? *Rural and Remote Health, 6*(3), 560–571.

Laverty, M., McDermott, D. R., & Calma, T. (2017). Embedding cultural safety in Australia's main health care standards. *Medical Journal of Australia, 207*(1),15–16. https://doi.org/10.5694/mja17.00328.

MacLean, S., Ritte, R., Thorpe, A., Ewen, S., & Arabena, K. (2017). Health and wellbeing outcomes of programs for Indigenous Australians that include strategies to enable the expression of cultural identities: A systematic review. *Australian Journal of Primary Health, 23*(4), 309–318. https://doi.org/10.1071/PY16061.

McKivett, A., Paul, D., & Hudson, N. (2018). Healing conversations: Developing a practical framework for clinical communication between Aboriginal communities and healthcare practitioners. *Journal of Immigrant and Minority Health, 21*(3), 596–605. https://doi.org/10.1007/s10903-018-0793-7.

McLeod, K., Thakchoe, S., Hunter, M. A., Vincent, K., Baltra-Ulloa, A. J., & MacDonald, A (2020). Principles for a pedagogy of unlearning. *Reflective Practice, 21*(2), 183–197. https://doi.org/10.1080/14623943.2020.1730782.

McNair, R. P., Hegarty, K., & Taft, A. (2012). From silence to sensitivity: A new identity disclosure model to facilitate disclosure for same-sex attracted women in general practice consultations. *Social Science & Medicine, 75*(1), 208–216. https://doi.org/10.1016/j.socscimed.2012.02.037.

Mead, N., & Bower, P. (2000). Patient-centredness: A conceptual framework and review of the empirical literature. *Social Science & Medicine, 51*(7), 1087–1110. https://doi.org/10.1016/s0277-9536(00)00098-8.

Mercer, S. W., Fitzpatrick, B., Gourlay, G., & Vojt, G. (2007). More time for complex consultations in a high-deprivation practice is associated with increased patient enablement. *British Journal of General Practice. 57*(545), 960–966. https://doi.org/10.3399/096016407782604910.

Newman, C. E., Prankumar, S. K., Cover, R., Rasmussen, M. L., Marshall, D., & Aggleton, P. (2020). Inclusive health care for LGBTQ+ youth: Support, belonging, and inclusivity labour. *Critical Public Health*, 1–10. https://doi.org/10.1080/09581596.2020.1725443.

Newman, L., Javanparast, S., Baum, F., & Hutchinson, C. (2015). *Evidence review: Settings for addressing the social determinants of health inequities.* Victorian Health Promotion Foundation. https://www.vichealth.vic.gov.au/-/media/ResourceCentre/PublicationsandResources/Health-Inequalities/Fair-Foundations/Full-reviews/HealthEquity_Settings-evidence-review.pdf?la=en&hash=A010F43C3ED329BE99C535A12BE535BCD6322532.

Nguyen, H.T. (2008). Patient centred care: Cultural safety in Indigenous health. *Australian Family Physician, 37*(12), 990–994.

Nursing Council of New Zealand. (2011). *Guidelines for cultural safety, the Treaty of Waitangi and Maori health in nursing education and practice.* https://www.nursingcouncil.org.nz/Public/Nursing/Standards_and_guidelines/NCNZ/nursing-section/Standards_and_guidelines_for_nurses.aspx.

Pallok, K., De Maio, F., & Ansell, D. A. (2019). Structural racism: A 60 year old African-American woman with breast cancer. *New England Journal of Medicine, 380*(16), 1489–1493. doi. 10.1056/NEJMp1811499.

Paradies, Y., Ben, J., Denson, N., Elias, A., Priest, N., Pieterse, A., Gupta, A., Kelaher, M., & Gee, G. (2015). Racism as a determinant of health: A systematic review and meta-analysis. *PLoS One, 10*(9), 1–48. https://doi.org/10.1371/journal.pone.0138511.

Persson, A., Newman, C. E., Rasmussen, M. L., Marshall, D., Cover, R., & Aggleton, P. (2020). Queerying notions of difference among two generations of Australians who do not identify heteronormatively. *Sexuality & Culture, 24*, 54–71. https://doi.org/10.1007/s12119-019-09625-3.

Ramsden, I. (1993). Cultural safety and nursing education in Aotearoa. *Nursing Praxis in New Zealand. 8*(3), 4–10.

Ramsden, I. (2002). Cultural safety and nursing education in Aotearoa and Te Waipounamu. [Doctoral dissertation, Victoria University of Wellington]. https://croakey.org/wp-content/uploads/2017/08/RAMSDEN-I-Cultural-Safety_Full.pdf.

Richardson, F., & MacGibbon, L. (2010). Cultural safety: Nurses' accounts of negotiating the order of things. *Women's Studies Journal*, *24*(2), 54–65.

Russell, L. M., Anstey, M. H. R., & Wells, S. (2015). Hospitals should be exemplars of healthy workplaces. *Medical Journal of Australia*, *202*(8), 424–426. https://doi.org/10.5694/mja14.01437.

Sahin, H., & Akyol, A. D. (2010). Evaluation of nursing and medical students' attitudes towards people with disabilities. *Journal of Clinical Nursing*, *19*(15–16), 2271–2279. https://doi.org/10.1111/j.1365-2702.2009.03088.x.

Shahid, S., & Thompson, S. (2009). An overview of cancer and beliefs about the disease in Indigenous people of Australia, Canada, New Zealand and the US. *Australian New Zealand Journal of Public Health*, *33*(2), 109–118. https://doi.org/10.1111/j.1753-6405.2009.00355.x.

Shannon, C., Carson, A., Atkinson R. C. (2006). The manager. *Medical Journal of Australia*, *184*(10), 530–531. https://doi.org/10.5694/j.1326-5377.2006.tb00354.x.

Tang, S., McBride, S., Potts, K. (2019). Social prescribing: Surely, we are not just going to prescribe tea and biscuits. *Journal of Paramedic Practice*, *11*(7), 294–295. https://doi.org/10.12968/jpar.2019.11.7.294.

Taylor, J., Jones, R. M., O'Reilly, P., Oldfield, W., & Blackburn, A. (2010). The Station Community Mental Health Centre Inc: Nurturing and empowering. *Rural and Remote Health*, *10*(3), 1–12.

Taylor, K., & Guerin, P. (2019). *Health care and Indigenous Australians: Cultural safety in practice* (3rd ed.). Palgrave Macmillan.

Thorne, S. 2018. Confronting bias in health care. *Nursing Inquiry*, *25*(2), 1–2. https://doi.org/10.1111/nin.12240.

Van Herk, K. A., Smith, D., & Andrew, C. (2011). Examining our privileges and oppressions: Incorporating an intersectionality paradigm into nursing. *Nursing Inquiry*, *18*(1), 29–39. https://doi.org/10.1111/j.1440-1800.2011.00539.x.

van Ryn, M., Burgess, D. J., Dovidio, J. F., Phelan, S. M., Saha, S., Malat, J., Griffin, J. M., Fu, S. S., Perry, S. (2011). The impact of racism on clinical cognition, behaviour, and clinical decision making. *Du Bois Review: Social Science Research on Race*, *8*(1), 199–218. https://doi.org/10.1017/S1742058X11000191.

Vukic, A., Jesty, C., Mathews, V., & Etowa, J. (2012). Understanding race and racism in nursing: Insights from Aboriginal nurses. *ISRN Nursing*, *2012*, 1–9. https://doi.org/10.5402/2012/196437.

Walter, M., & Baltra-Ulloa, J. (2016). The race gap: An Indigenous perspective on whiteness, colonialism, and social work in Australia. *Social Dialogue*, *4*(15), 29–32.

Warner, D., & Brown, T. (2011). Understanding how race/ethnicity and gender define age-trajectories of disability: An intersectionality approach. *Social Science & Medicine*, *72*(8), 1236–1248. https://doi.org/10.1016/j.socscimed.2011.02.034.

Williams, R. (1999). Cultural safety: What does it mean for our work practice? *Australian and New Zealand Journal of Public Health*, *23*(2), 213–214. https://doi.org/10.1111/j.1467-842X.1999.tb01240.x.

Wilson, A. M., Kelly, J., Magarey, A., Jones, M., & Mackean, T. (2016). Working at the interface in Aboriginal and Torres Strait Islander health: Focussing on the individual health professional and their organisation as a means to address health equity. *International Journal for Equity in Health*, *15*(1), 187. https://doi.org/10.1186/s12939-016-0476-8.

Zubrzycki, J., Shipp, R., & Jones, V. (2017). Knowing, being, and doing: Aboriginal and non-Aboriginal collaboration in cancer services. *Qualitative Health Research*, *27*(9), 1316–1329. https://doi.org/10.1177/1049732316686750

Part III

Working with diverse populations

7 Aboriginal and Torres Strait Islander Australians

Liesa Clague, Janelle Trees and Rob Atkinson

Learning outcomes

After working through this chapter, students will be able to:

1. Recognise and understand the cultural diversity within and between Aboriginal and Torres Strait Islander peoples.
2. Identify Aboriginal and Torres Strait Islander histories from pre-penal contact to present, including the impact that marginalisation and oppression have on health and wellbeing.
3. Explore the cultural, social, economic and environmental determinants of health relating to Aboriginal and Torres Strait Islander peoples.
4. Identify the various roles of Aboriginal and Torres Strait Islander health professionals and the importance of having an increased Aboriginal and Torres Strait Islander presence in the health workforce.
5. Understand the history of and the rationale for Aboriginal Medical Services (AMS), including Aboriginal Community Controlled Health Organisations (ACCHOs) and the key role of the National Aboriginal Community Controlled Health Organisation (NACCHO).
6. Identify culturally safe practice, including strategies and resources to contribute to improved health outcomes for Aboriginal and Torres Strait Islander peoples.

Key terms

Aboriginal Community Controlled Health Organisations (ACCHOs): A non-profit incorporated Aboriginal Community Controlled Organisation that provides wholistic and culturally appropriate Primary Health Care and Aboriginal health-related services to the community it serves. An ACCHO is governed by an Aboriginal board of management elected by a local Aboriginal community membership.
Aboriginal Health & Medical Research Council of NSW (AHMRC of NSW): Aboriginal Health & Medical Research Council of NSW was established in 1985. Members are ACCHOs led by their respective Aboriginal Communities to deliver comprehensive and culturally appropriate primary health care services.
Aboriginal Medical Service (AMS): First established in 1971 in Redfern (Redfern AMS). There are now around 140 Aboriginal Medical Services across Australia.
Aboriginal: The first peoples of this land now called Australia are the Aboriginal peoples; however, they also have other names that they use to refer to themselves: Goori, Koori, Arrernte, Kamilaroi, Yungl, Yaegl and so on.

Australian Health Practitioner Regulation Agency (Ahpra): The national association of 15 professional boards that regulate and enforce standards in health.
Australian Institute of Aboriginal and Torres Strait Islander Studies (AIATSIS): An independent government statutory authority for research, collection, and publication. A premier resource for Aboriginal and Torres Strait Islander peoples learning and record-keeping.
Colonisation: In this chapter, colonisation refers to a group of people seeking to extend their territories through the subjugation of other people in a new territory.
Cultural safety: In this chapter, cultural safety encompasses respect for intellectual property of the Aboriginal and Torres Strait Islander peoples, their stories and lived experiences.

The Australian Indigenous Doctors Association (AIDA) definition is:

> Cultural safety refers to the accumulation and application of knowledge of Aboriginal and Torres Strait Islander values, principles and norms. It is about overcoming the cultural power imbalances of places, people, and policies to contribute to improvements in Aboriginal and Torres Strait Islander health and increasing numbers within, and support for, the Aboriginal and Torres Strait Islander medical workforce. [...] AIDA views cultural safety on a continuum of care with cultural awareness being the first step in the learning process and cultural safety being the final outcome. This is a dynamic and multidimensional process where an individual's place in the continuum of care can change depending on the setting. For example, [in] Aboriginal and Torres Strait Islander community-controlled health services, hospitals or communities.
>
> (AIDA Cultural Safety Fact Sheet https://www.aida.org.au/wp-content/uploads/2018/07/Cultural-Safety-Factsheet_08092015.docx.pdf)

Invasion: An occasion when a country and its army uses force to enter and take control of another country.
National Aboriginal Community Controlled Health Organisation (NACCHO): The peak body representing 143 Aboriginal Community Controlled Health Organisations (ACCHOs) across the country on Aboriginal health and wellbeing issues. It has a history extending back to a meeting in Albury in 1974.
Penal colony: A type of prison, especially one that is far away from other people, as Australia was set up by the British.
Torres Strait Islanders: Torres Strait Islanders are a seafaring peoples, whose traditional countries are in the Torres Strait, off the Australian mainland's northern-most point. The region has over 270 islands in the strait of ocean between the northern tip of Queensland, Cape York, and the south-east coast of Papua New Guinea.
Wholistic: Placing a "w" in front of holistic makes us reflect that the process, design, and collaboration would look at the whole approach—not a hole that the approach could fall or sink into. It would be circular in its wholeness, which conceptualises the way we have grown up and the cycle of life, including our connection to land and country.

Chapter summary

Aboriginal and Torres Strait Islander peoples, their families and communities have survived and subsisted for well over 60,000 years. This highlights the strength and resilience of nations of peoples who survived with the environment, thrived throughout millennia with their appropriate and sustaining use and treatment of the fauna and flora (Muller, 2003, p. 33; Watson, 1997). Today, our peoples' health has been impacted, changed and our society pulled apart.

As a health professional, you have the capacity to gain knowledge and use it to the best effect by including Aboriginal and Torres Strait Islander ways of knowing, being and doing to work with our people and alongside us. We need to work together to build positive lasting change. We will encourage you to advocate for Aboriginal and Torres Strait Islander peoples, learn from each other, and challenge depictions you may have heard, experienced or seen in the media and other forms of information that are negative or derogatory.

The aim of this chapter is to explore the history of Aboriginal and Torres Strait Islander peoples of Australia, by introducing the reader to pre-penal colonial and Australia's penal colonial history and the impact of these historical events on Aboriginal and Torres Strait Islander peoples. We will look at some of the issues around marginalisation, oppression and dispossession, and what those experiences meant to culture, identity, power and human rights. Immediate consequences included displacement and economic exploitation of Aboriginal labour and resources, such as land and water.

Misused power and racism in their many forms can and have shaped policy and agendas of organisations like government departments and educational, health, religious and cultural institutions. We will show that we have a long way to go before change is meaningful.

Despite this, there has been substantial progress and growth. A human rights-based approach to strengths-based, *wholistic* care and cultural safety is embedded now in health delivery. For example, the idea of cultural safety is now embodied in medical, nursing and midwifery codes of conduct and standards for practice. This has been won through struggle and learning.

In this chapter you will learn from case studies that draw on the lived experiences of some Aboriginal nurses and doctors. It recognises the role of dominant societies and privilege. New arrivals need increased awareness that the environment we are living in is changing. We discuss racism that has been allowed to go on for hundreds of years: at a personal level, as well as institutional racism, conscious and unconscious biases. We invite you not to walk past behaviour that you would not accept if applied to those you care about. This chapter and the associated reading will empower you to reflect on history and subsequent behaviour that has been shaped by that history.

A key aspect of healing for Aboriginal and Torres Strait Islander peoples is acknowledging the significant grief in our communities, primarily due to the ongoing effects of colonisation. It is important to build a healthy workforce that includes Aboriginal and Torres Strait Islander peoples who are involved in decision making and partnership, building on autonomy and self-determination. Aboriginal and Torres Strait Islander peoples need allies in this endeavour.

Finally, in this chapter you will find evidence-based resources encouraging you to reflect on your learning, helping you to present and build good models and practices of care around good communication. This is to better understanding, culturally safe ways of doing, knowing and being that will guide your learning and your practice.

As Sister Alison Bush OA stated in 2018, "I only do my job and try to help people to understand each other."

Aboriginal and Torres Strait Islander peoples

The first peoples of this land we call Australia are the *Aboriginal* and *Torres Strait Islander* peoples; however, they also have other specific names that they use to refer to themselves, depending on where they are from and where they are connected. Palawa, Nyoongar, Goori, Koori, Yungl,

Yaegl: these are just a few of the many names. We want you to learn that when you are working or caring for Aboriginal and Torres Strait Islander peoples, acknowledging their preferred names links them to Country and their connection to their peoples.

Aboriginal peoples

As a civilisation that has lasted more than 60,000 years (Pascoe, 2014, p. 9), Aboriginal peoples survived environmental changes, including an Ice Age 20,000 years ago, traded among themselves and interacted and traded with people of other lands. Northern Australian Aboriginal people traded and travelled with people from present-day Sulawesi in Indonesia for at least a hundred years before the British arrived in Australia. In another powerful example, ochres from Lake Mungo, used ceremonially in burial over 26,000 years ago, were traded from sources distant to the site (Edwards, 1988).

More than 250 languages, including over 800 dialects, prospered on the Australian mainland and Torres Strait Islands before the establishment of the *penal colony* (Australian Institute of Aboriginal and Torres Strait Islander Studies, 2019a, 2019b).

Aboriginal people survived and flourished as conscious, well-learned (fully familiar—by routinely learning by means of repetition) and knowledgeable people, caring for themselves and their lands. The land was managed with fire and water. Resources were husbanded to remain sustainable. Aboriginal people domesticated plants, sowed, irrigated, and harvested grain, and stored foods. Pascoe (2014) argues that Australian Aboriginal people were the first humans to make bread.

Aboriginal peoples have a rich cosmology based on the creation and maintenance of the Land that cares for their people. Aboriginal peoples' Dreamtime is the understanding of the world and the stars, telling stories of connections. Dreamtime is where knowledge begins, including laws/lores for survival. Dreamtime knowledge guides our relationship to our surroundings and all living creatures.

Torres Strait Islanders

Torres Strait Islanders are seafaring peoples, whose traditional countries are in the Torres Strait off the Australian mainland's northern-most point. The region has over 270 islands in the strait of ocean between the northern tip of Queensland, Cape York, and the south-east coast of Papua New Guinea. The Torres Strait is the only part of Australia that borders another country.

There are 17 inhabited islands and 2 communities located at the tip of Cape York that are classified as a part of the Torres Strait. The Torres Strait Islander people traded with the people of Papua New Guinea. As ocean explorers, they were renowned for their seafaring, including their ability to navigate by the stars, as in the story of the great warrior, Tagai.

Tagai was a "cult hero" who became a huge star constellation that can be seen in the night sky. The Torres Strait Islander peoples use the stars along with the changing seasons to know when to plant crops, when to harvest, as well as to stay on-course when at sea (Hamacher, 2013).

There are two main traditional languages in the Torres Strait Islands: Meriam Mer, of the Eastern Islands, and Kalaw Lagaw Ya, of the near Western Islands. Three other dialects are spoken today to a much lesser extent in the Torres Strait Islands (Hamacher, 2013).

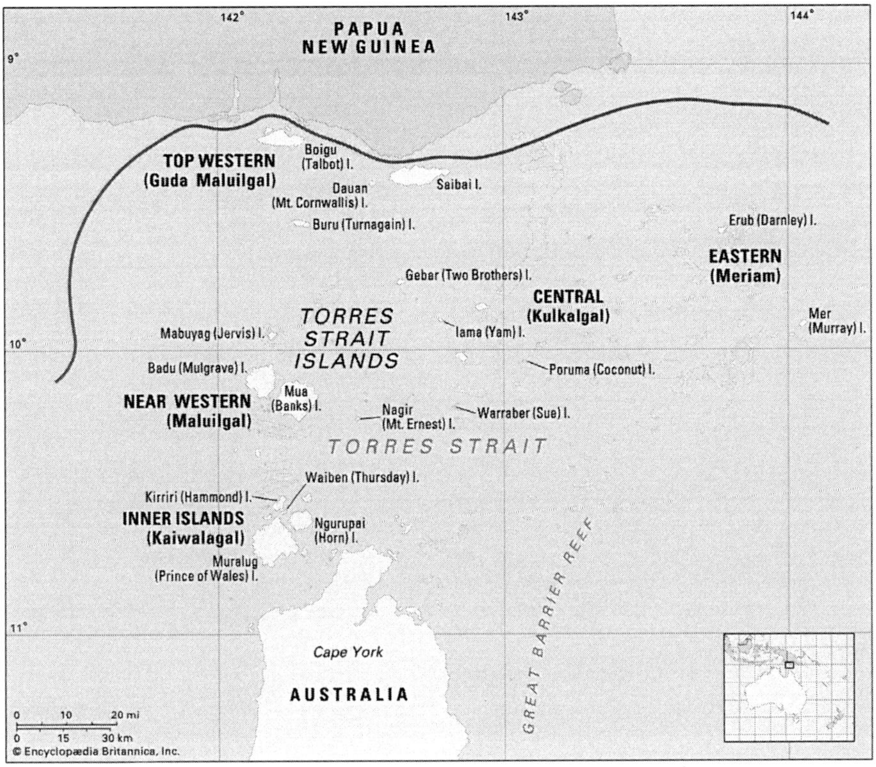

Figure 7.1 Torres Strait

> ### Box 7.1 Reflection—Aboriginal and Torres Strait Islander histories and cultures
>
> Think about facts and ideas in this section that are new to you. Discuss them with a colleague or friend.
>
> Use the resources in this chapter to learn more about aspects of Aboriginal and Torres Strait Islander histories and cultures that interest you.
>
> Learning about these cultures is a lifelong journey that enriches your experience of the world, as you learn to give better care to your Aboriginal and Torres Strait Islander clients, and grow in respect and understanding for your colleagues, health professionals who are Aboriginal and/or Torres Strait Islander.

The East Coast of Australia: First arrival of the British (including convicts from Ireland, Wales, Scotland and England) in the Sydney Basin

Thousands of kilometres south of the Torres Strait, on the east coast of Australia, Sydney is the present-day name of the Country where the British first arrived and laid claim to Aboriginal lands. Despite the devastation of the occupation, and witnessing overwhelming loss, descendants of the Aboriginal clans of the Sydney region continue to be connected to their Country (Reynolds, 1972, 1981, 1987).

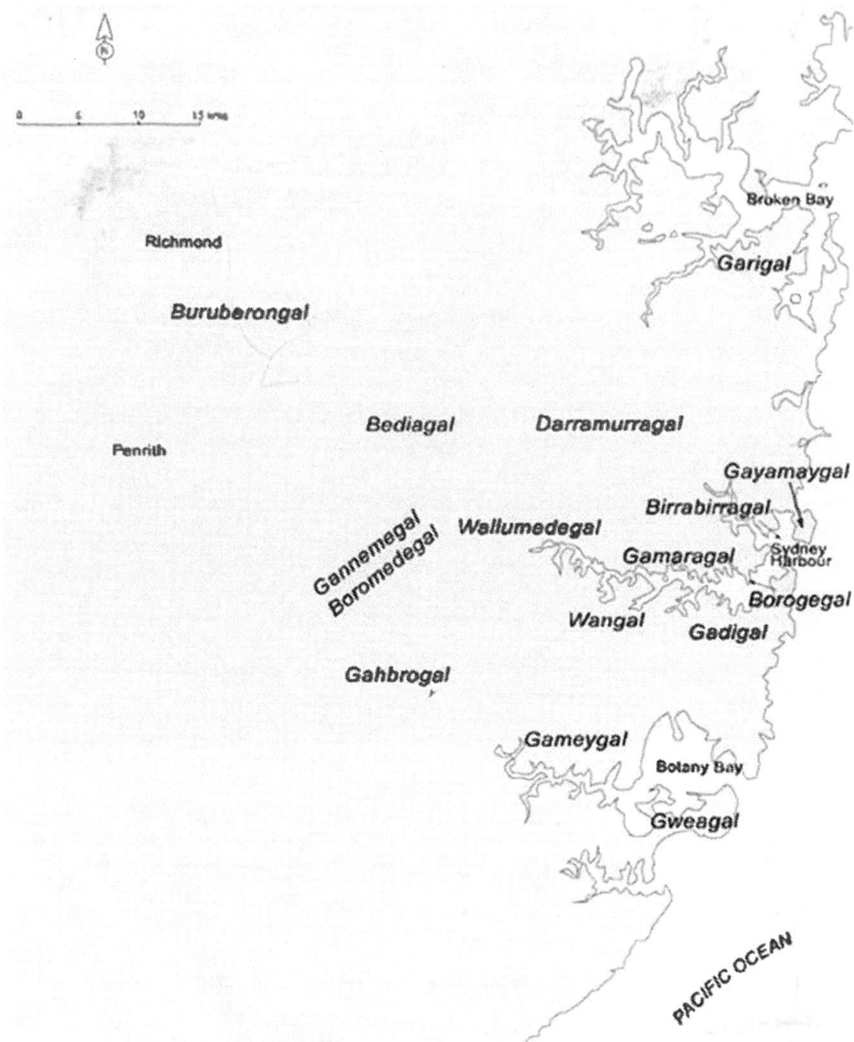

Figure 7.2 Clan in the Sydney region—courtesy of Dr Val Attenbrow (2010)

Aboriginal and Torres Strait Islander peoples from other parts of Australia have also come to live there, for the same reasons people all over the world flock to cities: opportunity, vitality and education. Today, Sydney has the nation's largest population of Aboriginal and Torres Strait Islander peoples.

We use Sydney as an example because it is where the *invasion* started. And it serves to show the persistence of Aboriginal land and culture in even the most urban environment (Figure 7.2).

What do we know about Aboriginal peoples from the Sydney Basin before the penal colony was established and invasion of land, resources, culture and society of Aboriginal peoples?

The Sydney basin was occupied by different Aboriginal clans prior to the arrival of Europeans. The Aboriginal peoples were self-sufficient. Because they lived harmoniously with the land, they were rich in resources. They fished, hunted, and harvested food from the surrounding bush. For more historical information, refer to the Aboriginal Heritage Office (Aboriginal Heritage Organisation, 2006, p. 25).

Many Aboriginal peoples domesticated plants, which they sowed, irrigated, harvested and stored as foods and medicines (Pascoe, 2014). The food the Aboriginal people ate was a nutrient-dense diet, high in fibre and low in fat and refined carbohydrates. They were muscular people with healthy skin, hair and teeth. In tune with their environment in a way that most of the invading Europeans could not see, the Aboriginal people did not take more than what was necessary from their gathering or hunting grounds (Whalan et al., 2017, p. 579). Captain Phillip, after spending three days exploring Port Jackson (now Sydney Harbour), was impressed by the "confidence and manly behaviour" of a group of Aboriginal people in the northern reaches of the harbour—hence the name *Manly Cove* (Attenbrow, 2010; Stralia Web's Regional Network, 2001).

There was much to learn from the Aboriginal people. However, that was not generally the attitude of the invaders from England. Most wanted to destroy the people of the land and consume all the resources: land, water and food for their livestock and for themselves as convicts and settlers. They did not come to trade but take over and destroy what they could of the society constructed by the Aboriginal peoples. Respect and trust were not elements of the invasion of Australia.

This behaviour was new to the Aboriginal and Torres Strait Islander peoples as they had traded and welcomed other peoples from within the islands of present-day Australia, as well as people from other lands, such as the Macassans from present-day Indonesia. Aboriginal and Torres Strait Islander peoples had long histories of travel to areas of South-East Asia and the Pacific, long before the penal colony was settled.

There is much to learn about the history and society of some of the Aboriginal nations around Sydney, but that should not stop health professionals negotiating culturally safe practices and behaviour towards Aboriginal and Torres Strait Islander peoples (Figure 7.3).

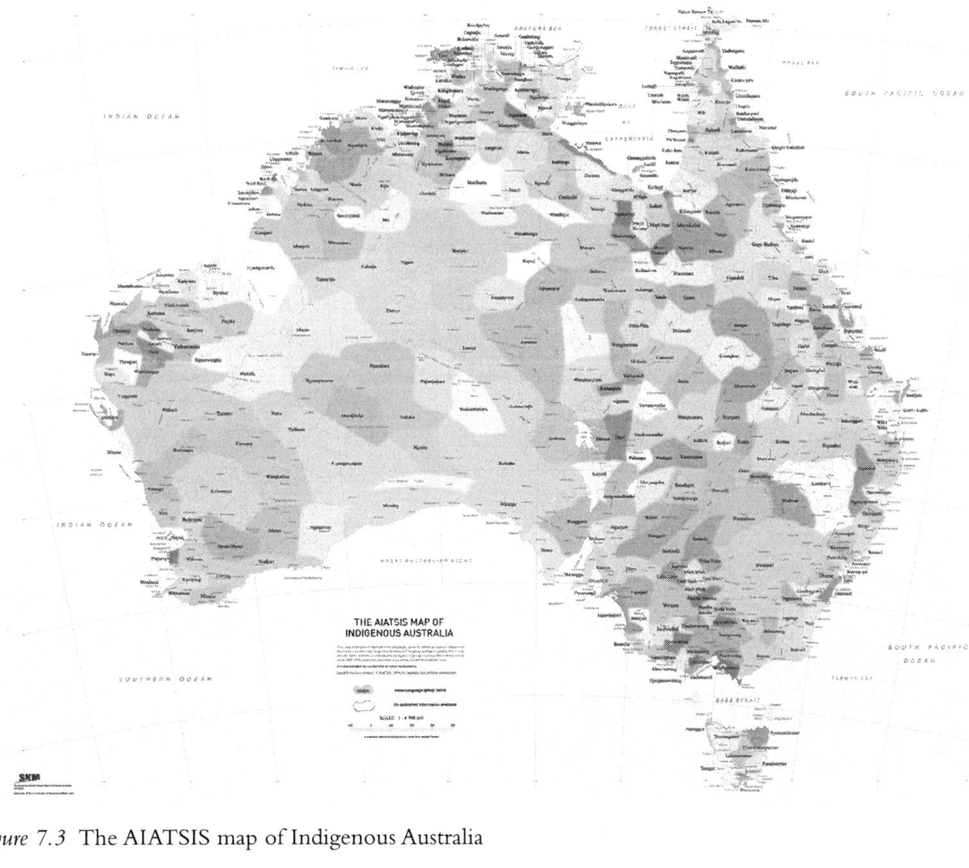

Figure 7.3 The AIATSIS map of Indigenous Australia

Box 7.2 Reflection—The AIATSIS map of Indigenous Australia

On the map find a place you have been to. Do you know the Aboriginal or Torres Strait Islander language group of that place? If not, find it on the map. Do you know any facts about the language group or their Dreamtime stories?

From your browsing on the net, find an interesting fact or Dreamtime story. Tell your colleagues about the fact or dreamtime story. What does the dreamtime story demonstrate to you about learning about and understanding through the world of creation stories?

Examples include: *How Frogmouth Found Her Home* (Kwaymullina, 2013), *Dunbi the Owl* (Utemorrah & Lofts, 2004) and *The Rainbow Serpent* (Roughsey, 1992)

Do you have creation stories in your culture? Do they have similar messages of learning? Why? Why not?

Impacts of invasion and the establishment of a penal colony in Australia: Breakdown of societies

In 1787 before departing England, Phillip's instructions of 17 April 1787 included the following:

> You are to endeavour by every possible means to open intercourse with the natives, and to conciliate their affections, enjoining all our subjects to live in amity and kindness with them. And if any of our subjects shall wantonly destroy them or give them any unnecessary interruption in the exercise of their occupation, it is our will and pleasure that you do cause such offenders to be brought to punishment according to the degree of the offence.
>
> (McRae, Nettheim, & Beacroft, 1997, p. 33)

These instructions were not followed, and the notion of Terra Nullius was created. The great south land was considered wasteland, unoccupied, and belonging to no one. Despite common belief, there was immediate and ongoing resistance by Aboriginal peoples.

Amongst its human cargo, the First Fleet brought with it many illnesses. Dental disease was relatively rare among Aboriginal people; smallpox, influenza, measles, whooping cough, tuberculosis, leprosy and syphilis were unknown (Sangha, Le Brocque, & Costanza, 2015). This all changed from 1788 onwards as the Aboriginal and Torres Strait Islander peoples were terrorised and coerced by the European invaders into a world unnatural to their existence (Attenbrow, 2010; Grieves, 2009; Irish, 2017; Whitehouse, Watkin Lui, Sellwood, Barrett, & Chigeza, 2014).

This happened differently in different time frames across the country.

Tasmanian Aboriginal people were brutally invaded during the so-called Black War from the mid-1820s until 1832.

The invasion began in Sydney in 1788, but even in New South Wales, the Dainghutti clan were not dispossessed until the early 1900s, partly because their mountainous land was not suitable for English agriculture, but also because of the people's continuous opposition.

In contrast, Walpiri, Anmatyerre and Kaytetye peoples of the present-day Northern Territory were massacred in 1928, in the last government-sanctioned mass-killing of Aboriginal people.

The military conquest and dispossession of Aboriginal and Torres Strait Islander peoples took over a century. Some argue that we were never conquered. Certainly, sovereignty was never ceded.

Box 7.3 Reflection—Aboriginal people of coastal Sydney

Go to Australian museum site: https://australianmuseum.net.au/learn/cultures/atsi-collection/sydney/

Look at the time frame of events and at how the information is linked to documents and transcriptions of diaries and ledgers written by different people who came to the penal colony.

After reading consider:

- What did you learn? Write a few dot points.
- How do you see the impact of the writing? Did you pick up any biases, or misunderstanding of the culture of the Aboriginal peoples being written about? What were they?
- What did you feel after reading what the First Fleet wrote about Aboriginal people? Write down a list of your feelings, and explain why you felt that way to your group or explain why you may agree or disagree with the Englishmen's comments.

How did the writer use the words to express their disregard for the cultures of the Aboriginal peoples? Write down the words used, then change the words into more positive words, respectful of the culture.

The establishment of the penal colony and the British settlement introduced widespread warfare with destruction of the local people, their culture and society. Land was subject to ownership; food and water sources were polluted and destroyed. There was mass destruction of Aboriginal populations by introduced diseases such as smallpox, measles, influenza, syphilis, alcoholism and others.

Box 7.4 Reflection—Exploring the impact of disease introduced into Australia

These resources and readings tell of the diseases introduced into Australia during and after the time the penal colony was being established:

- Dowling, P.J. (1997). *A great deal of sickness: Introduced diseases among the Aboriginal people of colonial Southeast Australia* [Doctoral dissertation, Australian National University]. At Open Research https://openresearch-repository.anu.edu.au.
- Goldsmid, J. M. (1989). Imported disease in Australia: An ongoing problem. In R. Steffen, H. O. Lobel, J. Haworth, & D. J. Bradley (Eds.), *Travel Medicine* (pp. 45–49). Springer.
- Warren, C. (2014, April 17). Was Sydney's smallpox outbreak of 1789 an act of biological warfare against Aboriginal tribes? *Australian Broadcasting Corporation.* https://www.abc.net.au/radionational/programs/ockhamsrazor/was-sydneys-smallpox-outbreak-an-act-of-biological-warfare/5395050
- And: Smallpox: 1789 Biological warfare against First Nations (Warren, 2019) at http://nationalunitygovernment.org/content/was-sydneys-smallpox-outbreak-1789-act-biological-warfare-against-aboriginal-tribes
- Watch 'The First Australian Fight Back-John Pilger-The Secret Country, on YouTube.

Box 7.5 Reflection—A brief Aboriginal history

What are three major causes of devastation to the Aboriginal clans of the Sydney area?

Go to this website: https://www.aboriginalheritage.org/history/history/

Read the quote, and write down how would you feel, if put into the same situation.

There is a quote from Judge Advocate David Collins (1798) that his friend Colebee's tribe had been reduced to only three people. Those witnessing could not remain unmoved.

> The colonists had destroyed within months a way of life that had outlasted British history by tens of thousands of years, and the people soon realised that the trespassers were committed to nothing less than total occupation of the land.

The negative effects of invasion and establishment of the penal colony for the Aboriginal and Torres Strait Islanders peoples still have an impact today, often in severe ways. Dispossession and alienation, poverty and oppression are still keenly felt (Concilia Ltd, 2017). Learning about this terrible history and its contemporary consequences is vital to ongoing learning and safety as a health worker in Australia. Beyond this chapter's Learning Outcomes, you are on a path of lifelong learning.

Being positive, what does this history mean for Aboriginal and Torres Strait Islander peoples?

- Their continuing resilience in the face of such adversity and strength shows there is much to gain through their knowledge of being, doing and knowing,
- Acknowledging the past events and learning to survive in such difficult times entailed adapting, learning and holding onto ancient knowledges and ways, despite the invasion of their lands, sea and water ways.
- To build better outcomes for future generations is a significant and meaningful goal for Aboriginal and Torres Strait Islander peoples, and especially in relation to themselves, their family connections, and community networks as a whole.

Health in Australia cannot be seen outside of, or apart from, the role of government. The government was the instrument of dispossession and colonisation. The federal government maintains control of how health services are delivered to Aboriginal and Torres Strait Islander peoples.

Government policies

Government policies over time have had a lasting impact for Aboriginal and Torres Strait Islander peoples, even if they address problems created by the past, that does not erase the past. The history of forced resettlement on reserves, missions, and the placing of many thousands of children in institutions, and the loss of land linking the deviation to breakdown in culture, are evident in the oppression still experienced by many Aboriginal and Torres Strait Islander people today (Stanner, 1979; von Sturmer, 1984).

Box 7.6 Reflection—Impacts of settlement on Aboriginal people

Go to this website: https://www.alrc.gov.au/publication/recognition-of-aboriginal-customary-laws-alrc-report-31/3-aboriginal-societies-the-experience-of-contact/impacts-of-settlement-on-aboriginal-people/

By reading and viewing this resource, you are hearing from the Australian Law Reform Commission about the extent of distress and terror inflicted on Aboriginal and Torres Strait Islander children. You will also deepen your understanding of the various legal and other requirements and stressors affecting and impacting on Aboriginal and Torres Strait Islander peoples, their health, customs, culture, language, spiritual connection to Country and other aspects of their lives.

In the article *Reducing the Health Disparities of Indigenous Australians: Time to Change Focus* by Durey and Thompson (2012), the authors looked at interviews with non-Indigenous medical practitioners in Western Australia who worked closely with Indigenous health. What they found was that racism emerged as a key issue. They concluded,

> Current health policies and practices favour standardised care where the voice of those who are marginalised is often absent. Examining the effectiveness of such models in reducing health disparities requires health providers to critically reflect on whether policies and practices promote or compromise Indigenous health and wellbeing—an important step in changing the discourse that places Indigenous people at the centre of the problem.
>
> (p. 1)

Box 7.7 Reflection—Reflecting on the experiences of Aboriginal and/or Torres Strait Islander peoples

Take a moment to think about how you would feel being taken away at a young age, away from your parents, close family and friends, customs, being forbidden to speak your language, made to eat different foods, dress differently, live differently in a dormitory with other people who were the same as you—but different.

- What are some of the feelings? Write them down.
- How long would you have those feeling, if it were for a week living in this new environment?
- If that time frame changed to 5–10 years, what kind of long-term impact would that have on some people? Write them down on paper
- What services are available to support the impact of long-term trauma, depression and heartbreak and loss of family, culture, language, and other losses? Write them down. What do you see or feel as you reflect on the lessons learnt?
- In your group, discuss the health effects of grief, sadness, anger, resilience or other feelings and emotions.

Box 7.8 Reflection—Government policies and acts

Following is a diagram of some of the policies over time that impacted Aboriginal and Torres Strait Islander peoples negatively as well as positively.

Chose a policy and research how it affected Aboriginal and Torres Strait Islander peoples' health. Taking a wholistic view, draw a diagram or write a paragraph about the benefits and adverse results of the policy.

Think about how you would feel if you were affected, influenced, or changed by the policy.

Would this impinge on you as a person, your character, and rights in society? How would you view the health system? Why or why not? (See Figure 7.4.)

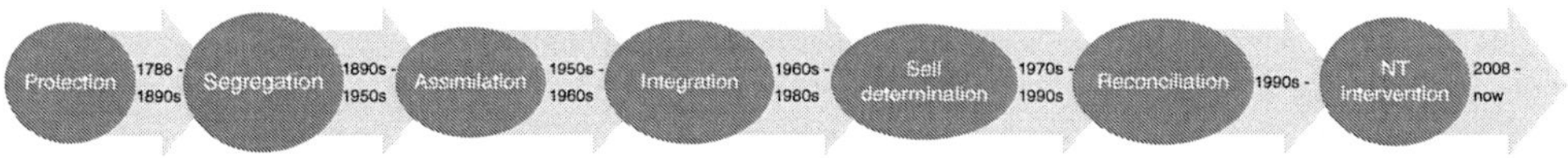

Figure 7.4 Diagram of some of the policies over time that have impacted Aboriginal and Torres Strait Islander peoples

In contrast, there have been policies affecting Aboriginal and/or Torres Strait Islander people that were made in consultation with the people and their needs. For example, the 1983 government definition of Aboriginal and Torres Strait Islander identity came from consultation with community representatives.

If a person is of Aboriginal and/or Torres Strait Islander descent, identifies as an Aboriginal and/or Torres Strait Islander person and is accepted as such by the Aboriginal and/or Torres Strait Islander community in which they live, then they are identified by the government as Aboriginal and/or Torres Strait Islander (Gardiner-Garden, 1996).

Being aware of these policies means you can discuss and research what they may mean for Aboriginal and Torres Strait Islander peoples, whether they agree or do not agree with the government definition. This discussion is sometimes a difficult one, reflecting painful history. However, knowing who you are and where you come from (and being accepted and understood as such) is vital to health and wellbeing for Aboriginal and Torres Strait Islander people, families and communities.

Box 7.9 Reflection—Australian Human Rights Commission

Visit the Human Rights website: https://humanrights.gov.au/our-work

The website has several case studies to draw from and strategies to develop practical outcomes.

List some strategies you would use.

A key concern discussed in Chapter 4 is privilege and White privilege.

What do these words express?

What does this feel like, and why would it impact Aboriginal and Torres Strait Islander people today?

Australia is a multicultural society, but if you think about equality and equity we still see, Aboriginal and Torres Strait Islander peoples still experience, inequality and inequities in treatment, as well as oppressive behaviours and attitudes by other cultures that are new to Australia.

Aboriginal and Torres Strait Islander peoples and their health

In Australia, approximately half of all Aboriginal and Torres Strait Islander peoples now live in major cities and inner regional areas, with implications for planners, policymakers and service providers. The move to these areas for many Aboriginal peoples has complex effects on health.

There are differences between circumstances from urban and regional, to living in rural and remote areas. Aboriginal and Torres Strait Islander peoples in very remote areas have much more disadvantage and difficulty relative to non-Aboriginal people, and even compared to urban Aboriginal people, across a range of socio-economic indicators, including high unemployment, decreased economic development, less education and inadequate access to food (Marrone, 2007; World Health Organisation, 2008).

Box 7.10 Reflection—Understanding inequalities experienced by Aboriginal and/or Torres Strait Islander peoples

Look at the following resources, and choose one. As you explore it, write down some differences and similarities in living and health conditions for Aboriginal communities and/or Torres Strait Islander urban, rural and remote communities.

- HealthInfoNet 2019: https://healthinfonet.ecu.edu.au/
- McCormack, L. A., McBride L. A., & Paasche-Orlow, M. K. (2016). Shifting away from a Deficit Model of Health Literacy. *Journal of Health Communication, 21*(sup 2), 4–5.
- The National Rural Health Alliance (2016) fact sheet: https://www.ruralhealth.org.au/sites/default/files/publications/nrha-factsheet-about-us-jan-2020.pdf
  The Vision of the National Rural Health Alliance, as the peak non-government rural and remote health organisation is good health and wellbeing in rural and remote Australia.
- Wakeman, J., & Humphreys, J. S. (2019). Better health in the bush: Why we urgently need a national rural and remote health strategy. *Medical Journal of Australia, 210*(5), 202–203.

Disparities in health between Aboriginal and Torres Strait Islander peoples and other Australians are shown in many reports, including the annual Close the Gap report and the Australian Institute of Health and Welfare (AIHW) biannual Australia's Health. Reasons for such inequalities include structural inequity, intergenerational trauma, racism and the economic consequences of dispossession (Aboriginal and Torres Strait Islander Social Justice Commissioner, 2005; Australian Institute of Health and Welfare, 2017; Dodson, 1994; Garey, Towney, McPhee, Little, & Kerridge, 2003; Howard-Wagner, Bargh, & Altamirano-Jiménez, 2018).

Box 7.11 Reflection—Exploring reasons for inequalities experienced by Aboriginal and/or Torres Strait Islander peoples

Using the resources in Reflection 7.10, choose the top 10 reasons, as you see them, for the inequalities faced by Aboriginal and Torres Strait Islander peoples today.

You will learn more from the Table of Health Disparity near the end of this chapter. One of the ways Aboriginal people and their supporters have begun to address these problems and grown to care for themselves, their families and each other is by developing a radically different model of health care.

Aboriginal Community Controlled Health Organisations (ACCHOs) and Aboriginal Medical Services (AMS): A wholistic model of primary health care

The first *Aboriginal Medical Service* (AMS) was founded in Redfern, in 1971. As a Community Controlled Health Service, it was the first of its kind in Australia run by Aboriginal and Torres Strait Islander and non-Aboriginal people.

Federal government funding was made available in 1972, a year after its establishment and opening. Today, it has grown into a multidisciplinary health service consisting of a range of clinics; allied health services such as optometry and dentistry; primary health services and health promotional activities; early childhood programs and midwifery, women's health and much more. Aboriginal medical services have been established as community-controlled health services for Aboriginal and Torres Strait Islander communities across the country.

Aboriginal Community Controlled Health Organisations (ACCHOs) have a strong team approach to patient care that has evolved with the services in response to each community's needs. ACCHOs encompass a large range of providers in a unique model of primary health care and often have a less hierarchical culture than a hospital might have. Working with other health professionals in an ACCHOs is a great way to immerse yourself in Aboriginal and Torres Strait islander cultures and learn about our understanding of health. This does not mean that there are not challenges. However, ACCHOs used a primary health care model before it was termed *Primary Health Care* by the World Health Organisation to describe the performance of a broad range of activities and services. They do an excellent job in health promotion, treatment and prevention of disease as well as management of acute and chronic conditions and have been at the forefront of developing the concept and practice of cultural awareness and *cultural safety* by servicing the Aboriginal community's needs and employing Aboriginal health workers who bring their lived experiences, knowledge and understanding of culture.

The importance of understanding health

Health professionals are diverse people. This shows in how each of us views health and defines health. Health and well-being for Aboriginal and Torres Strait Islander peoples has changed dramatically since the invasion and colonisation of Australia.

Our nations are still being disrespected, by other peoples of the many nations that come to our country. We continue to hold a wholistic approach to health and wellbeing.

The fundamental learning, getting to know the diversity of our peoples, is by knowing, doing and being. By getting to know the peoples of the land, working in partnership and collaboration and being respectful, you will have a chance to listen and think about the ways communication flows. Life will lead you to understand culturally safe practices and care. Be guided by our understanding of health:

> Aboriginal health means not just the physical well-being of an individual but refers to the social, emotional and cultural well-being of the whole community in which each individual is able to achieve their full potential as a human being, thereby bringing about the total well-being of their community. It is a whole-of-life view and includes the cyclical concept of life-death-life.
>
> (National Aboriginal Health Strategy [NAHS], 1989a; see also Gee, Dudgeon, Schultz, Hart, & Kelly, 2014, p. 56)

Ten years later the same body (National Aboriginal Health Strategy Working Party, 1989b) stated that

> Health to Aboriginal peoples is a matter of determining all aspects of their life, including control over their physical environment, of dignity, of community self-esteem and of justice. It is not merely a matter of the provision of doctors, hospitals, medicines or the absence of disease and incapacity.
>
> Health care services should strive to achieve the state where every individual is able to achieve their full potential as a human being and thus bring about the total well-being of their community.

These Aboriginal definitions exemplify a strengths-based approach to health. Connection to friends and family, community, environment and cultures increases health and resilience in all people. Aboriginal and Torres Strait Islander peoples can help maintain psychological strength by focussing on what they do well to stay healthy.

Culture is an important determinant of health

Professor Ngiare Brown at the 2013 NACCHO summit said: 'It's time to move away from the deficit model that is implicit in much discussion about the social determinants of health, and instead take a strengths-based cultural determinants approach to improving the health of Aboriginal and Torres Strait Islander people' (Sweet, 2013). The deficit model looks at defining communities and individuals in terms such as negativity, deficiency and failure (Fforde, Bamblett, Lovett, Gorringe, & Fogarty, 2013; Fogarty, Bulloch, McDonnell, & Davis, 2018).

Professor Brown also stressed "the importance of a focus on resilience, and the value of the Aboriginal Community Controlled Health sector as a national network for promoting cultural revitalisation and sustainable intergenerational change".

This has come about because of the lived experience of Aboriginal and Torres Strait Islander peoples, saying health is much more than this, and we need to work with our own worldview and lived experience to adapt and develop the concept. This also includes areas such as racism, oppression, marginalisation and the experienced impact and grief of establishing a penal colony and the treatment of a population group (Aboriginal and Torres Strait Islander peoples) who are still impacted today (Brown & Brown, 2007).

The following show a much broader approach to looking at the social determinants of health and how Aboriginal and Torres Strait Islander peoples are building on what Sir Michael Marmot has brought to the public health arena and World Health Organisation publication of *The Solid Facts* (Wilkinson & Marmot, 2003).

Strong culture and wellbeing are central to the health of Aboriginal and Torres Strait Islander peoples as Professor Brown suggests:

> We represent the oldest continuous culture in the world, we are also diverse and have managed to persevere despite the odds because of our adaptability, our survival skills and because we represent an evolving cultural spectrum inclusive of traditional and contemporary practices. At our best, we bring our traditional principles and practices—respect, generosity, collective benefit, and collective ownership—to our daily expression of our identity and culture in a contemporary context. When we are empowered to do this, and where systems facilitate this reclamation, protection and promotion, we are healthy, well and successful and our communities thrive.
>
> (Brown, 2012, May 20–May 31)

Making the link to AMSs and ACCHOs, Melissa Sweet commented that:

> Key to a social and cultural determinants approach to addressing Aboriginal and Torres Strait Islander health is empowering Aboriginal and Torres Strait Islander services and communities.
>
> (Sweet, 2013)

Box 7.12 Reflection—Considering culture

Discuss individually or in groups what Professor Brown is highlighting about building on determinants of health. Draw a *mind map* showing how as a group you would develop a program to introduce the benefits of including cultural well-being, respect, generosity, collective collaboration, and ownership to the community you are doing the program with.

The *Close the Gap—Progress and Priorities report* (Close the Gap Campaign Steering Committee, 2017) discussed social and cultural determinants of health this way:

> For Aboriginal and Torres Strait Islander peoples, social determinants formed by societal structures and inequalities can be added to the historical impact of colonisation and its contemporary impacts, including the perseverance of racism and the dynamics of cultural misconnection. Hence the term "social and cultural determinants of health" provides a more focused and contextually appropriate means to understanding the nature of the issues faced regarding health equality in Australia.
>
> (Close the Gap Campaign Steering Committee for Indigenous Health Equality, 2017, p. 25)

Box 7.13 Reflection—The establishment of Aboriginal Medical Services (AMS)

Listen to the video and read the blog post by Professor Brown or read the article by Campbell, Hunt, Scrimgeour, Davey, and Jones (2017).

Consider the rationale for the establishment of Aboriginal Medical Services. Why do they work, or not?

Listen to Professor Brown: Winnunga AMS ACT Aboriginal Health in Aboriginal Hands on YouTube.

Or read 'Culture is an important determinant of health, Professor Ngiare Brown at the WHO Summit' at https://blogs.crikey.com.au/croakey/2013/08/20/culture-is-an-important-determinant-of-health-professor-ngiare-brown-at-naccho-summit/

Changes happening for health professional bodies such as Ahpra

In May 2018, the *Australian Health Practitioner Regulation Agency* (Ahpra) (2018) included a comprehensive description of cultural safety for Aboriginal and Torres Strait Islander peoples in *The National Scheme's Aboriginal and Torres Strait Islander Health and Cultural Safety Strategy 2020–2025*, as well as in the Nursing and Midwifery Board of Australia's (2018) *Code of Conduct for Nurses and Midwives*.

It says that regarding

> Aboriginal and Torres Strait Islander health, cultural safety provides a de-colonising model of practice based on dialogue, communication, power sharing and negotiation and the acknowledgement of white privilege.

3.1 Aboriginal and/or Torres Strait Islander peoples' health

Australia has always been a culturally and linguistically diverse nation. Aboriginal and/or Torres Strait Islander peoples have inhabited and cared for the land as the first peoples of Australia for millennia, and their histories and cultures have uniquely shaped our nation. Understanding and acknowledging historic factors such as colonisation and its impact on Aboriginal and/or Torres Strait Islander peoples' health helps inform care. In particular, Aboriginal and/or Torres Strait Islander peoples bear the burden of gross social, cultural and health inequality. In supporting the health of Aboriginal and/or Torres Strait Islander peoples, nurses must:

a. provide care that is wholistic, free of bias and racism, challenges belief based upon assumption and is culturally safe and respectful for Aboriginal and/or Torres Strait Islander peoples
b. advocate for and act to facilitate access to quality and culturally safe health services for Aboriginal and/or Torres Strait Islander peoples, and
c. recognise the importance of family, community, partnership and collaboration in the health care decision-making of Aboriginal and/or Torres Strait Islander peoples, for both prevention strategies and care delivery.

(Nursing and Midwifery Board of Australia, 2018, p. 9)

There is a need to remember that cultural safety grew from a colonised experience (from Maori nurses in New Zealand). Non-Indigenous health professionals who have not had the experience of being colonised and who reap the benefits and privileges of the dominant society need to safeguard that they do not colonise or inhibit cultural safety. For Aboriginal peoples, cultural safety has been talked about for some time; however, they have used different words to express the process.

Cultural safety underpins all nursing practice. The Congress of Aboriginal and Torres Strait Islander Nurses and Midwives (CATSINaM) endorse the NZ Aotearoa model of cultural safety and believe this model should be implemented in Australia in ways that are empowering (Congress of Aboriginal and Torres Strait Islander Nurses and Midwives (CATSINaM), 2014a, 2014b, 2019; Congress of Aboriginal and Torres Strait Islander Nurses and Midwives (CATSINaM) & Nursing and Midwifery Board of Australia, 2018).

Box 7.14 Case study—The seeds of good health in Sydney

Kathleen teaches in a primary school. Her children attend the school, and her husband works at the Aboriginal Medical Service (AMS). At a training course, Kathleen heard about a program called Being Healthy in Mind, Body and Spirit. The program helped Aboriginal and Torres Strait Islander children do better at school. Kathleen is inspired.

She contacts the local Aboriginal Medical Service to talk to them about setting up the program. Maybe health staff could come out to the school, taking time with students to do some health checks? She talks to Kim, the health promotion officer at the AMS, about the program.

Kathleen meets with clinic staff and visiting doctors. They work on putting together their own local program to do hearing checks and three- or four-year-old child health checks. There is a high incidence of hearing problems in the community. There are other health problems, too, including child obesity and lack of good nutrition.

The school has a high proportion of Aboriginal students. They decide to form a working group of people from the AMS, the school and the local Aboriginal community, including local students, to find out what their priorities are. A few of the older students attend the meeting with their parents.

Previously, a nurse thought that it would be good to introduce vitamin tablets to students. But after two weeks of trying to get students to eat the tablets, Kathleen gave up on that.

Kathleen talks with the AMS staff about supplying the school with fruits and vegetables to eat during recess. The response from the students is overwhelming. They happily eat all the fruit supplied.

A committee is established. Teachers, the principal of the school and local parents work together to build raised garden beds and grow eatable native plants around the school.

The school approaches the local council to obtain funding to establish a school garden and bush tucker garden. The committee also gains support from a local nursery.

This leads to the whole community being involved in addressing a need. The project builds physical, mental and spiritual health in students. Teachers use the school garden in curriculum development.

This project brings the community together on several levels to help change the health outcomes of young people. More importantly it brings the diverse community together in a common agenda, to address the needs of their children (Clague, Harrison, Stewart, & Atkinson, 2018).

Box 7.15 Reflection—Questions for discussion

In groups discuss the following. Write down your ideas. Come back to the bigger group to discuss the ideas you gleaned.

- What would be some of the objectives the working group had for the health checks? Why?
- Why would the working group establish a committee?

- Can you think of other ways to get funding and resources to implement the program?
- As a health professional being an advocate is vital. How does it help the client? How does it benefit you?
- How did the working group/committee advocate on behalf of the school students? What were the long-term goals and outcomes?
- The *National Aboriginal Community Controlled Health Organisation* (NACCHO) is the national governing body for the Aboriginal Health Services (AMS). Do you know other Aboriginal health services you can source resources from in each state and the territories?
- Can you evaluate the program? How would you do this? Why would this be important to the community and other stakeholders?

Disparities in health

As a health professional, it is important to understand research and health data such as that shown in Table 7.1. You need to be able to research and apply data from your local area or the community. This will help you establish a basis to run a program with the community, for example, a health-promotion activity, working with the community for better outcomes, via partnership, support, and shared knowledge.

You will be part of building the knowledge base of the community, while learning yourself. This can lead to increased opportunities for positive outcomes linked to health promotion activities. Data is relevant for a whole range of reasons: from funding to developing health promotion activities to understanding a community's needs and demographics (Aboriginal and Torres Strait Islander Social Justice Commissioner, 2005; Durey & Thompson, 2012; Williams, Lawrence, & Davis, 2019).

Use Table 7.2 and the following Activity to learn about applying data to be useful to the community.

Box 7.16 Reflection—Researching best practice health-promotion activities

Using Table 7.2, fill in the spaces by researching best practice health promotion activities, working with Aboriginal and Torres Strait Islander peoples within their communities.

Think about what you have learnt thus far about cultural safety and ways to enhance and embrace partnership, collaboration and use cultural safety with service providers. It may be also good to link to the skills of people in the community such as artists, dancers, elders, youth who are creative in engaging their community, families and individuals so you reach different age-groups, genders, demographics of the community to get the health promotion activity to work. "Think outside the circle" (Clague et al., 2018).

Scenario: Torres Strait

You are a male Remote Area Nurse on an exceedingly small, remote island in the Torres Strait. Three times a week the power goes off all over the island. With every power failure you must take all the vaccines out of the fridge and put them in eskies with frozen bricks to keep them

Table 7.1 Disparity in health between Aboriginal and Torres Strait Islander people and other Australians

Comparing:	*In which States and Territories?*	*For Aboriginal & Torres Strait Islander people (age-adjusted):*
Diabetes (both types)	National	3.5 times more likely to have diabetes 2012–2013.[1] Diabetic deaths are six times higher.[2]
End-stage kidney disease	National	6.8 times the rate 2011–2015.[3]
Cancer	NSW, Qld, SA, WA, NT	1.1 times incidence rate. Death rate 1.4 times higher 2009–2013.[4]
Rheumatic heart disease	NT clearest data Problem is national	98% of cases (NT) Aboriginal or Torres Strait Islander patients.[5]
Tuberculosis	National	Nine times higher 2010–2014.
Smoking	National	Three times higher rate of smoking 2012–2014. National rate has declined by 10% since 2002.[6]
Obesity	National	Second-highest contributor to disease burden after smoking. Six percent higher rate of obesity and overweight than other Australians.[7]
Education	National	Year 12 completed 26% in 2014, up from 17% in 2002; Australia overall: 78% in 2010.[8]
Racism	National	One in three experience racial discrimination 2014.
Poverty	Income Gap is widening in rural and remote areas, closing in urban areas (but the gap persists)	Disposable household income: urban & remote Aboriginal and Torres Strait Islander versus Non-Indigenous income: about 80 and 30 percent, respectively.[9]
Incarceration	Nationally	13 times higher rate of imprisonment.[10]
Infant mortality	NSW, QLD, SA, WA, NT	Twice as high (2015–2017)
Maternal mortality	Nationally	31.6 deaths per 100k women: almost five times higher (4.6 x in 2012–2016).
Death by intentional self-harm	NSW, Qld, SA, WA, NT	Twice as high. Age-adjusted 2017. Suicide is leading cause of death by external cause.[11]

1 Australian Indigenous HealthInfoNet. (2019). *Overview of Aboriginal and Torres Strait Islander health status 2018*. Perth: Australian Indigenous HealthInfoNet

2 https://www.pmc.gov.au/sites/default/files/publications/indigenous/Health-Performance-Framework-2014/tier-1-health-status-and-outcomes/123-leading-causes-mortality.html

3 Healthinfonet. *Op. cit.* 2018.

4 Healthinfonet. *Op. cit.* 2018.

5 Australian Institute of Health and Welfare 2013. Rheumatic heart disease and acute rheumatic fever in Australia: 1996–2012. Cardiovascular disease series. Cat. no. CVD 60. Canberra: AIHW.

6 Australian Bureau of Statistics 2016; National Aboriginal and Torres Strait Islander Social Survey 2014–15 (Released 28 April 2016). Cat. No. 4714.0 Health Risk Factors.

7 Australian Institute of Health and Welfare. Australian Burden of Disease Study 2011: Impact and causes of illness and death in Aboriginal and Torres Strait Islander people (AIHW Cat. No. BOD 7; Australian Burden of Disease Study Series No. 6). Canberra: AIHW, 2016.

8 https://www.abs.gov.au/AUSSTATS/abs@.nsf/Lookup/4102.0Main+Features40Mar+2011. Accessed April 2019.

9 Markham, F., & Biddle, N. (2016). *Income, poverty and inequality*. 2016 Census Paper No. 2ISSN 1442-3871. http://caepr.cass.anu.edu.au/sites/default/files/docs/CAEPR_Census_Paper_2.pdf. Accessed April 2019.

10 Australian Bureau of Statistics Prisoners in Australia 2018 https://www.abs.gov.au/ausstats/abs@.nsf/mf/4517.0. Accessed April 2019.

11 Aboriginal and Torres Strait Islander Health Performance Framework 2014 Report, 1.23 2014.

Table 7.2 Utilising data and information to develop health promotion activities for communities, families and individuals

Health and well-being lens from Aboriginal and / or Torres Strait Islander perspectives on topics such as:	**Health promotion activities that work remember: Focus of engagement by listening What the community wants Bring services to community Build capacity of the community Funding**	**Primary, secondary, tertiary prevention: services to use local/regional, state/ territories, national government and non-government build resources to enhance knowledge**
Diabetes (both types)	Using the Australian Indigenous Health*Info*Net https://healthinfonet.ecu.edu.au/learn/health-topics/diabetes/ Teaching Social Justice Using a Pedagogy of Engagement (Belknap, 2008)	Aboriginal Medical Services may have a diabetes educator/ community nurse specialist that works in diabetes treatment
End-stage kidney		
Cancer		
Rheumatic heart disease		

cold, to preserve them. And then you have no water, so you must keep buckets filled with water to make sure you have water to flush the toilet.

There is a new clinic slowly being built.

The island has a short landing strip, so evacuations of critical patients are done by helicopter. One helicopter serves 16 clinics in the Torres Strait. It takes up to 72 hours for the helicopter to come.

Your team is a single nurse and a Torres Strait Islander Health Worker: Suzie. You can call the doctor for help when you need it. The doctors usually rotate through the roster, so they do not know the staff well.

You have done Remote Isolated Practice Training. You understand the local terrain better than the doctor on the phone. The burden of chronic disease and the severity and complexity of chronic disease is huge. There is poverty on the island with very few opportunities for employment.

One night in the Wet Season a car pulls up in front of the clinic. You have done a long day's work. You have had two hours of sleep.

The patient is a 38-year-old Torres Strait Islander woman called Mary. Her son Leo drove her. Mary is working really hard to breathe. Mary is well known by staff. She has renal disease with complications.

Now think about culturally safe practice in this situation:

Observations

"Mary's creatinine is always far too high. Her kidneys are struggling," Suzie explained. She has treated Mary before in these crises. Mary never wanted to know about her condition or taking medicine. Mary needs a wheelchair into the clinic from the car.

In the clinic, on the exam table, you hook her up to the monitor. Her respiratory rate is 60 breaths per minute—amazingly fast.

Her oxygen saturation is 82% on room air. She is not getting the oxygen she should. Blood pressure is about 80 systolic. You think, *"Her heart's not pumping effectively. The blood's not moving around like it should."* You notice that Mary looks frightened. *"Her skin is so tight you could bounce a coin off it. Mary is massively overloaded with fluid."*

> **Box 7.17 Reflection—Torres Strait**
>
> Reflect on the preceding scenario. Even if you do not know what is happening clinically, think about the following questions:
>
> As a health professional on an island, what are you worried about?
>
> What cultural, social, economic and environmental determinants of poor health have you acknowledged and become aware of?
>
> What kind of pressures do these determinants place on the Torres Strait Islander Health Worker? And on you as the other team member?

Your patient is well and truly in cardiac failure (which means her heart is unable to pump effectively).

Her son Leo is angry, with red eyes from being upset.

You have got her on the bed. Then the power goes off. It is dark. The rain's roaring on the tin roof. Suzie is with you. As you are about to cannulate Mary, Leo says, "If you don't get that cannula in, I'll bash ya."

You feel his breath on your neck. Suzie growls at him in Kriol, but he keeps scowling at you.

Mary body is swollen from the excess fluid. It is difficult to palpate her vein.

> **Box 7.18 Reflection—Potential concerns**
>
> Take a moment: What is important to reflect here? Ask yourself these questions:
>
> Apart from the medicines being given to Mary, what else would be on the Health Worker's mind?
>
> What would you be worrying about? How is this likely to affect your work?

Story continues

With the right medicines, Mary starts to improve. You have to put a urinary indwelling catheter (IDC) in her.

> **Box 7.19 Reflection—Cultural sensitivities**
>
> Take a moment: What is important to consider now?
>
> Ask yourself this question: From a cultural point of view, this is a sensitive situation. Why?
>
> NOTE: In these circumstances tapping into your senses: listening, touch and smell, with careful observation, will enhance your practice of care and your own safety as well as that of those around you.

You have a careful talk to Leo. Suzie is a real help.

You explain, *"Look, we've got your mum this far. I need to put the catheter in to empty her bladder. We have to get the fluid out of her so she can breathe. The medicine will move it out of her. But if urine accumulates in her bladder, it will cause her pain. It could really hurt her. The distress could make her sicker."*

Suzie interprets. Mary is well enough now to consent to the procedure. Leo holds her hand.

Suzie holds Mary's other hand. You place the IDC in under torchlight.

Next, you have to get Mary into the helicopter and to the mainland hospital.

On the phone to the doctor far away, he asks, *"What's Mary's chest sound like?"*

"Mary has got very fine crackles. She's got a wheeze—cardiac asthma."

The doctor asks, *"What does cardiac asthma sound like?"*

You describe Mary's wheeze—which is a sign of heart failure.

In the helicopter, Mary grabs Suzie's hand and your hand and says, *"Thank you for saving my life."*

You are all emotional.

From the hospital Mary is transferred to the Dialysis Unit in town on the mainland.

Mary makes a full recovery.

Scenario summary

Mary was known to the clinic for being very obstinate. She did not want to go to town for dialysis. She did not want to leave the island. She did not want to leave her Country.

But she was not ready to die, either. Because of this incident, Mary was forced to take measures to change and take responsibility for her illness—medically. She accepted that.

It took an enormous amount of work to earn the respect of Mary and Leo. It took time and teamwork, constantly learning, to earn Suzie's respect, also.

Mary came back to visit the island regularly, taking the hour-and-a-half flight. You saw Leo on a number of occasions at the local shop in town. He came over one time to say, *"Oh, thanks for looking after my mum."*

Box 7.20 Reflection—Questions for personal reflection

Take a moment: What is important to think about here? Ask yourself these questions:

What do you know about risk factors for heart failure and kidney disease? Which of these risk factors affect Torres Strait Islander people?

Why was Mary not taking her medicines? What was she afraid of?

How would you help or support Mary if you were living on the island? Or visiting?

Think about how this would have been if you had only arrived three months previously. You and the community are just getting to know each other. What are the lessons learnt, including the cultural protocols as a male or female, in your role as a health professional?

This scenario tells you a story of what can happen in an actual setting. Aboriginal and Torres Strait Islander health professionals (AHPs or AHWs) work 24/7 in their communities. They are a great source of guidance and support; listen to them.

Some settings have resources, and others do not, as shown in this example from a small island in the Torres Strait. Health professionals need to think about the environment and economic situation that form the reality for most communities.

The challenge is, to be challenged:

- To be the safest person you can be in the circumstances you work in.
- Follow the standards of your profession and code of conduct and ethics.
- Keep learning about cultural safety and Aboriginal and Torres Strait Islander people's lived experiences (which is an aspect of their Intellectual Property) as is part of cultural safety.

(Australian Indigenous Doctors' Association, 2013; Brascoupe & Waters, 2009; NSW Ministry of Health, 2019; Smye & Browne, 2002; Thomas, Bainbridge, & Tsey, 2014)

Learn more about this topic

Aboriginal and Torres Strait Islander people affected by cardiovascular risk accounted for 12% of total deaths in Australia in 2017. Compared with non-Aboriginal Australians, Aboriginal and Torres Strait Islander peoples were 70% more likely to die from circulatory diseases.

Renal failure: Aboriginal and Torres Strait Islander peoples experience a disease burden two and a half times higher than in the non-Aboriginal Australian population.

https://www.heartfoundation.org.au/about-us/what-we-do/heart-disease-in-australia/cardiovascular-risk-profile-of-aboriginal-and-torres-strait-islander-peoples

https://kidney.org.au/advocacy/guidance-and-tools/indigenous-health/health-statistics

As Horace Mann famously stated, "A different world cannot be built by indifferent people".

Conclusion

There is still much we need to learn, and also much to accept that we will never know, about the history and society of some of the Aboriginal and Torres Strait Islander nations around Australia.

This continuing learning is no barrier to health professionals learning to change their actions and attitudes in ways that embody and express culturally safe practices and respectful behaviour towards Aboriginal and Torres Strait Islander peoples. We acknowledge the work of health organisations such as Aphra who have worked to embed cultural safe practices in their ethics and standards of care for nurses and midwives practice.

We need to be mindful and respectful of the lived experiences of Aboriginal and Torres Strait Islander peoples. Accessing and using health care can trigger negative reactions that lead to trauma for individuals, families and the whole community.

So, we need to be compassionate, conscientious and mindful to:

- Advocate for, and to be culturally sensitive to, the needs of population groups such as Aboriginal and Torres Strait Islander peoples.
- Call out individual and institutional racism within health care settings and among service providers.
- Acknowledge our own biases. The way we communicate needs to be open and honest to make a difference in the care of Aboriginal and Torres Strait Islander people and their health outcomes.
- Acknowledge the diversity within Aboriginal and Torres Strait Islander populations.
- Look for best practice in health-promotion and primary health care activities.

- Collaborate with health service providers and network with Aboriginal communities with respect and openness to benefit all stakeholders in our quest for better health.
- Take time to build trust in relationships for long-lasting outcomes and change for the good.

Box 7.21 Reflection—Chapter review questions

Aboriginal and Torres Strait Islander people are the first nation peoples of Australia. What makes them uniquely different from what you have learnt and understood from the chapter activities and information?

The federal government legislated an *Aboriginal and Torres Strait Islander Act* to people who identified themselves as Aboriginal and or Torres Strait Islander under the Aboriginal Lands Right Act as a person. Who satisfied what criteria? When did Aboriginal and Torres Strait Islander peoples become citizens of their country?

Compare and contrast the World Health Organisation definition of "health" to the National Aboriginal and Islander Health Organisation (NAIHO) "health" definition developed in 1979.

Explain your understanding of the Close the Gap report's (2017) discussion on the cultural and social determinants of health.

Box 7.22 Reflection—Questions for discussion

If you could apply Professor Brown's cultural and social determinants of health definition, as described in the **Culture Is an Important Determinant of Health** section—what area would you address as a group to campaign, canvas or raise awareness?

As a group, design a diagram to explain the concept of Aboriginal Community Controlled Health Organisations (ACCHO) or Aboriginal Medical Services (AMS) and their role in servicing Aboriginal and Torres Strait Islander peoples.

How best would you explain to someone from overseas the health of Aboriginal and Torres Strait Islander peoples and why they have life expectancy so different from the general population?

Design an image or diagram that expresses an aspect (or several aspects) of Aboriginal and Torres Strait Islander health and embed a health promotion activity that is working.

Useful website resources

- Explore the website of the National Aboriginal Community Controlled Health Organisation https://www.naccho.org.au/ or the Australian Institute of Health and Welfare Cultural safety in health care for Indigenous Australians: monitoring framework at https://www.aihw.gov.au/reports/indigenous-australians/cultural-safety-health-care-framework/contents/summary

Search YouTube for these videos:

- Understanding the concept of privilege
- What is Privilege?
- Macklemore & Ryan Lewis feat. Jamila Woods – White Privilege II

Reading

- Get the news. Read and subscribe to NACCHO Aboriginal Health News Alerts https://nacchocommunique.com/
- Go to https://www.quora.com/ and do a quick search to read the discussion of: 'Why is the concept of 'privilege' useful, above and beyond 'racism' and 'discrimination?'
- The Beyond Blue website has great resources to expand your understanding of mental health and illness in Aboriginal experience. Do a search for 'Aboriginal' on https://beyondblue.org.au/
- Measuring Inequity: A Systematic Review of Methods Used to Quantify Structural Racism (Australian Human Rights and Equal Opportunity Commission, 2017; Australian Human Rights and Equal Opportunity Commission. and Dodson., 1993; Groos, Wallace, Hardman, & Theall, 2018)
- And see the NMBA and CATSINaM joint statement on culturally safe care 2018 at https://www.nursingmidwiferyboard.gov.au/Codes-Guidelines-Statements/Position-Statements/joint-statement-on-culturally-safe-care.aspx

Data

- https://www.aihw.gov.au/reports/life-expectancy-death/deaths/contents/life-expectancy
- https://www.abc.net.au/news/2018-02-08/closing-the-gap/9407824

Map

- https://commons.wikimedia.org/wiki/File:TorresStraitIslandsMap.png

References

Aboriginal and Torres Strait Islander Social Justice Commissioner. (2005). *Social justice report 2005.* Human Rights and Equal Opportunity Commission. https://humanrights.gov.au/sites/default/files/content/social_justice/sj_report/sjreport05/pdf/SocialJustice2005.pdf.

Aboriginal Heritage Organisation. (2006). *Aboriginal Heritage Office.* http://www.aboriginalheritage.org/.

Attenbrow, V. (2010). *Sydney's Aboriginal past: Iinvestigating the archaeological and historical records.* University of New South Wales Press.

Australian Health Ministers' Advisory Council's National Aboriginal and Torres Strait Islander Health Standing Committee. (2016). *Cultural respect framework 2016–2026 for Aboriginal and Torres Strait Islander health: A national approach to building a culturally responsive health system. Australian Health Ministers' Advisory Council.* http://www.coaghealthcouncil.gov.au/Portals/0/National Cultural Respect Framework for Aboriginal and Torres Strait Islander Health 2016_2026_2.pdf.

Australian Health Practitioners Regulation Agenc IAHPRA)y. (2018). *The National Scheme's Aboriginal and Torres Strait Islander health and cultural safety strategy 2020–2025.* https://nacchocommunique.files.wordpress.com/2020/02/aboriginal-and-torres-strait-islander-cultural-health-and-safety-strategy-2020-2025-1.pdf.

Australian Human Rights and Equal Opportunity Commission (2017). *Institutional racism [Conference presentation].* The Alfred Deakin Insitute for Citzenship and Globalisation's Institutional Racism Conference, Melbourne. https://humanrights.gov.au/about/news/speeches/institutional-racism.

Australian Human Rights and Equal Opportunity Commission, & Dodson, M. (1993). *Aboriginal and Torres Strait Islander Social Justice Commission: First report 1993.* https://humanrights.gov.au/our-work/aboriginal-and-torres-strait-islander-social-justice/publications/social-justice-reports.

Australian Indigenous Doctors' Association. (2013). *Cultural safety factsheet: Position paper cultural safety for Aboriginal and Torres Strait Islander doctors, medical students and patients.* https://www.aida.org.au/wp-content/uploads/2018/07/Cultural-Safety-Factsheet_08092015.docx.pdf.

Australian Indigenous HealthInfoNet. (2019). *Australian Indigenous HealthInfoNet.* https://healthinfonet.ecu.edu.au/.

Australian Institute of Aboriginal and Torres Strait Islander Studies. (2019a). *Australian Institute of Aboriginal and Torres Strait Islander Studies.*

Australian Institute of Aboriginal and Torres Strait Islander Studies. (2019b). *Australian Institute of Aboriginal and Torres Strait Islander Studies (AIATSIS).* https://aiatsis.gov.au/explore/articles/indigenous-australian-languages.

Australian Institute of Health and Welfare. (2017). *The health & welfare of Australia's Aboriginal & Torres Strait Islander people.* https://www.aihw.gov.au/reports-data/health-welfare-overview/indigenous-health-welfare/overview.

Belknap, R. A. (2008). Teaching social justice using a pedagogy of engagement. *Nurse Educator, 33*(1), 9–12. https://doi.org/10.1097/01.NNE.0000299499.24905.39.

Brascoupe, S., & Waters, C. (2009). Cultural safety: Exploring the applicability of the concept of cultural safety to Aboriginal health and community wellness. *Journal of Aboriginal Health, 5*(2), 6–40.

Brown, A., & Brown, N. J. (2007). The Northern Territory intervention: Voices from the centre of the fringe. *Medical Journal of Australia, 187*(11–12), 621–623.

Brown, N. (2012, May 20–May 31). *Pacific Caucus Intervention to the 12th Session of the United Nations Permanent Forum on Indigenous Issues.* UNPFII Twelfth Session, United Nations, New York. https://www.un.org/development/desa/indigenouspeoples/unpfii-sessions-2/unpfii-twelfth-session.html.

Campbell, M. A., Hunt, J., Scrimgeour, D. J., Davey, M., & Jones, V. (2017). Contribution of Aboriginal Community-Controlled Health Services to improving Aboriginal health: An evidence review. *Australian Health Review, 42*(2), 218–226.

Clague, L., Harrison, N., Stewart, K., & Atkinson, C. (2018). Thinking outside the circle: Reflections on theory and methods for school-based garden research. *The Australian Journal of Indigenous Education, 47*(2), 139–145. https://doi.org/10.1017/jie.2017.21.

Close the Gap Campaign Steering Committee. (2017). *Close the gap report—Progress and priorities report 2017.* https://humanrights.gov.au/sites/default/files/document/publication/Close the Gap report 2017.pdf.

Concilia Ltd. (2017). *Australians together.* https://australianstogether.org.au/discover/australian-history/get-over-it/.

Congress of Aboriginal and Torres Strait Islander Nurses and Midwives (CATSINaM). (2014a). *Cultural safety position statement.* https://www.catsinam.org.au/static/uploads/files/cultural-safety-endorsed-march-2014-wfginzphsxbz.pdf.

Congress of Aboriginal and Torres Strait Islander Nurses and Midwives (CATSINaM). (2014b). *Towards a shared understanding of terms and concepts: Strengthening nursing and midwifery care of Aboriginal and Torres Strait Islander peoples.* https://www.catsinam.org.au/static/uploads/files/catsinam-cultural-terms-2014-wfwxifyfbvdf.pdf.

Congress of Aboriginal and Torres Strait Islander Nurses and Midwives (CATSINaM). (2019). *Midwifery cultural safety training standards: Background document.* https://www.midwives.org.au/sites/default/files/uploaded-content/website-content/20190416_catsinam_endorsed_background_document_-_midwifery_cultural_safety_training_standards_.pdf.

Congress of Aboriginal and Torres Strait Islander Nurses and Midwives (CATSINaM), and Nursing and Midwifery Board of Australia. (2018). *NMBA and CATSINaM joint statement on culturally safe care.*

https://www.nursingmidwiferyboard.gov.au/codes-guidelines-statements/position-statements/joint-statement-on-culturally-safe-care.aspx.

Dodson, M. (1994). *The end in the beginning: Re(de)finding Aboriginality* [Paper presentation]. The Wentworth Lecture, Australian Aboriginal Studies. https://aiatsis.gov.au/sites/default/files/docs/presentations/1994-wentworth-dodson-michael-end-in-the-beginning.pdf.

Dowling, P. J. (1997). *A great deal of sickness: Introduced diseases among the Aboriginal people of colonial Southeast Australia 1788–1900 [Doctoral Dissertation, Australian National University]*. Open Research. https://open-research-repository.anu.edu.au/handle/1885/7529.

Durey, A., & Thompson, S. C. (2012). Reducing the health disparities of Indigenous Australians: Time to change focus. *BMC Health Services Research*, *12*(151), 1–11. https://doi.org/10.1186/1472-6963-12-151.

Edwards, W. H. (1988). *An introduction to Aboriginal society*. Social Science Press.

Fforde, C., Bamblett, L., Lovett, R., Gorringe, S., & Fogarty, B. (2013). Discourse, deficit and identity: Aboriginality, the race paradigm and the language of representation in contemporary Australia. *Media International Australia, Incorporating Culture and Policy*, *149*(1), 162–173. https://doi.org/10.1177/1329878X1314900117.

Fogarty, W., Bulloch, H., McDonnell, S., & Davis, M. (2018). *Deficit discourse and Indigenous health: How narrative framings of Aboriginal and Torres Strait Islander people are reproduced in policy*. The Lowitja Institute & National Centre for Indigenous Studies. https://www.lowitja.org.au/content/Document/Lowitja-Publishing/deficit-discourse.pdf.

Gardiner-Garden, J. (1996). *The Definition of Aboriginality [Paper presentation]. The Aboriginal Citizenship Conference*, Australian National University, Canberra. http://www.aph.gov.au/LIBRARY/pubs/rn/2000-01/01RN18.htm.

Garey, G., Towney, P., McPhee, J. R., Little, M., & Kerridge, I. H. (2003). Is there an Aboriginal bioethic? *Journal of Medical Ethics*, *30*, 570–575. https://doi.org/10.1136/jme.2002.001529.

Gee, G., Dudgeon, P., Schultz, C., Hart, A., & Kelly, K. (2014). Aboriginal and Torres Strait Islander social and emotional wellbeing. In P. Dudgeon, H. Milroy, & R. Walker (Eds.), *Working together: Aboriginal and Torres Strait Islander mental health and wellbeing principles and practice* (pp. 55–68). Commonwealth of Australia. https://www.telethonkids.org.au/globalassets/media/documents/aboriginal-health/working-together-second-edition/working-together-aboriginal-and-wellbeing-2014.pdf.

Goldsmid, J. M. (1989). Imported disease in Australia: An ongoing problem. In R. Steffen, H. Lobel, J. Haworth, & D. J. Bradley (Eds.), *Travel medicine* (pp. 45–49). Springer. https://doi.org/10.1007/978-3-642-73772-5_7.

Grieves, V. (2009). *Aboriginal spirituality: Aboriginal philosophy, the basis of Aboriginal social and emotional wellbeing, Discussion Paper No. 9*. Cooperative Research Centre for Aboriginal Health. https://www.lowitja.org.au/content/Document/Lowitja-Publishing/DP9-Aboriginal-Spirituality.pdf.

Groos, M., Wallace, M., Hardman, R., & Theall, K. (2018). Measuring inequality: A systematic review of methods used to quantify structural racism. *Journal of Health Disparities Research and Practice*, *11*(2), 190–206.

Hamacher, D. W. (2013). *A shark in the stars: Astronomy and culture in the Torres Strait*. The Conversation. https://theconversation.com/a-shark-in-the-stars-astronomy-and-culture-in-the-torres-strait-15850.

Howard-Wagner, D., Bargh, M., & Altamirano-Jiménez, I. (2018). *The neoliberal state, recognition and indigenous rights: New paternalism to new imaginings*. Australian National University Press.

Irish, P. (2017). *Hidden in plan view: The Aboriginal people of coastal Sydney*. NewSouth Publishing.

Kwaymullina, A. (2013). *How frogmouth found her home*. Fremantle Press.

Marrone, S. (2007). Understanding barriers to health care: A review of disparities in healthcare services among indigenous populations. *International Journal of Circumpolar Health*, *66*(3), 188–198.

McCormack, L. A., McBride, C. M., & Paasche-Orlow, M. K. (2016). Shifting away from a deficit model of health literacy. *Journal of Health Communication*, *21*(sup2), 4–5. https://doi.org/10.1080/10810730.2016.1212131.

McRae, H., Nettheim, G., & Beacroft, L. (1997). "Phillip's Instructions" Barton (1889). *Indigenous legal Issues: Commentary and Materials*, *2*, 33.

Muller, S. (2003). Towards decolonisation of Australia's protected area management: The Nantawarrina Indigenous protected area experience. *Australian Geographical Studies*, *4*(1), 29–43.

National Aboriginal Health Strategy Working Party. (1989a). *National Aboriginal health strategy*. National Aboriginal Health Strategy Working Party.

National Aboriginal Health Strategy Working Party. (1989b).*National Aboriginal Health Strategy (NAHS)*. https://www.atns.net.au/agreement.asp?EntityID=757.

NSW Ministry of Health. (2019). *Aboriginal cultural activities policy*. https://www1.health.nsw.gov.au/pds/ActivePDSDocuments/PD2019_025.pdf - page=4.

Nursing and Midwifery Board of Australia. (2018). *Code of conduct for nurses*. https://www.nursingmidwiferyboard.gov.au/codes-guidelines-statements/professional-standards.aspx.

Pascoe, B. (2014). *Dark emu black seeds: Agriculture or accident?* Magabala Books.

Reynolds, H. (1972). *Aborigines and settlers: The Australian experience, 1788–1939*. Cassell Australia.

Reynolds, H. (1981). *The other side of the frontier: Aboriginal resistance to the European invasion of Australia*. University of New South Wales Press.

Reynolds, H. (1987). *Frontier: Aborigines, settlers and land*. Allen & Unwin.

Roughsey, D. (1992). The rainbow serpent. *HarperCollins Publishers*.

Sangha, K., Le Brocque, A., & Costanza, A. (2015). Ecosystems and indigenous well-being: An integrated framework. *Global Ecology and Conservation*, *4*, 445–458.

Smye, V., & Browne, A. (2002). Cultural safety and the analysis of health policy affecting aboriginal people. *Nurse Researcher*, *9*(3), 42–46.

Stanner, W. (1979). Durmugan: A Nangiomeri (1959). In. W. Stanner (Ed.), *White man got no dreaming: Essays 1938–1973* (pp. 67–105). Australian National University Press.

Stralia Web's Regional Network. (2001). *Manly and Northern Beaches*. https://www.manlyaustralia.com.au/info/history/.

Sweet, M. (2013). *Culture is an important determinant of health: Professor Ngiare Brown at NACCHO Summit*. Croakey. https://croakey.org/culture-is-an-important-determinant-of-health-professor-ngiare-brown-at-naccho-summit/.

The National Rural Health Alliance. (2016). *Food security and health in rural and remote Australia (Publication No. 16/053)*. Rural Industries Research and Development Corporation. https://www.agrifutures.com.au/wp-content/uploads/publications/16-053.pdf.

Thomas, D. P., Bainbridge, R., & Tsey, K. (2014). Changing discourses in Aboriginal and Torres Strait Islander health research, 1914–2014. *Medical Journal of Australia*, *201*(1), S15–S18. https://doi.org/10.5694/mja14.00114.

von Sturmer, J. (1984). The different domains. In Australian Institute of Aboriginial Studies (Ed.), *Aborigines and Uranium: Consolidated report on the social impact of uranium mining on the Aborigines of the Northern Territory* (pp. 218–237). Australian Government Publishing Service. https://nla.gov.au/nla.obj-1826856247/view?partId=nla.obj-1832276824#page/n0/mode/1up.

Utemorrah, D., & Lofts, P. (2004). *Dunbi the owl*. Scholastic Press.

Wakerman, J., & Humphreys, J. S. (2019). Better health in the bush: Why we urgently need a national rural and remote health strategy. *Medical Journal of Australia*, *210*(5), 202–203. https://doi.org/10.5694/mja2.50041.

Warren, C. (Producer). (2019). *Smallpox: 1789 biological war fare against First Nations*.

Watson, I. (1997). Indigenous peoples' law-ways: Survival against the colonial state. *Australian Feminist Law Journal*, *8*(1), 39–58. https://doi.org/10.1080/13200968.1997.11077233.

Whalan, S., Farnbach, S., Volk, L., Gwynn, J., Lock, M., Trieu, K., Brimblecombe, J., & Webster, J. (2017). What do we know about the diets of Aboriginal and Torres Strait Islander peoples in Australia? A systematic literature review. *Australian and New Zealand Journal of Public Health*, *41*(6), 579–584. https://doi.org/10.1111/1753-6405.12721h.

Whitehouse, H., Watkin Lui, F., Sellwood, J., Barrett, M. J., & Chigeza, P. (2014). Sea country: Navigating Indigenous and colonial ontologies in Australian environmental education. *Environmental Education Research Journal*, *20*(1), 56–69.

Wilkinson, R., & Marmot, M. (2003). *Social determinants of health: The solid facts*. World Health Organisation. https://www.euro.who.int/__data/assets/pdf_file/0005/98438/e81384.pdf.

Williams, D., Lawrence, J., & Davis, B. (2019). Racism and health: Evidence and needed research. *Annual Review of Public Health*, *40*, 105–125.

World Health Organisation. (2008). Australia's disturbing health disparities set Aboriginals apart. *Bulletin of the World Health Organisation*, *86*(4), 241–320.

8 Culturally and linguistically diverse Australians

Rocco Cavaleri, Virginia Mapedzahama, Rashmi Pithavadian, Rubab Firdaus, David Ayika and Amit Arora

Learning outcomes

After working through this chapter, students should be able to:

1. Understand Australia's past migration policies and the ways in which they shaped Australian society and culture.
2. Explain the contemporary implications of Australia's migration history for culturally and linguistically diverse Australians.
3. Understand the meaning of the term *culturally and linguistically diverse* (CALD) and critically assess the challenges of using this term.
4. Describe the influence of culture on health and wellbeing.
5. Acknowledge the challenges of culturally safe health care provision among a culturally and linguistically diverse population.

Key terms

Asylum: The right to international protection within a particular country. An "asylum seeker" describes someone who is seeking such protection but whose claim for refugee status has not yet been determined.

Culturally and linguistically diverse (CALD): A term adopted in Australia to describe people with a cultural heritage differing from that of the Anglo-Australian majority. This term includes diversity in terms of country of birth, preferred language, English proficiency and other ethnocultural characteristics such as year of arrival in Australia, religious affiliations and birthplace of parents.

Culture clash: Conflict or tension arising between individuals attributable to dissimilarities in cultural values and practices.

Culture shock: A sense of disorientation or unfamiliarity when experiencing a new cultural environment.

Discrimination: Occurs when a person is excluded from benefits generally available to other members of a society because of a perceived difference or a stigmatised identity.

Ethnicity: A category or group of people who identify with each other, usually on the basis of presumed similarities such as common language, geography, ancestry, history, society, culture and/or social treatment.

Ethnocentrism: Evaluation of other cultures according to preconceptions originating in the standards and customs of one's own culture.

Migration: The movement of people from one place to another with the intention of settling.

Prejudice: A preconceived belief regarding another individual based upon their membership, affiliation or affinity with a particular group or cultural identify.
Race: A socially constructed grouping of humans based on shared physical categories generally viewed as distinct by a society.
Racism: A socially constructed grouping of humans based on shared physical categories generally viewed as distinct by a society..
Refugee: An individual who is forced to leave their country of origin and is unable to return due to the threat of persecution or harm. Refugees have been formally recognised under the *1951 Convention Relating to the Status of Refugees.*

Chapter summary

This chapter will develop students' understanding of Australia's migration history. There will be a brief discussion of migration that occurred following the arrival of the first Europeans through to the mid-1970s, marking the end of the White Australia Policy. Australia's contemporary migration history (including refugees and asylum seekers) will be discussed in more depth, and students will be introduced to the concept of "multiculturalism" as it has been understood across this century. These discussions will be framed by debates around how race and ethnicity are understood in contemporary Australia. Again, links to power, racism, prejudice, discrimination, culture shock and culture clash will be examined. Exploration of these concepts will enable readers to develop an appreciation for the experiences and difficulties associated with migrating. Through cases that span Australia's migration history, students will be able to reflect on their own ancestry and the roles and impact migration has had on health and wellbeing. The concept of CALD Australians will be critically discussed, and the complications inherent in this term will be explored. The health and wellbeing needs of a variety of CALD Australian groups will be discussed such that students are able to develop an understanding of the diversity within and across CALD groups. In doing so, students will engage in activities to explore their perceptions of themselves, others who are not like them and the implications of these differences on their future interactions with people from cultures or language groups not like their own.

Introduction

Australia has a unique history that has shaped the ethnocultural diversity of its people. Over a relatively short time frame, the nation has transitioned from a society predicated on mono-cultural British values to one that embraces and celebrates diversity. Indeed, Australia now represents one of the most culturally and linguistically diverse populations in the world. Approximately 75% of people in Australia identify with an ancestry other than Australian, and over one-quarter of the population were born overseas (Australian Bureau of Statistics, 2016). This transition to multiculturalism has not been without challenges, and multiple iterations to Australian immigration policies have been required to reveal diversity as a necessity for the nation's growth and prosperity.

With increasing diversity comes a broader set of belief systems regarding health and illness. Culture greatly influences health practices and help-seeking behaviours (Knipscheer & Kleber, 2008). Achieving equitable health outcomes for culturally and linguistically diverse communities is therefore complex, requiring consolidated efforts across political, organisational, and professional levels of health care. Multiple barriers must be overcome to ensure that all individuals are able to access equitable and effective care, irrespective of their beliefs or affiliations.

This chapter introduces students to the concept of *culturally and linguistically diverse* (CALD) Australians. The discussion is introduced through the socio-historical context of Australia's *migration* policies, which have profoundly influenced the nation's ethnocultural landscape. The diversity of Australia's population is highlighted, along with some of the challenges that multiculturalism has presented over time. The inextricable link between health and culture is then explored, along with the current barriers CALD populations face in achieving equitable access to health care. The chapter concludes with practical tips and strategies that may be employed to promote cultural responsiveness within the health care setting.

Australia's migration policies—A brief history

With a history dating approximately 70,000 years and comprising over 700 language groups, Indigenous Australians represent the nation's first inhabitants and the oldest continuous culture on Earth (Mence, Gangell, & Tebb, 2017). In 1788, policies arising from colonisation subjected approximately three-quarters of a million of Australia's First Peoples to violence and dispossession (O'Dowd, 2011). Australian society has since been shaped by successive changes to government policy. Accordingly, the ethnocultural composition of Australia has changed greatly over the last 250 years.

Australia's first migrant populations were predominately from the United Kingdom, driven by early colonisation throughout the 1700s (Mence et al., 2017). Australia was used by Britain initially as a means by which to ameliorate prison overcrowding, with approximately 165,000 convicts being transported to Australia by 1868 (Richards, 1987). During this time, free settlers also arrived from Britain and Ireland to farm and occupy land, often without authority or payment (Richards, 1987). Non-European migration began throughout the 18th and 19th centuries due to the "gold rush" and demand for labour. Racial hostilities ensued, with the British majority exhibiting a preference for a homogenous, "white" Australia (Jayasuriya, 1996; Mence et al., 2017). Indeed, a primary impetus for the Australian federation in 1901 was the desire for a unified immigration policy (Mence et al., 2017).

The *White Australia Policy* was instituted via legislative amendments from federation until the late 1950s, with some elements of the policy continuing as late as the 1970s (Mence et al., 2017). This policy sought to prevent immigration into Australia from non-European countries. The primary mechanism by which people were excluded from Australia was the *dictation test* (Palfreeman, 1958). This test, instituted between 1901 and 1958, required a person seeking entry into Australia to write out a passage dictated to them in any European language, at the discretion of an immigration officer. In a fundamental example of racial exclusion and *discrimination*, the test was applied selectively to non-European migrants and always in a language that the applicant was known not to speak (McNamara, 2009). The White Australia policy excluded all non-European immigration into Australia, resulting in a largely British-European culture. Following World War II, Australian governments expressed the belief that Australia must increase its population to avoid the threat of future invasion. The Assisted Passage Migration Scheme was created in 1945 as part of a newly developed "Populate or Perish" policy (Burnley, 2001; Mence et al., 2017). However, societal expectations were still grounded in assimilation, with the belief that migrants should adopt the English language and "Australian values" (Burnley, 2001; Mence et al., 2017). Eventually, Australia began accepting *refugees* who were seeking *asylum*. From World War II until 1954, over 180,000 people were sponsored by the International Refugee Organisation to resettle from Europe to Australia on humanitarian grounds (Stats, 2014). From 1964, Australia began to transition towards policies favouring integration over assimilation, promoting a greater level of cultural and linguistic diversity (Van Krieken, 2012). Integration policies encouraged migrants to adopt Australian values while also retaining their own unique languages and customs.

With the abolition of the White Australia Policy, and the eventual introduction of the Racial Discrimination Act in 1975, migration patterns shifted from Southern Europeans in the 1960s to people from South-East Asia and the Middle East between the 1970s and 1980s (Mence et al., 2017; Phillips, Klapdor, & Simon-Davies, 2010). The Racial Discrimination Act made racially based selection criteria unlawful, and Australia began to transition from policies promoting integration towards those appreciating "multiculturalism". The government-led promotion of multiculturalism represented the official acceptance of diversity as a necessity for Australia's growth and prosperity.

Contemporary Australia and cultural diversity

Despite considerable initial shortcomings, ongoing iterations to Australia's migration policies have seen the establishment of a rich and diverse society. Australia is now represented by over 300 distinct ancestries, and approximately 21% of Australians speak a language other than English on a day-to-day basis (Australian Bureau of Statistics, 2016). Migration is Australia's largest source of population growth today, with nearly one-fifth of the overseas-born Australian population arriving in the last decade (Australian Bureau of Statistics, 2019). These data highlight why Australia is now celebrated as one of the most ethnoculturally diverse countries in the world. Indeed, with over one-quarter of Australians being born overseas, the nation ranks third globally in terms of the number of international migrants relative to its population (International Organization for Migration, 2019).

Who are culturally and linguistically diverse Australians?

The term *culturally and linguistically diverse* (CALD) has been used in Australia since the 1990s when referring to non-Indigenous people with a cultural heritage differing from that of the English-speaking, Anglo-Saxon majority (Adusei-Asante & Adibi, 2018). Indigenous Australians are generally not included when referring to CALD communities during research or policy discourse because their experiences and needs as First Nation peoples are considered to differ significantly from other ethnocultural groups (Sawrikar & Katz, 2009).

Over a relatively short time frame, Australia has transitioned from a society that valued cultural homogeneity to one that embraces and celebrates diversity. Even a quick perusal of Australia's 2016 census data reveals the incredible diversity present amongst individuals living in Australia (Table 8.1). Apart from English (73%), languages commonly spoken at home include Mandarin (2.5%), Arabic (1.4%), Cantonese (1.2%), Vietnamese (1.2%) and Italian (1.2%) (Australian Bureau of Statistics, 2016).

Table 8.1 The diverse Australian population—Country of birth (COB)

Country of birth (COB)	*Australian population*	*Predominant religion in COB*	*Predominant language in COB*
England	907,570	Christianity	English
New Zealand	518,466	Christianity	English
China	509,555	Atheist	Mandarin
India	455,389	Hinduism	Hindi
Philippines	232,386	Christianity	Tagalog
Vietnam	219,351	No religion (or Vietnamese folk religion)	Vietnamese
Italy	174,042	Christianity	Italian

Data integrated from Australian Bureau of Statistics (2016) and Munro (2017).

As multiculturalism has grown throughout Australia, so, too, have discussions regarding the most appropriate way to refer to these "diverse" groups. The CALD label replaced the term *Non-English Speaking Background* (NESB), which had been used since the 1970s (Adusei-Asante & Adibi, 2018; Sawrikar & Katz, 2009). This was because NESB was considered to have conflicting meanings and did not adequately identify the many cultural and linguistic groups in Australia (Adusei-Asante & Adibi, 2018; Sawrikar & Katz, 2009). NESB also eventually developed negative connotations because it distinguished people based on their *non*-English heritage, promoting a sense of exclusion and portraying people of diverse backgrounds as not entirely *Australian* (Adusei-Asante & Adibi, 2018; Sawrikar & Katz, 2009). Conversely, CALD does not assign a stereotypical characteristic from which minority groups deviate. The term also subtly highlights potential barriers faced by individuals of differing cultural and linguistic characteristics and is flexible enough to be inclusive of all ethnic groups (Sawrikar & Katz, 2009). Despite these benefits, there exists contention regarding the definition and appropriateness of the CALD label. Accordingly, for the purpose of this chapter, we define CALD as a term adopted in Australia to describe people with a cultural heritage differing from that of the Anglo-Australian majority. This term includes diversity in terms of country of birth, preferred language, English proficiency, and other ethnocultural characteristics such as year of arrival in Australia, religious affiliations, and birthplace of parents (Australian Bureau of Statistics, 2014).

Although CALD is now the preferred term in Australia, it is important to note that the term is indeed uniquely Australian, and no other countries have formally adopted this label. Additionally, like the term NESB before it, the CALD label has been highly criticised by some scholars. For example, current definitions of CALD exclude people of Anglo-Saxon origin, implying that their cultural or linguistic diversity is not present or "sufficiently" diverse (Adusei-Asante & Adibi, 2018; Sawrikar & Katz, 2009). It has been argued that celebrating multiculturalism more broadly, including the Anglo-Saxon majority, would allow cultural diversity to become more of an intrinsic part of the Australian identity (Sawrikar & Katz, 2009). Further, CALD does not acknowledge that racial difference may also contribute to disparity and exclusion. Several alternate terms have therefore been proposed, each with their own unique set of advantages and disadvantages.

Notwithstanding the imperfections of the CALD label, its sentiment reflects the remarkable journey Australia has taken towards embracing and promoting diversity. Australian governments have celebrated this journey as a triumph in overcoming division and promoting multicultural cohesion. However, multiculturalism is not without challenges. One pressing challenge is the capacity of health care providers and authorities to meet the needs of a culturally diverse population. Achieving equitable health outcomes for CALD communities is complex and multifaceted, requiring consolidated efforts across political, organisational, and professional levels of health care.

The relationship between culture and health

Culture and health practices are inextricably linked, and belief systems greatly influence our perceptions of health and illness. In Australia, the dominant institutional health belief system is underpinned by the "biomedical" model. This model is grounded in physiological processes, focusing upon objective analysis and responding to illness (Holland, 2017). The biomedical model holds individuals responsible for their health and considers clinicians to be knowledgeable and respectable (Holland, 2017; Zwi, Woodland, Kalowski, & Parmeter, 2017). However, this Western-originated model does not necessarily align with those present throughout a culturally and linguistically diverse society. For example, the "spiritual" belief system, common among North African and Middle Eastern cultures, considers illness to be beyond individual control

(Holland, 2017). Under this model, health and prosperity is influenced by supernatural forces, and prevention of illness requires respect to be paid to family, friends and ancestors. The "traditional" belief system emphasises the relationship between the human body, our surroundings and the supernatural world (Holland, 2017). In traditional Chinese and Ayurvedic medicines, illness is prevented by maintaining balance and harmony, with the individual actively contributing to the maintenance of their own health and wellbeing (Zwi et al., 2017). Understandably, the dominance of the biomedical model in Australia has been cited as a common source of "*culture shock*" among individuals with differing health beliefs (Zwi et al., 2017). This culture shock refers to a sense of disorientation or unfamiliarity when experiencing a new cultural environment (Xia, 2009).

Box 8.1 Reflection—Your cultural identity

How would you describe your cultural identity? Consider the following:

- The foods you eat
- The clothing you wear
- Celebrations, festivals or holidays in which you participate
- Music and dance with which you engage
- The language you speak at home and at school or work
- Your religious beliefs
- Anything else that is important to you and your cultural group

What is "health" in your culture?

Think about the ways in which you would describe a healthy individual. Do you think that any of your health practices might conflict with those practiced under a biomedical model?

There is a plethora of ways in which culture may alter our response to any given health encounter. Certain diagnoses may not be recognised or accepted across all health belief models, and what constitutes *illness* may vary. For example, in Western countries, mental illnesses are most commonly attributed to either sociological or biological causes (Furnham & Wong, 2007). Conversely, in rural China, supernatural phenomena, such as witchcraft or evil spirits, are also considered to be important causes of mental health problems (Furnham & Wong, 2007). Where one individual may seek treatment, another may suppress their symptoms due to cultural stigma or fear of spiritual repercussions, and yet another may not consider their current state to reflect illness at all. People can draw upon multiple health belief models and may alter their practices and expression of beliefs during times of adversity. Such complexity poses a number of challenges for the Australian health care system, and difficulty responding to these cultural requirements has been identified as a key driver of health disparities (Johnstone & Kanitsaki, 2007).

The "healthy migrant effect"

The health profile of migrant communities throughout Australia is generally considered to be favourable. Indeed, migrant populations demonstrate 15% lower mortality rates than Australian-born individuals and show a lower prevalence of many lifestyle-related risk factors (Australian Institute of Health and Welfare, 2018). This health profile has seen the development of a theory known as the "healthy migrant effect". According to this theory, migrants possess a better health status than host communities because of pre-migration health screening, as well as self-selection, where only healthy migrants have the financial capacity to relocate (Moullan & Jusot, 2014). However, these data do not take into account differences between English- and non-English-speaking migrants or account for families that experience a decline in their health status over time due to acculturation and environmental changes. Acculturation describes the process in which individuals of one cultural group adopt the beliefs of another group over time (Delavari, Sønderlund, Swinburn, Mellor, & Renzaho, 2013). Previous research suggests that older generations tend to maintain more traditional belief systems, while young adults and children more readily adopt new languages and belief systems (Delavari et al., 2013; Thomson & Hoffman-Goetz, 2009). Migrant morbidity and mortality data is also likely skewed because many individuals who become unwell choose to return to their countries of origin to rest or die among family and friends (Wallace & Kulu, 2018).

Health disparities

In support of the "healthy migrant effect", Australians arriving from English-speaking counties typically demonstrate high quality of life scores and reduced risk of chronic disease (Australian Institute of Health and Welfare, 2018). However, when migrants are examined based upon country of birth, a far more variable health profile emerges. For example, individuals from the Middle East have lower rates of physical activity and a higher rate of chronic disease compared to Australian-born communities (Dassanayake, Dharmage, Gurrin, Sundararajan, & Payne, 2011). Communities from South-East Asia, Southern Europe and Eastern Europe also have a higher risk of sedentary behaviours (Dassanayake et al., 2011). Interestingly, previous research has demonstrated that both English- and non-English-speaking migrants may be at a higher risk of mental health issues, particularly depression (Straiton, Grant, Winefield, & Taylor, 2014). However, findings regarding mental health are mixed, with other studies showing no difference between overseas- and Australian-born individuals (Liddell, Nickerson, Sartor, Ivancic, & Bryant, 2016).

Box 8.2 Case study—Social and cultural context of the mental health of Filipinas in Queensland

Extracted from Thompson, Manderson, Woelz-Stirling, Cahill, & Kelaher (2002)

Filipina women say that the family is the main source of emotional and instrumental support in the Philippines, whereas in Australia, in the absence of family, it is the individual. Separation from family is often exacerbated by the unmet expectation that the husband will be the main confidant and source of emotional support in Australia. It is this absence of support, rather than the presence of additional stressors, that nearly all of the Filipinas interviewed in this study see as the main cause for depression and emotional problems. For example, problems in raising children are not seen as a contributor to stress; instead it is the lack of support in the absence of extended family in assisting with the task. Women say that depression and emotional problems are uncommon in the Philippines because an individual always has a family member to whom they can talk and who will support them:

> Depression is not common in the Philippines. It is non-existent. They can always relate to someone else. They can always have someone to talk to and support them. There is no such thing as depression.

Depression in Australia is therefore seen as the result of an absence of family:

> We're more depressed here because I don't think I am happy because my family's not around here. I have to go on with my life with only my husband and my daughter. If I'm living in the Philippines I have my sister there and I can say my problem.

Self-Reflection Task:

1. Who are key confidants and sources of emotional support for you?
2. Think about a friend or a person who you know who is from a culturally and linguistically diverse background. What may be some emotional support mechanisms for him/her?
3. Are these similar to you, or are they different? Why may they be similar or different?

Barriers to CALD health care

There are several barriers to accessing equitable and effective care throughout a diverse population. Health care services and belief models may differ greatly in an individual's country of origin. Expectations regarding the accessibility and effectiveness of services may also influence help-seeking behaviour, which has been shown to be lower among migrant populations (Knipscheer & Kleber, 2008). Additionally, the individualistic nature of Australian health care provision may generate concern among people from more collectivist cultures, such as those present in African American or Indian societies (Zwi et al., 2017). In collectivist cultures, groups, families and religious leaders are consulted before making decisions that may affect one's health or community. Such individuals may feel pressured by certain clinicians to make decisions without being offered this opportunity for broader consultation, often leading to feelings of helplessness (McLaughlin & Braun, 1998; Roberts, Jadalla, Jones-Oyefeso, Winslow, & Taylor, 2017).

Another one of the most apparent barriers to health care is limited English proficiency. Although professional interpreters have been shown to improve health outcomes among non-English-speaking individuals, their utilisation is not without challenges, and there remains an unmet need for interpreters across many health systems (Flores, Abreu, Barone, Bachur, & Lin, 2012; Gill, Beavan, Calvert, & Freemantle, 2011; Phillips & Travaglia, 2011). Patients may be reluctant to share sensitive information with an interpreter present, and there may be difficulties ensuring all parties understand medical or colloquial terminology (Hunt & de Voogd, 2007). Translated health education material may also not be adequate, as it typically assumes a high degree of health literacy and understanding of Western medical concepts (Arora, Liu, Chan, & Schwarz, 2012).

Box 8.3 Reflection—Practical tips for working with interpreters

- Try to identify cultural differences in yourself and your patients. Be self-aware of biases and values that you may be bringing into the situation.
- Use a trained interpreter rather than a family member to translate.

- Familiarise yourself with the professional interpreter.
- Speak with the interpreter before each appointment to clarify expectations.
- Arrange for triangular seating, so everyone present can see nonverbal cues.
- Introduce everyone who is present in the setting.
- Look at family members as you speak, and try to speak directly with them.
- Be aware of differences in communication styles (e.g., verbal and nonverbal).
- Consider the role of silences in each interaction. They may represent discomfort with a topic or uncertainty about a question being asked.
- Use the interpreter to ensure the patient understands the key take-home messages.
- Use the interpreter to arrange the next appointment and confirm commuting arrangements.
- Use the interpreter to ensure the patient understands how to cancel or change appointments if anything changes.
- Debrief with interpreter afterward to ensure communications were fully translated.

Beyond language itself, communication styles vary across cultures and have been shown to influence patient satisfaction and health outcomes (Williams, Weinman, & Dale, 1998). In some cultures, including English, the content of an exchange is considered to be more important than the context in which it is delivered (Hall, 1959). Addressing specific questions is prioritised in the health care setting, and achieving a particular task may be emphasised more than relationship building (Zwi et al., 2017). Conversely, in other cultures, such as Indigenous Australian, Chinese and Arabic, communication is heavily influenced by context (Hall, 1959). Relationship building may be emphasised before a particular task is attempted, and non-verbal communication and the social status of the speaker are given particular consideration (Kim, Pan, & Park, 1998). These varying styles may present difficulties in the health care setting and have been cited as a common source of "*culture clash*" (Roberts, 2008). A culture clash refers to conflict or tension arising between individuals attributable to dissimilarities in cultural values and practices (Ngo, 2008). For example, context-based communicators may view those who do not value context as rude or abrupt. Conversely, some people may view context-based communicators as verbose or lacking respect for people's time.

Box 8.4 Case study—Barriers accessing mental health services among Culturally and Linguistically Diverse (CALD) immigrant women in Australia: Policy implications

Extracted from Wohler & Dantas (2017).

CALD immigrant women voiced their difficulties in communicating with service providers due to lack of proficiency in English. Fear of being judged, of not being understood, of losing their job, of being hospitalised and of community and family's reactions were major concerns. Many women were uncomfortable discussing personal issues in a foreign language. In some cases, culture-specific syndromes or daily emotional stressors related to acculturation could not be clearly articulated in English. Hence, daily living stress can potentially lead to misinterpretation and misdiagnosis. Even though interpreters could be requested for assistance, many women were concerned about confidentiality, especially if they came from a small ethnic group. Some doctors were reported to be reluctant to use interpreters, and researchers suggested that health practitioners may view refugee women as a source of income rather than a person requiring assistance. The use of interpreters often impacted on the duration of the consultation, reducing the number of appointments available to the general public.

Self-Reflection Task:

1. Why is communication important in health care?
2. What are some ways in which you could potentially reduce communication barriers with your patients?

Ethnocentrism, both conscious and unconscious, has also been shown to impact health care delivery (Capell, Dean, & Veenstra, 2008). Ethnocentrism refers to the tendency of individuals to view the world and people of other cultures through the lens of their own cultural group. Clinicians may perceive their views to be the "correct" one, limiting exploration or understanding of patient perspectives. Likewise, patients may not be willing to accept advice given to them by clinicians whose broader belief systems do not align with their own.

Box 8.5 Case study—Sikh from India refused to have his hair removed prior to heart catheterisation

Extracted from Galanti (2014).

Raj Singh, a 72-year-old Sikh from India, had been admitted to the hospital after a heart attack. He was scheduled for a heart catheterisation to determine the extent of the blockage in his coronary arteries. The procedure involved running a catheter up the femoral artery, located in the groin, and then passing it into his heart, where special x-rays could be taken. His son was a cardiologist on staff and had explained the procedure to him in detail.

Susan, his nurse, entered Mr. Singh's room and explained that she had to shave his groin to prevent infection from the catheterization. As she pulled the razor from her pocket, she was suddenly confronted with the sight of shining metal flashing in front of her. Mr. Singh had a short sword in his hand and was waving it at her as he spoke excitedly in his native tongue. Susan got the message. She would not shave his groin.

She put away her "weapon", and he did the same. Susan, thinking the problem was that she was a woman, said she would get a male orderly to shave him. Mr. Singh's eyes lit up again as he angrily yelled, "No shaving of hair by anyone!"

Susan managed to calm him down by agreeing. She then called her supervisor and the attending physician to report the incident. The physician said he would do the procedure on an unshaved groin. At that moment, Mr. Singh's son stopped by. When he heard what had happened, he apologized profusely for not explaining his father's Orthodox Sikh customs.

Self-Reflection Task:

1. Do you have beliefs or customs that may not resonate with Western medicine?
2. Have you ever experienced "culture clash" within or beyond the health care setting?

Culturally safe health care with CALD communities

Appreciating the influence of culture on an individual's health is integral in promoting equitable health care delivery. Developing culturally safe professional practice requires a concerted effort at all levels of the health care system. Practical approaches such as cultural safety training and case management across health care providers and community leaders have been shown to enhance access and effectiveness (Joshi et al., 2013; Zwi et al., 2017). In some cultures, offering gender-specific clinicians or the option to preferentially select providers has also been shown to improve outcomes (Joshi et al., 2013). Beyond these steps, clinicians should be encouraged to reach a mutual understanding of their patient's presentation, health beliefs, assumptions, support networks, and treatment preferences. Rather than assuming the traditional biomedical role of an "expert" seeking to educate, it is often beneficial to first understand the patient's perspective and generate a therapeutic relationship.

Continually seeking information regarding differing health belief systems and adopting an empathetic cultural approach is helpful when interacting with people throughout a multicultural community. Clinicians focused on client cultural safety will appropriately consider the clinical environment and utilise open-ended questions combined with active listening. However, it is also important to acknowledge that developing culturally safe approaches is an iterative process, and people will inevitably face misunderstandings or make mistakes. An important way of mitigating such issues is ensuring that the patient and their family are made aware that the health care provider's intention is to provide the best care possible (Zwi et al., 2017). When explicitly unified in this goal, errors or misunderstandings are more likely to be understood and forgiven.

It is important to reflect consistently on the ways in which cultural issues may impact particular interactions. Zwi et al. (2017) provide a number of practical tips for maintaining culturally safe practice, including adapting processes to improve communication and responding to signs indicating that a patient or their family have withdrawn or disengaged. Frameworks, such as the LEARN model, are also useful in exploring health beliefs and developing collaborative health care plans (Berlin & Fowkes, 1983).

Box 8.6 Reflection—The LEARN model (Berlin & Fowkes, 1983)

Listen with empathy.

Explain your understanding of a particular problem.

Acknowledge and discuss similarities or differences in perspectives, explaining the reasoning behind your own recommendations.

Recommend a patient-centred health care plan.

Negotiate and collaboratively agree upon a course of action.

Self-Reflection Task:

1. In your health profession, you see a 10-year-old girl developing some hints of depression and oppositional behaviour. You ask her mother about these behaviours and find that she is not sharing much information. You ask the child, "How are things going at home?" Your question is greeted by silence. Her mother looks away. How would you apply LEARN model in the above case?
2. In your health profession, you are seeing Asma, a 40-year-old woman who has recently arrived as a refugee from Iraq and mainly speaks Arabic. Asma is expressing concerns regarding her youngest daughter, Zahra. Asma's eldest son, Fariz,

> a 13-year-old, agrees to translate for you. Using the LEARN model, you start by asking open-ended questions about the family's migration history and their prior and current living conditions. Fariz tells you most of the story without asking his parents questions. When you ask about challenges with acculturation, Fariz replies that the family is "doing fine." You later learn that his younger sister Zahra, aged 5, says only a few words. You wonder how you might gain a clearer understanding of the issues contributing to Zahra's developmental delay. How would you approach this situation?

Health practitioners may wonder about where to go to find guides to support culturally safe health care practice. Some practitioners have found useful information about how to develop health-promoting therapeutic relationships by utilising tools such as the Cultural Awareness Tool. Although there has been limited evaluation of their effectiveness, such tools provide a foundational step towards cultural safety and provide lists of questions to ask of patients so the health care provider can better understand their expectations, priorities and beliefs (Wright, Seah, Tilbury, Rooney, & Jayasuriya, 2003). Providers can also seek feedback from patients regarding their provision of cultural safety using checklists such as the Iowa Cultural Understanding Assessment–Client Form (Center for Substance Abuse Treatment, 2014) or reflect upon their own level of cultural safety using tools provided by the National Center for Cultural Competence (https://nccc.georgetown.edu/). Indeed, health care providers have the responsibility to adapt their practice to achieve culturally safe practice and optimise health care delivery for all individuals throughout Australia's rich and diverse population.

Conclusion

This chapter has introduced students to socio-political factors that have shaped Australia's cultural and linguistic diversity and presented some of the challenges associated with health care delivery in this context. Students should now have an appreciation for the broad policy changes that have transformed Australia into a multicultural nation over time. The chapter also highlighted the link between culture, health and wellbeing, and presented a number of health belief models beyond the mainstream biomedical model employed throughout Australia. Upon completing this chapter, students should now have an appreciation for the health disparities present throughout CALD communities, and have a framework from which to develop strategies to enhance their own cultural responsiveness. Addressing the health care gap among CALD communities requires a concerted effort among all providers, and the knowledge acquired throughout this chapter represents the first step in ensuring equitable and effective care for all Australians moving forward.

References

Adusei-Asante, K., & Adibi, H. (2018). The culturally and linguistically diverse (CALD) label: A critique using African migrants as exemplar. *The Australasian Review of African Studies, 39*(2), 74.

Arora, A., Liu, M. N., Chan, R., & Schwarz, E. (2012). English leaflets are not meant for me: A qualitative approach to explore oral health literacy in Chinese mothers in southwestern sydney, Australia. *Community Dentistry and Oral Epidemiology, 40*(6), 532–541.

Australian Bureau of Statistics. (2014). *Cultural and linguistic diversity (CALD) characteristics (no. 4529.0.00.003)*. https://www.abs.gov.au/ausstats/abs@.nsf/Lookup/by Subject/4529.0.00.003~2014~Main Features~Cultural and Linguistic Diversity (CALD) Characteristics~13.

Australian Bureau of Statistics. (2016). *Census quickstats*. https://quickstats.censusdata.abs.gov.au/census_services/getproduct/census/2016/quickstat/036.

Australian Bureau of Statistics. (2019). *Australian demographic statistics, Dec 2019* (no. 3101.0). https://www.abs.gov.au/Ausstats/abs@.nsf/7d12b0f6763c78caca257061001cc588/fa9c11f1913bdafcca25765100098359!OpenDocument.

Australian Institute of Health and Welfare. (2018). *Australia's health 2018*. https://www.aihw.gov.au/getmedia/7c42913d-295f-4bc9-9c24-4e44eff4a04a/aihw-aus-221.pdf.aspx?inline=true.

Berlin, E. A., & Fowkes Jr, W. C. (1983). A teaching framework for cross-cultural health care: Application in family practice. *The Western Journal of Medicine*, *139*(6), 934–938.

Burnley, I. H. (2001). *The impact of immigration on Australia: A demographic approach*. Oxford University Press.

Capell, J., Dean, E., & Veenstra, G. (2008). The relationship between cultural competence and ethnocentrism of health care professionals. *Journal of Transcultural Nursing*, *19*(2), 121–125. https://doi.org/10.1177/1043659607312970.

Center for Substance Abuse Treatment. (2014). Improving cultural competence. Substance Abuse and Mental Health Services Administration.

Dassanayake, J., Dharmage, S. C., Gurrin, L., Sundararajan, V., & Payne, W. R. (2011). Are Australian immigrants at a risk of being physically inactive? *International Journal of Behavioral Nutrition and Physical Activity*, *8*(1), 53. https://doi.org/10.1186/1479-5868-8-53.

Delavari, M., Sønderlund, A. L., Swinburn, B., Mellor, D., & Renzaho, A. (2013). Acculturation and obesity among migrant populations in high income countries. A systematic review. *BMC Public Health*, *13*(1), 458. https://doi.org/10.1186/1471-2458-13-458.

Flores, G., Abreu, M., Barone, C. P., Bachur, R., & Lin, H. (2012). Errors of medical interpretation and their potential clinical consequences: A comparison of professional versus ad hoc versus no interpreters. *Annals of Emergency Medicine*, *60*(5), 545–553. https://doi.org/10.1016/j.annemergmed.2012.01.025.

Furnham, A., & Wong, L. (2007). A cross-cultural comparison of British and Chinese beliefs about the causes, behaviour manifestations and treatment of schizophrenia. *Psychiatry Research*, *151*(1), 123–138. https://doi.org/10.1016/j.psychres.2006.03.023.

Galanti, G.-A. (2014). *Caring for patients from different cultures* (5th ed.). University of Pennsylvania Press.

Gill, P. S., Beavan, J., Calvert, M., & Freemantle, N. (2011). The unmet need for interpreting provision in UK primary care. *PLoS One*, *6*(6), 1–6. https://doi.org/10.1371/journal.pone.0020837.

Hall, E. T. (1959). *The silent langauge*. Doubleday.

Holland, K. (2017). *Cultural awareness in nursing and health care: An introductory text* (3rd ed.). Routledge.

Hunt, L. M., & de Voogd, K. B. (2007). Are good intentions good enough? Informed consent without trained interpreters. *Journal of General Internal Medicine*, *22*(5), 598–605. https://doi.org/10.1007/s11606-007-0136-1.

International Organization for Migration. (2019). *World immigration report 2020*. https://www.un.org/sites/un2.un.org/files/wmr_2020.pdf.

Jayasuriya, L. (1996). Immigration and settlement in Australia: An overview and critique of multiculturalism. In N. Carmon (Ed.), *Immigration and integration in post-industrial societies: Theoretical analysis and policy-related research* (pp. 206–226). Springer.

Johnstone, M.-J., & Kanitsaki, O. (2007). An exploration of the notion and nature of the construct of cultural safety and its applicability to the Australian health care context. *Journal of Transcultural Nursing*, *18*(3), 247–256. https://doi.org/10.1177/1043659607301304.

Joshi, C., Russell, G., Cheng, I.-H., Kay, M., Pottie, K., Alston, M., Smith, M., Chan, B., Vasi, S., Lo, W., Wahidi, S., & Harris, M. F. (2013). A narrative synthesis of the impact of primary health care delivery models for refugees in resettlement countries on access, quality and coordination. *International Journal for Equity in Health*, *12*(1), 88.

Kim, D., Pan, Y., & Park, H. S. (1998). High- versus low-context culture: A comparison of Chinese, Korean, and American cultures. *Psychology and Marketing*, *15*(6), 507–521. https://doi.org/10.1002/(SICI)1520-6793(199809)15:6<507::AID-MAR2>3.0.CO;2-A

Knipscheer, J. W., & Kleber, R. J. (2008). Help-seeking behavior of West African migrants. *Journal of Community Psychology*, *36*(7), 915–928. https://doi.org/10.1002/jcop.20264.

Liddell, B. J., Nickerson, A., Sartor, L., Ivancic, L., & Bryant, R. A. (2016). The generational gap: Mental disorder prevalence and disability amongst first and second generation immigrants in Australia. *Journal of Psychiatric Research, 83*, 103–111. https://doi.org/10.1016/j.jpsychires.2016.08.011.

McLaughlin, L. A., & Braun, K. L. (1998). Asian and Pacific Islander cultural values: Considerations for health care decision making. *Health and Social Work, 23*(2), 116–126. https://doi.org/10.1093/hsw/23.2.116.

McNamara, T. (2009). The spectre of the dictation test: Language testing for immigration and citizenship in Australia. In G. Extra, M. Spotti, & P.V. Avermaet (Eds.), *Language testing, migration and citizenship: Cross-national perspectives on integration regimes* (pp. 224–241). Continuum. http://hdl.handle.net/11343/31111.

Mence, V., Gangell, S., & Tebb, R. (2017). *A history of the department of immigration: Managing migration in Australia*. Department of Immigration and Border Protection. https://www.homeaffairs.gov.au/news-subsite/files/immigration-history.pdf.

Moullan, Y., & Jusot, F. (2014). Why is the healthy immigrant effect different between European countries? *European Journal of Public Health, 24*(suppl_1), 80–86. https://doi.org/10.1093/eurpub/cku112.

Munro, K. (2017). A brief history of immigration to Australia. *SBS News*. https://www.sbs.com.au/news/a-brief-history-of-immigration-to-australia.

Ngo, B. (2008). Beyond "culture clash" understandings of immigrant experiences. *Theory into Practice, 47*(1), 4–11. https://doi.org/10.1080/00405840701764656.

O'Dowd, M. (2011). Australian identity, history and belonging: The influence of white Australian identity on racism and the non-acceptance of the history of colonisation of indigenous Australians. *International Journal of Diversity in Organisations, Communities & Nations, 10*(6), 29–44. https://doi.org/10.18848/1447-9532/CGP/v10i06/38941.

Palfreeman, A. C. (1958). The end of the dictation test. *The Australian Quarterly, 30*(1), 43–50.

Phillips, C. B., & Travaglia, J. (2011). Low levels of uptake of free interpreters by Australian doctors in private practice: Secondary analysis of national data. *Australian Health Review, 35*(4), 475–479. https://doi.org/10.1071/AH10900.

Phillips, J., Klapdor, M., & Simon-Davies, J. (2010). *Migration to Australia since federation: A guide to the statistics*. Department of Parliamentary Services. https://www.aph.gov.au/binaries/library/pubs/bn/sp/migrationpopulation.pdf.

Richards, D. (1987). Transported to New South Wales: Medical convicts 1788–1850. *British Medical Journal, 295*(6613), 1609–1612. https://doi.org/10.1136/bmj.295.6613.1609.

Roberts, C. (2008). Intercultural communication in healthcare settings. In H. Kotthoff & H. Spencer-Oatey (Eds.), *Handbook of intercultural communication* (pp. 243–262). De Gruyter Mouton. https://doi.org/10.1515/9783110198584.

Roberts, L. R., Jadalla, A., Jones-Oyefeso, V., Winslow, B., & Taylor, E. J. (2017). Researching in collectivist cultures: Reflections and recommendations. *Journal of Transcultural Nursing, 28*(2), 137–143. https://doi.org/10.1177/1043659615623331.

Sawrikar, P., & Katz, I. (2009). *How useful is the term "culturally and linguistically diverse" (CALD) in Australian research, practice, and policy discourse? 11th Australian Social Policy Conference, An Inclusive Society*. http://unsworks.unsw.edu.au/fapi/datastream/unsworks:39250/bin47a64732-6a49-49aa-aad2-39aa4f68bf76?view=true.

Stats, K. (2014). Characteristically generous? Australian responses to refugees prior to 1951. *Australian Journal of Politics and History, 60*(2), 177–193. https://doi.org/10.1111/ajph.12053.

Straiton, M., Grant, J. F., Winefield, H. R., & Taylor, A. (2014). Mental health in immigrant men and women in Australia: The North West Adelaide health study. *BMC Public Health, 14*(1), 1–15. https://doi.org/10.1186/1471-2458-14-1111.

Thompson, S., Manderson, L., Woelz-Stirling, N., Cahill, A., & Kelaher, M. (2002). The social and cultural context of the mental health of Filipinas in Queensland. *Australian and New Zealand Journal of Psychiatry, 36*(5), 681–687. https://doi.org/10.1046/j.1440-1614.2002.01071.x.

Thomson, M. D., & Hoffman-Goetz, L. (2009). Defining and measuring acculturation: A systematic review of public health studies with hispanic populations in the United States. *Social Science and Medicine, 69*(7), 983–991.

Van Krieken, R. (2012). Between assimilation and multiculturalism: Models of integration in Australia. *Patterns of Prejudice*, *46*(5), 500–517. https://doi.org/10.1016/j.socscimed.2009.05.011.

Wallace, M., & Kulu, H. (2018). Can the salmon bias effect explain the migrant mortality advantage in England and Wales? *Population, Space and Place*, *24*(8), 1–18. https://doi.org/10.1002/psp.2146.

Williams, S., Weinman, J., & Dale, J. (1998). Doctor–patient communication and patient satisfaction: A review. *Family Practice*, *15*(5), 480–492. https://doi.org/10.1093/fampra/15.5.480.

Wohler, Y., & Dantas, J. A. (2017). Barriers accessing mental health services among culturally and linguistically diverse (CALD) immigrant women in Australia: Policy implications. *Journal of Immigrant and Minority Health*, *19*(3), 697–701. https://doi.org/10.1007/s10903-016-0402-6.

Wright, B., Seah, E., Tilbury, F., Rooney, R., & Jayasuriya, P. (2003). The cultural awareness tool (CAT): An assessment tool to assist practitioners in assessing and planning treatment for clients from CALD background. https://researchrepository.murdoch.edu.au/id/eprint/20780/.

Xia, J. (2009). Analysis of impact of culture shock on individual psychology. *International Journal of Psychological Studies*, *1*(2), 97–101. https://doi.org/10.5539/ijps.v1n2p97.

Zwi, K. J., Woodland, L., Kalowski, J., & Parmeter, J. (2017). The impact of health perceptions and beliefs on access to care for migrants and refugees. *Journal of Cultural Diversity*, *24*(3), 63–72.

9 Religious diversity in Australia

Douglas Ezzy

Learning outcomes

After working through this chapter, students should be able to:

1. Describe the diversity of religions in Australia and how this is changing both in the general population and in health care settings.
2. Discuss some of the ways that religious and spiritual beliefs can impact on people's experiences of health and illness and what they consider appropriate behaviour.
3. Explain why consideration of people's religious and spiritual beliefs is important in health care.
4. Outline culturally safe health care practice for patients' religious/spiritual needs.

Key terms

Culturally safe health care practice: Health care that aims to be guided by the recipient of the health care, noting in particular what they consider to be important and appropriate practices and beliefs, and respecting these.
Death bed visions: The experience of a person who is dying. They see loved ones and family members who have already died.
Methodological agnosticism: A way of thinking that makes no judgement on the truth or falsity of religious beliefs and practices, but that still allows the individual to have their own views on these matters. Their practice is agnostic, although the health care worker themselves may not be an agnostic.
Nonreligion: People who do not identify with any particular religion. This includes atheists (who reject religion), agnostics (who are not sure about religion), people who are just not very interested in religion, and people who are "spiritual but not religious".
Religion: Ritual practices, typically as part of a community, that draw on symbols and beliefs that guide how people behave and relate.
Religious diversity: The variety of religious and not religious people in Australia. Australia's changing religious diversity includes the rising numbers of people who are not religious, the decline of traditional Christianity and the increasing ethnic diversity within Christianity, the growing numbers of Buddhists, Muslims, Hindus, and Sikhs, mostly as a result of migration, the growth of Pentecostals, and the rise of alternative spiritualities such as the New Age and meditation.
Respect: "An essential component of a high-performance organization. It helps to create a healthy environment in which clients feel cared for as individuals, and members of health care

teams are engaged, collaborative and committed to service. Within a culture of respect, people perform better, are more innovative and display greater resilience. On the contrary, a lack of respect stifles teamwork and undermines individual performance. It can also lead to poor interactions with clients. Cultivating a culture of respect can truly transform an organization, and leaders set the stage for how respect is manifested." (James, 2018).

Spirituality: The individual experience of ritual practices, symbols and beliefs that guide behaviour and relationships. Individual spirituality may be part of a person's participation in a religious group, or may be completely separate from organised religion.

Chapter summary

This chapter will explore religious diversity and how religion can impact delivery of health services. Students will be introduced to the main religious groups in Australia and explore how the different religions interact and are impacted by the dominant Christian beliefs in Australia. The chapter will discuss how spirituality can assist people to find a sense of meaning or purpose in their lives in a way that is strongly influenced by cultural heritage. Students will be guided through activities to explore how religious beliefs adopted by people influence the way that individuals, families and community groups respond to significant life events like birth, illness, death and dying. Case studies will be provided as a basis for discussion about how health professionals can respond sensitively toward the beliefs and values of diverse religious groups in their care.

Introduction

Understanding how to best respect religious diversity in health care settings is an important part of health care work. Hence, it is important to understand the diversity of religion in Australia and the impact it has on people who are ill or suffering. Religion in Australia is changing, and this chapter provides an overview of those changes, introducing the variety of religions found in contemporary Australia. The chapter also explains the concept of "respect" as a key method for negotiating relationships with people of various religious and secular backgrounds. This is part of health care practice that emphasises cultural safety. The chapter is organised in three sections: (1) What is religion? (2) Religion in Australia; and (3) Culturally safe health care practice for patients' religious and spiritual needs.

What is religion?

What constitutes "religion" is difficult to define. While many people think of it as attending church, mosque, or temple, religion is much broader than this. For some people their "religion" is the very core of their being. For others it is something they do once a year, or at weddings or funerals, and rarely considered at other times. Both of these forms of "religion" are equally legitimate, from the perspective of understanding society and health care. As health care workers, it is not up to us to judge which forms of religion are right or wrong. Although we may have personal opinions on this, they should not influence how people are treated in health care. For example, some people identified their religion as "Jedi" on the Census. While for some it was a joke, for many it pointed to how the things that give them a sense of meaning, purpose and community are to be found outside the traditional forms of religion, such as in raves (all-night dance parties), cosplay (where people dress up and act out roles of fictional characters) or online gaming. This might mean, for example, that they find listening to particular music comforting, or that the find it valuable to have a picture of a favourite character from a television show. These things might not seem "religious", but they can be spiritually comforting. In short, we need to be open minded about what might constitute "religion" and not assume that we know what that means.

"Religion" used to be defined as "belief in God." However, this definition is problematic for some forms of Buddhism that don't have deities. It also doesn't work very well for some animist Indigenous religions that often don't have deities, but rather understand this world as "enchanted" and for whom a relationship with "Country" is central (Harvey, 2005). Some people then defined religion as about belief in a "higher power" or "transcendence". This too is problematic because some religions are primarily about living in this world and are focused on ritual practices rather than belief. The religions of Japan, for example, are mostly religions of practice, with belief a secondary consideration that most people don't concern themselves with (Kasulis, 2004). In Japan, a religion is typically chosen for the ritual event: Shinto for a birth, Christianity for a wedding, Buddhism for a funeral. Given these considerations, religion can be defined as "a set of ritual practices that engage symbolic resources to provide an etiquette for relationships and an emotional and cognitive sense of self-worth and purpose" (Ezzy, 2014, p. 22). This definition emphasises that religion is about doing things (ritual), that religion shapes the way that people relate to the world (etiquette or ethics) and that it typically provides a sense of worth and purpose.

It is difficult to separate out "religion" from "culture" for some groups, such as some Indigenous Australians and some ethnic groups. For example, although many Indigenous Australians identify as Christians on the Census, and few identify as having "Aboriginal religion", for many there are elements of their culture that provide them with meaning, ritual and a sense of place in the world that guides their sense of right and wrong. For example, Derek McCarthy (2005) notes that for Aetorea New Zealand's Maori, a relationship to land is central to their spirituality. Australian Indigenous peoples tend to have a similarly strong relationship to "country" or "land". For Indigenous peoples, ill health may be intimately bound up with a sense of "dislocation from land, their home, their identity, and ultimately, their spirituality" (McCarthy, 2005, p. 176). While the ability to solve this dislocation may vary, demonstrating empathy for the "loss and grief" can be supportive. Similarly, from an Australian perspective, Garry Worete Deverell (2018) reflects on the intertwining of his Christian faith and his Tasmanian Aboriginal heritage, and Deborah Bird Rose explores the wisdom of "dingo stories" she heard, among others, from "old Tim" from the Layit clan whose land is demarcated by the Wickham River in Northern Australia (Rose, 2011). Both Deverell and Rose point to the importance of relationships with "land" or "country".

Religion and spirituality are about practices and relationships, as much as they are about belief. These practices might be traditional Christian prayer, but they also might be spending time on a person's "country" for Indigenous people, or they might involve wearing a t-shirt with a favourite television character for someone who does cosplay. The challenge for health care workers is to ask, listen and respect the things that matter to patients.

These can be defined as follows:

Religion—ritual practices, typically as part of a community, that draw on symbols and beliefs that guide how people behave and relate.

Spirituality—the individual experience of ritual practices, symbols and beliefs that guide behaviour and relationships. Individual spirituality may be part of a person's participation in a religious group, or may be completely separate from organised religion.

Religion is important in health care settings because respecting people's religion can have a major impact on their care and recovery. One of the reasons this is important is because religion can have a major impact on how people feel. For example, eating kosher food is very important for an observant Jew. While there may be little difference in the nutritional value of food that is kosher or not kosher, from the perspective of patient care, it can be crucial. "If [people] define situations as real, they are real in their consequences" (Thomas & Thomas, 1928, p. 572). If an observant Jew finds out that they have eaten food that is not kosher, this could cause extreme distress and delay a person's recovery. Note that the important word here is *observant*. The important question about a person's religion is not about what people believe, but about what they practice.

DeLaune et al. (2016, pp. 456–458) provide a useful list of dietary practices and health care beliefs for various religions. For example, for Muslims, pork is prohibited, meat needs to be ritually slaughtered and during Ramadan they fast during the daytime. However, as noted earlier, the degree to which a person will be observant may vary significantly. The question the health care practitioner needs to ask is about practices: Is it important to someone to eat kosher or halal food? Is it important that they pray at specified times? Would having a particular religious object on their bedside table be comforting, and if so, can a family member bring one in? Within the various religious traditions there is a wide variation in practices, and it is important to ask the individual person what matters to them.

Religion is also important when confronting bigger picture questions about meaning, worth and purpose, often associated with the end of life. The most common reason that nurses, doctors and social workers refer a patient to a religious chaplain is for end-of-life issues, such as "a pregnancy loss", "facing impending death", "unresolved grief" or "questions of the meaning of life" (Galek et al., 2007, p. 367). If someone wants assistance with an end-of-life issue, it is better to start this process as early, as soon as these sorts of issues are identified (Kellehear, 1999). Martins and Caldeira (2018) note that spiritual practices and beliefs can be important coping strategies in response to spiritual distress that often emerges for cancer patients.

As Australia becomes increasingly religiously diverse, it is increasingly likely that a health care practitioner will not know a great deal about a person's religion. Respect is the most useful way of thinking about the practices that are required in this context (Richardson-Self, 2015). Respect is integral to providing "culturally safe" health care (McCarthy, 2005). The idea of respect means that the person is seen as an equal member of society and therefore deserving of equal rights to other people. Some people talk about "tolerance" as a way to approach religious diversity. However, the idea of "tolerance" is problematic because it suggests that what is "tolerated" is somehow of less worth or inappropriate (Beaman, 2017). Aiming for "respect" suggests that we accept that there is a diversity of approaches to religion and nonreligion, and that we accept that other people will make different choices to our own. To respect someone's religion does not require that we ourselves agree with those religious beliefs or practices, only that we accept people's right to choose them.

For many people, religion remains a central part of their lives. Religious practices, stories, rituals, communities, and beliefs enable them to remain hopeful, to live through pain and suffering and to find ways of being generous and ethical in their relationships. As Karen Armstrong (2005, p. 3) puts it: mythology enables "us to live more intensely" within the world. "In mythology we entertain a hypothesis, bring it to life by means of ritual, act upon it, contemplate its effect upon our lives, and discover that we have achieved new insight into the disturbing puzzle of our world" (Armstrong, 2005, p. 10).

This can be defined as follows:

Respect—the idea that other people's religious and nonreligious practices and beliefs deserve equal rights, even though we ourselves may not agree with them.

Box 9.1 Case study—Death bed visions

This can be defined as follows:

Death bed vision—the experience of a person who is dying. They see loved ones and family members who have already died.

Respect of people's religious, or nonreligious beliefs is central to good health care. Twenty-five percent of people (that is, one in four people) who are conscious while they are dying are reported to experience death bed visions of pre-deceased relatives and other loved ones (Barbato, 2000). These visions are often very vivid, and the person experiences them as if they are real. People who have already passed on, such as parents, partners, and other loved ones, are seen to be really there in the room. These experiences are typically comforting for the person who is dying. They can even be profoundly joyful. However, they can be confusing for relatives, friends, and health care workers who are present. The challenge for health care professionals is to respect such experiences without feeling the need to either believe in them or to argue with them. Scientifically, there is considerable debate over exactly what causes such visions (Kellehear, 1999). The important thing from the point of view of a health professional is that they are comforting for the patient, and on that basis need to be respected.

Box 9.2 Reflection—How would you respond to someone having a death bed vision?

Imagine that you are part of a health care team for someone who is dying. Imagine you are present in the room with the dying person and they begin to describe a death bed vision of their now deceased parents, who they think are there to welcome them to the next life.

Questions for consideration:

- What are the range of possible responses that people might make to a death bed vision?
- It would be very unhelpful to try to convince the dying person that they are hallucinating. Why is it unhelpful?
- Death bed visions can be very comforting for a dying person. What might be some constructive things that a health care worker could do in this context?
- Another approach may be for the health care worker to simply continue doing whatever else is required as part of their normal work. How do you think this would make the dying person feel?

This can be defined as follows:

Religious diversity—the variety of religious and not religious people in Australia. Australia's changing religious diversity includes the rising numbers of people who are not religious, the decline of traditional Christianity and the increasing ethnic diversity within Christianity, the growing numbers of Buddhists, Muslims, Hindus, and Sikhs, mostly as a result of migration, the growth of Pentecostals, and the rise of alternative spiritualities such as the New Age and meditation.

Religion and the Australian census

If someone says that they regularly practise their religion, it is almost equally likely they are Anglican, Catholic, Pentecostal, Hindu, Buddhist, or Muslim. Census statistics can be deceiving (Table 9.1). On the 2016 Australian Census, approximately 3.1 million Australians identified as Anglicans and 250,000 identified as Pentecostals. However, we know that only 5% of people

Table 9.1 Religious identification in the 2016 Australian Census

No religion	30.1%	30.1%
Catholic	22.6%	
Anglican	13.3%	
Uniting Church	3.7%	
Christian (not further defined)	2.6%	
Presbyterian & Reformed	2.3%	
Eastern Orthodox	2.1%	
Baptist	1.5%	
Pentecostal	1.1%	
Lutheran	0.7%	
Other Protestant	0.5%	
Jehovah's Witnesses	0.4%	
Latter-day Saints	0.3%	
Seventh-day Adventist	0.3%	
Oriental Orthodox	0.2%	
Other Christian	0.5%	
All Christian		52.1%
Islam	2.6%	
Buddhism	2.4%	
Hinduism	1.9%	
Sikhism	0.5%	
Judaism	0.4%	
Other religions	0.3%	
Pagans	0.1%	
All other religions		8.2%
No response	9.6%	9.6%

Data was integrated from Australian Bureau of Statistics (2016) and Bouma and Halafoff (2017).

who identify as Anglicans attend church weekly, whereas 73% of Pentecostals attend church regularly (Bellamy & Castle, 2004). If that pattern still holds for the 2016 Census, then it means that on any given weekend there are more Pentecostals in church, approximately 180,000, than there are Anglicans, approximately 150,000. In other words, most of the people who say they are "Anglican" almost never go to church. Being "Anglican" may still be very important to them. They may still pray, or read the Bible, or value the guidance of a chaplain, or they might not. It is just a different way of being Anglican. It is probable that Muslims, Hindus, and Buddhists are also more likely to practice than Anglicans. This means that the people for whom religious practice is important are distributed over quite a wide range of religions.

Table 9.1 also includes "Pagans". Pagans are a quite small group at 0.1% of the population. However, there are many people who engage in spiritual practices that are part of the broader "New Age" for which there is no category on the Census. They might use crystals, or Tarot cards, celebrate the solstice, or have other more specific items or practices. To see these things as religious practices that can be respected can be helpful to the person. A crystal or a Tarot deck is not a substitute for proper medical care, but a crystal or a Tarot deck might make a person who is in hospital feel better. If this is the case, then it is worth respecting the person's desire to have them nearby.

Catholics and abortion

According to official Catholic teaching, abortion is morally wrong (Dixon, 2013). However, this does not mean that all people who identify as Catholics share this belief. Nearly half (45%) of the people who say they are Catholic in a national survey also say that "Women should be able to obtain an abortion readily when they want one" (Betts, 2009, p. 30). However, similar to Anglicans, many people who say they are Catholic do not actually attend Catholic Mass regularly. In a study focusing only on Catholics who attended Mass regularly, approximately one out of every five say that abortion is justified (Dixon, 2013, p. 446).

In other words, it is really important to ask an individual what is or is not acceptable to them. Just because someone says they are Catholic does not mean that you can predict their attitude towards abortion, homosexuality, or the use of contraception. There is a great deal of variation in the beliefs and practices of individual religious people, and it is very common that these may not conform to the official beliefs of the religion with which they identify.

Sometimes people claiming to represent Christians make statements that seem to imply that all Christians reject abortion, same-sex marriage or voluntary euthanasia. However, from national surveys and polling data, we know that of all the people who say they are Christian (including Catholics, Anglicans, Pentecostals, and others), that more than half support same-sex marriage, and even more support abortion and voluntary euthanasia (Maddox, 2014, p. 147). In other words, what is presented in the mainstream media as "the Christian view" of various moral and health issues is often quite different from what the majority of Christians actually think.

The rise of nonreligion

This can be defined as follows:

Nonreligion—people who do not identify with any particular religion. This includes atheists (who reject religion), agnostics (who are not sure about religion), people who are just not very interested in religion, and people who are "spiritual but not religious".

In recent years an increasing number of Australians say they have "no religion". As indicated in Table 9.1, the group of people who say they have "no religion" is now the largest religious "group" in Australia, at 30.1% of the population. That means that nearly one person in every three says that they do not have a religion. This is a major change over the last 50 years. In 1966, less than 1% of Australians said they had no religion, rising to 19% in the 2009 Census (Bouma & Halafoff, 2017). The rise in nonreligion is also occurring in other countries around the world, with 37% with no religion in New Zealand, 21% in the UK and 16% in the USA.

It is important not to assume that if a person says that they have "no religion" that it is clear what this means. Among those who say they are "not religious", only a small minority are atheists. Atheists are confident that religion is wrong, that that there are no supernatural deities. People who have "no religion" might be an agnostic, who say they do not know what they believe. The category of "no religion" also includes people who are disinterested in religion and choose not to think about it. Even more confusingly, there is another category of people who say they have "no religion" but identify as "spiritual but not religious" (Beyer, 2015). These people may engage in occasional religious practices, or dislike the institutionalised aspects of religion. They may be quite willing to talk to religious chaplain, or want a religious icon or a crystal beside their bed, something that atheists would strongly reject. In short, the category of people who say they have "no religion" includes a very wide range of attitudes toward religion. Again, the important thing is to ask a person what they want, and to not assume that because they have identified as "not religious" that it is obvious what this means.

Religion in Australia

Religion and migration

Prior to 1970 there were very few identified Hindus, Buddhists or Muslims in Australia. However, we should note that in the 1800s there were significant numbers of Chinese Buddhists (mainly in the goldfields), Afghan Muslims (many of whom were camel caravanners in outback Australia) and others (Jupp, 2002). The White Australia Policy was implemented in 1901 and was

Table 9.2 Religion and migration

	1996	*2001*	*2006*	*2011*	*2016*
Islam	1.1	1.3	1.7	2.2	2.6
Buddhism	1.1	1.9	2.1	2.5	2.4
Hinduism	0.4	0.5	0.7	1.3	1.9

designed to restrict the people who could migrate to Australia, primarily favouring people from the UK. After the official end of the White Australia Policy in 1973, greater numbers of migrants from all around the world, including from Asia and India, were allowed. This has resulted in the progressive growth of the numbers of Buddhists, Muslims, and Hindus in Australia (Table 9.2).

However, many of these new migrants are also Christians. John Newton (2018) reports that the growth in the Pentecostal numbers in Australia since 2000 has largely been a result of Pentecostals migrating from Africa and Latin America. This illustrates a pattern that is common in Australia, where migrant communities form bonds and relationships with other ethnic groups as a result of joining existing religious groups in Australia. A similar pattern occurred with the post-war migrants from Italy in the 1950s and 1960s, who were predominantly Catholic and started attending Mass with the predominantly Irish Catholic congregations in Australia (Jupp, 2002).

Tasmania provides an interesting comparison of migration patterns that is similar to many rural and regional areas in Australia. Whereas 2.6% of Australians identified as Muslim, only 0.5% of Tasmanians identified as Muslim in 2016 (Australian Bureau of Statistics, 2016). This number is up from 2011, when only 0.2% of Tasmanians identified as Muslim. The numbers of Buddhists and Hindus in Tasmania follow a similar pattern. These low numbers of Muslims, Buddhist and Hindus also reflects migration flows. When migrants did move to Tasmania in the 1980s and 1990s, it was very difficult to find work, due to the weak economy, and they have typically relocated to Melbourne or Sydney were work is easier to find. The growing numbers of Muslims, Hindus and Buddhists in Tasmania reflects both increasing numbers of international university students attending the University of Tasmania and increasing numbers of migrants and refugees remaining in Tasmania.

Box 9.3 Reflection—Religious diversity in your suburb

Describe the types of religions that are visible in the suburb where you live or around the university campus.

Is this different if you grew up somewhere different to where you now live, such as in a regional area or overseas?

Box 9.4 Case study—Teenage witches

Although Pagans only make up 0.1% of the Australian population on the Census, there is good evidence that many more people, particularly young people, experiment with Paganism and Witchcraft. Paganism is an umbrella term that refers to a wide range of traditions including Witchcraft, Druidry, Heathens (who follow the Norse Gods and Goddesses) and a variety of others (Berger & Ezzy, 2007). There is significant variation, but Pagan religions tend to celebrate the passing of the seasons, including the solstices and equinoxes, in a ritual calendar referred to as the wheel of the year. Pagan religions tend to be quite individualistic. There are some organisations, but the majority of Pagans practice on their own or as part of small local groups.

The most common Christian prayers are about their health. The most common magical workings by teenage Witches are also about their health (Berger & Ezzy, 2007, p. 29). For example, Morgan was a 19-year-old American teenage Witch when we interviewed her. She told us that the first magical working she performed as a 17-year-old was for health issues: "I had a number of friends who were in very bad health situations, and I made them some sachets, and some herbal bags, and what not" (Berger & Ezzy, 2007, p. 50). There is no evidence that such magical practices can directly impact physical health issues. However, such magical practices can change the way that young people *feel*, and whether a person feels optimistic or despairing can have a major impact on their health.

The support of friends from religious communities can be an important part of some people's recovery from illness. Pagan religions, including Witchcraft, tend to be highly stigmatised. As a consequence, many Pagan communities are online communities—where it tends to be easier to remain anonymous, or to participate in a group without informing family or friends. Practising respect toward such beliefs and practices is an integral part of engaging in culturally safe health care work.

Culturally safe health care practice for patients' religious and spiritual needs

Respect and methodological agnosticism

One way of thinking about how best to practice respect as a health care worker is to think of practicing "methodological agnosticism". This term was originally used to describe how sociologists should approach studying religion (Berger, 1967). However, I suggest that it might also be a useful way for health care workers to think about their health care practice. Agnosticism is a way of thinking about religion where the person says they "do not know" whether religion is true or not. This means that the agnostic person is both open to hearing about religion and makes no judgement about the religion, leaving the conversation open. To add the term "methodological" to this creates "methodological agnosticism" and points to the idea that the method of practice, in this case health care practice, is agnostic, even though the individual health care worker themselves may have strongly held views on religion (for or against it).

Methodological agnosticism as a form of practice facilitates relationships of *respect*. Respect is the idea that other people's religious and nonreligious practices and beliefs deserve equal rights, even though we ourselves may not agree with them. If we are "methodologically agnostic" this means that we can interact with people who are religious, or not religious, without having to either convince them that they are wrong, or having to accept their religious ideas as correct of ourselves.

This can be defined as follows:

Culturally safe health care practice: Health care that aims to be guided by the recipient of the health care, noting in particular what they consider to be important and appropriate practices and beliefs, and respecting these.

Usher and associates (2017, p. 339) define culturally safe health care as "determined by the end users rather than the health care providers." This is exactly what practising respect means. It is not always possible to have a detailed understanding of the rules and expectations of particular religious, spiritual or cultural groups. However, health care workers can practice respect and openness that Usher et al. (2017, p. 340) describe as "cultural capability".

Box 9.5 Reflection—Methodological agnosticism

Agnosticism: The idea that you do not know whether a religion, or any religion, is true or not. Agnostics are just not interested in the question.
Methodological: The way you do something, your practice or method of working.
Methodological agnosticism as health care practice: Simply accepts statements about religious ideas or practices at face value. Makes no attempt to judge or correct religious ideas or beliefs.

This can be defined as follows:

Methodological agnosticism—a way of thinking that makes no judgement on the truth or falsity of religious beliefs and practices, but that still allows the individual to have their own views on these matters. Their practice is agnostic, although the health care worker themselves may not be an agnostic.

"Cults" and "dangerous" religions

It is important to not make assumptions about religious people because of images of them that may have been presented in the media. Members of minority religions (such as Scientology or The Jehovah's Witnesses) are often described as "cults", a word that is best avoided. James Richardson (1996) shows that many news outlets amplify the dangers of minority religions in their reporting in a way that is very biased (Ezzy, 2018). If a patient discloses that they are a member of a minority religion, the health care worker should aim to practice respect towards them. While we may have images of what this religion involves drawn from mainstream media, the important thing is to respond to the actual practices and requests of the patient, rather than the media images.

Box 9.6 Reflection—How would you respond to someone who was a Seventh Day Adventist?

Imagine that you are part of a health care team for someone who is a Seventh Day Adventist. You may have seen a television program about this group. One famous Seventh Day Adventist is Lindy Chamberlin, who was convicted and then found innocent of the murder of her child in central Australia (Richardson 1996). How would you deal with this?

Questions for consideration:

- Should you be more cautious in the way you interact with someone when they disclose they are a Seventh Day Adventist?
- Seventh Day Adventists are not that very different from other forms of Christianity except that they have their church services on Saturday instead of Sunday. They are quite similar to Baptists, for example, in many ways. Does this change the way you think about the person?
- How much does a fear of the "unknown" shape the way that people respond to members of religious minorities?

Religion and suffering

> Heather: "I was really sick … and I invoked the Goddess or evoked her and I just felt like Isis was with me wrapping her wings around me all sort of warm and feathery and I felt this incredible sense of peace. It was amazing. I just felt warm and comfortable and safe and there was no pain at all and I just went to sleep with this enormous grin on my face and I woke up the next morning dancing off the walls. It's happened again [since]—it's not the only time that I've had that experience."
>
> (Berger & Ezzy, 2007, p. 190)

Heather was a teenage Witch. Her Pagan prayers changed the way she felt. This enabled her to fall asleep more easily. Similar effects can be observed when members of all religions engage in familiar religious practices such as prayer or saying the rosary.

"In the intersection of religion and medicine, religion has played no greater role than that of providing consolation in sickness and death" (Ferngren, 2012, p. 8). Studies have found no evidence that people who are prayed for have better health outcomes (Roberts et al., 2009). However, prayer and other religious practices do enable people to deal with the suffering and grief that is often associated with illness. Think of a funeral. You may not want to go to a funeral because it is hard, and when you attend you may cry and feel very sad. However, the ritual does something important. It allows us to live with our grief and sadness so that they do not overwhelm us (Ezzy, 2014).

The important thing to note in both of these examples—the funeral and Heather's prayer—is that whether a person believes or not is not actually that important. The thing that changes the way the religious person feels is the performance of the ritual or the prayer. For religion to be effective, it typically involves doing or saying things, not just "believing" on its own. This is why it might be important to a Muslim to have an imam visit, or a Christian to be visited by a member of their congregation.

Religious diversity and self-confidence

According to Jackson (2009, p. 14), "the link is because, when we learn about different religions, you find out who you are … whether you're Christian, or some people don't want to be different things … you find out who you are inside".

The preceding quotation is from an interview with a school student after conducting some in-class study about the beliefs of Islam. Learning about diverse religious traditions can lead to constructive self-reflexivity that allows you to be more confident about your own beliefs and practices, or their absence. As people develop better understandings of the beliefs and practices of members of other religions, they develop better "religious literacy" (Jackson, 2009). Religious literacy can be thought of as part of culturally safe health care practice. The important thing is not that you understand every religion, but that you know enough about the diversity of religions to be able to ask a patient about their religious or spiritual practices and to respect what they say and request. The practices and beliefs of religious people become just another aspect of someone's life, rather than something surprising or strange.

It is easier to be open and respectful of people who are religious, or not religious, if you yourself have thought about and reflected on your own position. It may be that you are uninterested in religion, or that you are an atheist, or that you are a dedicated follower of a religion, or that you engage in yoga as a spiritual practice, or that you like to experiment with a range of spiritualities. All of these are responses to religion that are found in the community and therefore will be found among health care practitioners and the people they care for. "Methodological agnosticism" allows the practitioner to interact with people and focus on their health care work without having to worry about the person's views about religion.

Respect: Living well with religious diversity

Lori Beaman (2017) argues that equality for people of diverse religious and nonreligious traditions comes when negotiating religious differences becomes just an ordinary part of everyday practices. If a person's religion requires special food, kosher for a Jew, or halal for a Muslim, for example, then equality occurs when this requirement is negotiated with the minimum of fuss as if it is just an ordinary part of the person's life. "It is my contention that these micro-processes, or non-events, are exactly the place to begin reflecting on how deep equality is regularly accomplished" (Beaman, 2017, p. 23).

In health care settings this would mean that if a person is a Jehovah's Witness, a Hare Krishna, a devout Catholic, a young Witch, an atheist, or Buddhist, that this becomes just another piece of information similar to the suburb in which they live. It is noted, but not notable. A person's religion is used to inform care practices where the religion relates to their health care, but other than this, it is just another unremarkable aspect of a person's character and life.

There are a range of laws that vary across the states of Australia, requiring different degrees of respect of religion to ensure religious freedom. I argue that these laws can be important in protecting religious people from some of the more extreme forms of abuse and hatred (Ezzy, 2018). However, I also think that Beaman (2017) is right to argue that the most important form of respect shown to people who are religious or not religious is in everyday encounters where religious diversity becomes something that is celebrated and respected.

Conclusion

This chapter began discussing what constitutes religion. Religion is primarily about what people do, such as rituals or prayers, and their relationships. Beliefs are also part of religion, but they are less important in many religions. What this means in health care settings is that it is important to ask religious people what they want to do. This is an element of cultural safety in health care practice. It should not be assumed that because someone says they are religious that they will automatically follow the prescribed behaviours of that religion.

Next the chapter reviewed the very common occurrence of death bed visions. Dying people often have visions of pre-deceased relatives and loved ones. The best response to this is to simply accept the experience as something comforting and of value to the dying person. It would be a serious mistake to try to convince the dying person, or their relatives, that this was a hallucination.

The Australian Census statistics demonstrate that religion in Australia is changing. Traditional forms of Christianity are in decline, particularly Anglicanism. Non-Christian religions, such as Islam, Buddhism, Hinduism and Sikhism, are growing, mainly as a result of migration. The number of people identifying as having "no religion" is also rapidly growing.

Religious beliefs and practices, such as prayer and rituals, can be emotionally beneficial to people. The chapter discussed the detailed example of a teenage Witch's use of prayer. Members of other religions have similar practices.

"Methodological agnosticism" is a useful way of thinking about how to manage religion in a workplace and how to engage in culturally safe health care with people of diverse religious/spiritual identifications. Using this technique, a health care worker conducts themselves as if they are agnostic—that is to say the method of their work is agnostic. This does not, however, require that they themselves are actually agnostic. The worker may be religious, an atheist, or an agnostic.

"Respect" is the idea that other people's religious and nonreligious practices and beliefs deserve equal rights, even though we ourselves may not agree with them. By making respect a routine part of work practices, this can lead to a form of "deep equality". While there are formal rules and laws that require the respect of religious freedom, equality is best achieved when respect for religious diversity becomes something that is just an ordinary part of everyday life.

Box 9.7 Reflection—Chapter review questions

- What is meant by religion?
- What are the implications of a practice-oriented definition of religion for health care practice?
- What are the main religious groups as reported on the Australian Census, and how are these changing?
- Why are religious practices important to people in health care settings?
- What does it mean to respect someone's religion?

Box 9.8 Reflection—Questions for discussion

- Why is there increasing religious diversity in Australian health care settings?
- Why is it important for health care practitioners to respect someone's religion?
- What does it mean to be methodologically agnostic as a health care practitioner?
- What strategies could be used to promote respect for religious diversity in health care settings?

Box 9.9 Reflection—Questions for personal reflection

- What are your personal understandings of some of the religions discussed in this chapter, and how might this shape the way you respond to religious people in health care settings?
- What strategies can you employ to improve your religious literacy?
- How do you see your own professional responsibilities with regard to respecting religious diversity?

Useful website resources

Pew Forum's statistics on Global Religious Diversity: https://www.pewforum.org/2014/04/04/global-religious-diversity/

Prof Linda Woodhead: Most religious people are "normal": https://www.youtube.com/watch?v=Giv_XmOTr0w

Prof Robert Jackson's paper on understanding religious diversity: https://www.researchgate.net/publication/227107166_Understanding_Religious_Diversity_in_a_Plural_World_The_Interpretive_Approach

Harvard Divinity School project on Religious Literacy: https://rlp.hds.harvard.edu/

Anna Halafoff, Andrew Singleton, Gary D Bouma, Mary Lou Rasmussen about the importance of learning about religious diversity: https://theconversation.com/want-a-safer-world-for-your-children-teach-them-about-diverse-religions-and-worldviews-113025

References

Armstrong, K. (2005). *A short history of myth*. Canongate.

Australian Bureau of Statistics. (2016). *Australian standard classification of religious groups, 2016* (no. 1266.0). http://www.abs.gov.au/ausstats/abs@.nsf/mf/1266.0.

Barbato, M. (2000). Australians at the brink of death. In A. Kellehear (Ed.), *Death and dying in Australia* (pp. 208–222). Oxford University Press.

Beaman, L. (2017). *Deep equality in an era of religious diversity*. Oxford University Press.

Bellamy, J., & Castle, K. (2004). *NCLS occasional paper 3: 2001 church attendance estimates*. National Church Life Survey Research. http://www.ncls.org.au/default.aspx?sitemapid=2231.

Berger, H., & Ezzy, D. (2007). *Teenage witches*. Rutgers University Press.

Berger, P. L. (1967). *The sacred canopy: Elements of a sociological theory of religion*. Open Road Media.

Betts, K. (2009). Attitudes to abortion: Australia and Queensland in the twenty-first century. *People and Place, 17*(3), 25–39.

Beyer, P. (2015). From atheist to spiritual but not religious. In L. Beaman & S. Tomlins (Eds.), *Atheist identities: Spaces and social contexts* (pp. 137–152). Springer.

Bouma, G., & Halafoff, A. (2017). Australia's changing religious profile: Rising nones and pentecostals, declining British protestants in superdiversity: Views from the 2016 Census. *Journal for the Academic Study of Religion, 30*(2), 129–143. https://doi.org/10.1558/jasr.34826.

DeLaune, S. C., Ladner P. K., McTier, L., Tollefson, J., & Lawrence, J. (2016). *Fundamentals of nursing: Australian and New Zealand* (1st ed.). Cengage Learning.

Deverell, G. (2018). *Gondwana theology: A Trawloolway man reflects on Christian faith*. Morning Star Publishing.

Dixon, R. (2013). What do mass attenders believe? Contemporary cultural change and the acceptance of key Catholic beliefs and moral teachings by Australian mass attenders. *The Australasian Catholic Record, 90*(4), 439–458.

Ezzy, D. (2014). *Sex, death and witchcraft*. Bloomsbury.

Ezzy, D. (2018). Minority religions, litigation, and the prevention of harm. *Journal of Contemporary Religion, 33*(2), 277–289. https://doi.org/ 10.1080/13537903.2018.1469272.

Ferngren, G. B. (2012). Medicine and religion: A historical perspective. In M. R. Cobb, C. M. Puchlaski, & B. Rumbold (Eds.), *Oxford textbook of spirituality in healthcare* (pp. 2–11). Oxford University Press. https://doi.org/10.1093/med/9780199571390.001.0001.

Galek, K., Flannelly, K. J., Koenig, H. G., & Fogg, S. L. (2007). Referrals to chaplains: The role of religion and spirituality in healthcare settings. *Mental Health, Religion and Culture, 10*(4), 363–377. https://doi.org/10.1080/13674670600757064.

Harvey, G. (2005). *Animism: Respecting the living world*. Columbia University Press.

Jackson, R., (2009). Understanding religious diversity in a plural world: The interpretive approach. In M. De Souza, G. Durka, K. Engebretson, R. Jackson, & A. McGrady (Eds.), *International handbook of the religious, moral and spiritual dimensions in education* (pp. 399–414). Springer.

James, T. A. (2018). Setting the stage: Why health care needs a culture of respect. Harvard Medical School Lean Forward. https://leanforward.hms.harvard.edu/2018/07/31/setting-the-stage-why-health-care-needs-a-culture-of-respect/

Jupp, J. (2002). *From white Australia to Woomera: The story of Australian immigration*. Cambridge University Press.

Kasulis, T. (2004). *Shinto*. University of Hawaii Press.

Kellehear, A. (1999). *Health promoting palliative care*. Oxford University Press.

Maddox, M. (2014). Right-wing Christian intervention in a naïve polity: The Australian Christian lobby. *Political Theology*, *15*(2), 132–150. https://doi.org/10.1179/1462317X13Z.00000000071.

Martins, H., & Caldeira, S. (2018). Spiritual distress in cancer patients: A synthesis of qualitative studies. *Religions*, *9*(10), 285–302. https://doi.org/10.3390/rel9100285.

McCarthy, D. (2005). Spirituality and cultural safety. In D. Wepa (Ed.), *Cultural Safety in Aotearoa New Zealand*. Pearson.

Newton, J. K. (2018). Spiritual explosion: A review of the literature on the sudden growth of Pentecostalism in Australia. *Journal for the Academic Study of Religion*, *31*(1), 75–96. https://doi.org/10.1558/jasr.37176.

Richardson, J. T. (1996). Journalistic bias toward new religious movements in Australia. *Journal of Contemporary Religion*, *11*(3), 289–302. https://doi.org/10.1080/13537909608580776.

Richardson-Self, L. (2015). *Justifying same-sex marriage: A philosophical investigation*. Rowman & Littlefield Publishers.

Roberts, L., Ahmed, I., & Davison, A. (2009). Intercessory prayer for the alleviation of ill health. *Cochrane Database of Systematic Reviews*, *2*. https://doi.org/10.1002/14651858.CD000368.pub3.

Rose, D.B. (2011). *Wild dog dreaming: Love and extinction*. University of Virginia Press.

Thomas, W. I., & Thomas, D. S. (1928). *The child in America: Behaviour problems and programs*. Knopf.

Usher, K., Mills, J., West, R., & Power, T. (2017). Cultural safety in nursing and midwifery. In J. Daly, S. Speedy, & D. Jackson (Eds.), *Contexts of nursing* (5th ed.). Elsevier.

10 Australians with disabilities

Ellen Fraser-Barbour and Natalie Hamam

Learning outcomes

After working through this chapter, students should be able to:

1. Understand the diversity and prevalence of disability.
2. Define disability, and understand the differences between medical and social models of disability and how this influences our practice.
3. Recognise the overlap between disability and health conditions.
4. Explore how the social determinants of health impact people with disability.
5. Identify culturally safe health care for people with disability and some of the key barriers and facilitators to accessing health care.

Key terms

Ableism: Refers to attitudes and beliefs that infer ableness as superior and disability as inferior.
Accessibility: Mobility, environmental, information, communication and sensory access needs met with minimal effort or stress on the part of the individual with disability.
Disability: Disability is an umbrella term for impairments, activity limitations and participation restrictions (World Health Organisation, 2011). This chapter occasionally uses the phrase "people with disability", which is an example of person-first language and appropriate for professional writing. The chapter occasionally uses the phrase "disabled people" as an example of identity-first language. The phrase "disabled people" recognises the experience of disability as a core part of identity, equal to being identified as a gay woman, an African woman.
Discrimination: Occurs when a person is excluded from benefits generally available to other members of a society because of a perceived difference or a stigmatised identity
Impairments: Refers specifically to biological or psychological characteristics that impact on how a person functions.
Respect: "An essential component of a high-performance organization. It helps to create a healthy environment in which clients feel cared for as individuals, and members of health care teams are engaged, collaborative and committed to service. Within a culture of respect, people perform better, are more innovative and display greater resilience. On the contrary, a lack of respect stifles teamwork and undermines individual performance. It can also lead to poor interactions with clients. Cultivating a culture of respect can truly transform an organization, and leaders set the stage for how respect is manifested." (James, 2018).

Chapter summary

In this chapter students will continue to explore social determinants of health in order to gain a better understanding of disability and its incidence, prevalence and impact on disadvantaged populations. Students will explore models of disability and what it means to be disabled in Australia. The importance and reality of intersectional identities will be explored through students' engagement with online activities and class/tutorial tasks. These will assist students in understanding how multiple layers of identity and/or disadvantage can change health outcomes significantly and influence the incidence and/or management of disability. This will be accompanied by a review of current national policies and services (NDIS) aimed at supporting people living with a disability and their carers. Using case examples and research, students will investigate and develop an understanding of the ways health care professionals can work with people with disability.

Introduction

Although health care and disability services in Australia strive to be person-centred, various studies reveal that many people with disability experience barriers to accessing health care. Some of the barriers to accessing health care are physical and environmental, and others are social and cultural. Many people with disability report discrimination from health professionals and often feel judged, disrespected or unheard (Australian Institute of Health and Welfare, 2018). Health professionals sometimes hold assumptions that disability equals a lesser quality of life, and sometimes they inadvertently pass on these messages to the people they are working with (Fitzgerald & Hurst, 2017; Hammell, 2007). Indeed, many people with disability have described feeling as if their diagnosis is being used to define them in unhelpful ways, when in reality disability is one aspect of identity (Aston, Breau, & MacLeod, 2014; Linton, Krcek, Sensui, & Spillers, 2014).

If we are to promote the health and wellbeing of people with disability, it is vital to understand the effects of impairment on how people "do" daily life. This is the "functional" impact of disability. It is vital to not only understand how disability impacts on participation (World Health Organisation, 2011) in the social world around them. According to the International Classification of Functioning, Disability and Health (the ICF) developed by the World Health Organisation, disability is always an interaction between the individual and their broader social and political context (World Health Organisation, 2002). The ICF model uses the biopsychosocial model and highlights that whilst disability can be identified in terms of an individual's biological or psychological characteristics, it is also primarily a social phenomenon. Research tells us that people with disability experience significant social and cultural disadvantage, segregation, devaluation and poor treatment in all areas of community, including health care (Australian Institute of Health and Welfare, 2018). Consequently, a major focus in this chapter will be the social determinants of health for people with disability, as well as related barriers and facilitators to culturally safe health care.

Understanding disability

The Australian Bureau of Statistics' survey of *Disability, Aging and Carers* (2015) defines a person with *disability* as someone who has a permanent limitation, restriction or impairment that restricts their everyday activities. These *impairments* could be physical, mental, neurological, intellectual, or sensory. A disability could be a congenital condition, or a condition acquired later in life because of an injury, illness or a degenerative condition. The language used to describe disability has a profound impact on how people identify, communicate and understand the experience of disability.

Box 10.1 Reflection—Understanding disability

Take a moment to jot down all the words you think of when you hear the word *disability*.

- How might you group these words?
- Do they fall into categories?
- What might you name those categories?

You may have noted word categories such as these:

- Diagnostic and biological descriptors, e.g., "blind", "intellectual disability", "autism", "deaf";
- Deficit descriptors, e.g., "deformity", "lack of" "damaged" "handicapped" "suffers";
- Pejorative descriptors, e.g., "dumb", "incapacitated", "midget", "vegetable", "problem";
- Social descriptors, e.g., "experiences", "lives with ...", "has communication access needs"

These different types of descriptors reflect different cultural understandings of disability and can be seen in the way people portray disability more broadly in media and research. Language and labelling can help people find a sense of identity and connect people to communities and services. A formal diagnosis may also influence someone's eligibility for support. Adversely, labels may also stigmatise and devalue people, leading to *discrimination* and exclusion from society—particularly when these labels infer tragedy, negativity and a lesser quality of life.

The emphasis on classification and labelling is strongly rooted in the "medical model of disability" and is linked to the history of institutionalisation, incarceration and segregation of people with disability in the 19th and 20th centuries (Marks, 1997). It is worth noting that there are still many people with disability are over-represented in institutional settings such as correctional facilities, aged care nursing homes and hospital settings long term (Cadwallader, Spivakovsky, Steele, & Wadiwel, 2018). The medical model may be useful in providing descriptors and a language to communicate an individuals' biological functional capacity; however, the dominance of the medical model can be problematic and laden with negative assumptions and stereotype. It also often positions the health professional as the expert of disability, and people with disability as "recipients" of care, void of lived experience, knowledge, identity or citizenship. The medical model focuses on disability as "abnormal", "a tragedy" and problematises biology as an issue that needs to be cured and eradicated. These beliefs deeply infiltrated the ethos of health care, social care, institutional care, schools and what were previously called sheltered workshops prior to 1980s. It was typical for children to be viewed a burden to the family and therefore encouraged to be placed in institutions. One such example can be seen in the history of the Kew Cottages, an institution for children and adults with disability established in Victoria (Australia) with a long history of institutionalisation of both children and adults with disability and mental health issues. In Australia these large-scale accommodation settings were still operating well into the 1980s and early 1990s (Hallahan, 2010; Manning, 2009; Monk, 2010).

The "social model of disability", on the other hand, was a term coined by a disability studies scholar named Mike Oliver (1983). Oliver argued that the medical model, whilst useful in some respects, was failing people with disability because it did not consider the way in which a person's body interacted with the built and social world. Oliver offered the social model as a tool for health and social care professionals, which shifted attention to the social structures that impacted on people with disability. The social model has since been widely adopted by many researchers and advocates (Durell, 2014; Goering, 2015; Haegele & Hodge, 2016; Shakespeare, 2006).

Adopting the social model of disability as a framework helps us to better understand how disability is enacted when people engage with a social world that is not designed or accepting of their differences. Oliver has been clear that the social model of disability is not oppositional or in contrast to the medical model. Rather, it is a useful tool that builds on biological understandings of impairment, aiding our understanding of how disability can be imposed on by social and environmental barriers. Understanding this better can assist people with disability (Garden, 2010; Oliver, 2013).

The 2006 United Nations Convention on the Rights of People with Disability (CRPD) ascribes to the social model of disability and defines disability as an evolving concept, and that:

> ... disability results from the interaction between persons with impairments and attitudinal and environmental barriers that hinder their full and effective participation in society on an equal basis with others.
>
> (United Nations, 2006, p. 1)

Whilst it is important to have an understanding of how biology can change the way we function and negotiate the world, we must always be thinking about how the environment is designed, and how public attitudes and beliefs about disability impact social participation and citizenship of people with disability in the Australian context.

Box 10.2 Reflection—Disability in Australia

- What do you currently know about disability in Australia and the services provided to people with disability?
- What else do you think is important to know?

Australian context

People with disability account for 17.7% of Australia's population, with the prevalence of disability increasing with age (Australian Bureau of Statistics, 2018. According to the Australian Bureau of Statistics (2018), 11.6% of children and adults up to the age of 65 had a disability. By the time people reach the age of 65, this increases to 49.6% (one in two people). The prevalence of disability rapidly increased for ageing populations over the age of 80. These statistics illustrate that many of us may experience disability at some stage in our lives regardless of our upbringing and level of social and economic wealth (Australian Bureau of Statistics, 2015). If we do not have a disability ourselves, we will at the very least know someone else who has.

In recent years there has been critical social reform changing the landscape of disability services through the ratification of the United Nations Convention on the Rights of People with Disability (2009) and the introduction of the *National Disability Insurance Scheme Act* (2013). The National Disability Insurance Scheme (NDIS) funds disability specific supports for people with disability and their families and carers. It is governed by federal and participating state/territory governments.

The NDIS has changed the way the disability service sector has been funded, shifting funding away from block funding of services to individualised funding for consumers. In other words, it is the consumers (known as participants) who now receive funding packages to purchase and organise their own supports. NDIS participants can manage their funding in three ways:

- Self-managed: the national disability insurance agency provides the individual with access to funding, and the individual can manage a range of NDIS registered and unregistered supports that best achieve their goals. It is up to the individual or their designated nominee to negotiate prices, keep records and pay providers.
- Plan-managed: means the same as self-managed, but with the addition of an independent plan manager who pays providers at or below NDIS capped prices, assists with book keeping and records.
- NDIA-managed: means that the participant can use their funds to purchase supports and service only from NDIS registered providers at or below capped prices.

Allied-health providers (such as psychologists, dieticians, Disability Developmental Educators) will be able to register as disability-specific NDIS registered providers and offer service to participants regardless of how their plan funding is managed. Alternatively providers have the option of delivering services to self-managed participants as long as the transaction is legal. It is up to the participant to ensure the service or support meets certain requirements as outlined in Self-Management information from the NDIS.

Other health care services such as GP and hospital services are excluded from the NDIS. Such policy reform has particular relevance to health professionals who will be providing services within this new NDIS consumer-driven framework. It is also pertinent for general and specialist health care services to be aware of the NDIS (and other) interfaces. Sometimes the nature of people's support needs can be complex, requiring support from a range of disability, justice, child protection, housing and health care portfolios, among others. In these circumstances, people are at risk of falling through the cracks, with government agencies effectively "handballing" responsibility between departments.

Overlap between disability and health issues

According to data from the Australian Institute for Health and Welfare (2019) in 2017–18, an estimated 24% of adults with disability reported good or excellent health, compared to 65% for those without disability. People with disability were 10 times more likely to report poor physical health than those without disability. People with disability were also more likely to experience significant psychological distress and mental health issues across the life course (Australian Institute for Health and Welfare, 2019). There is also evidence to suggest that some types of disability are more likely to have issues with nutrition and physical health, correlating with specific types of secondary health conditions such as respiratory disorders, obesity, diabetes, oral health and digestive issues (Hatton & Emerson, 2015; Straetmans, van Schrojenstein Lantman-de Valk, Schellevis, & Dinant, 2007). Evidence also shows a high prevalence of age-related health conditions such as dementia among people with intellectual disability. Meanwhile children and adults with physical conditions such as spina bifida, cerebral palsy or spinal cord injury (to name a few) generally report higher levels of chronic pain, fatigue and respiratory and cardiovascular disease (Guy-Coichard, Nguyen, Delorme, & Boureau, 2008; Hadden & von Baeyer, 2005; Oddson, Clancy, & McGrath, 2006). Women with disability are more likely to experience barriers to appropriate health promotion information or access to reproductive and sexual health or cancer screening (Civil Society CRPD Shadow Report Working Group, 2019). There is a significant gap in life expectancy between people with and without disability, markedly so among people living in supported accommodation settings. The shorter life expectancy among people living in supported care is often preventable and attributable to untreated (preventable) illness and inadequate access to health care and prevention measures (Heslop, Blair, Fleming, Hoghton, Marriott, & Russ, 2013).

The medical model and the social model in health care

There is evidence that the medical model still tends to dominate views and understandings of disability in some areas of allied health, nursing and medical sciences. This can be seen in the prevalence of negative language and a strong focus on investigating, identifying and accurately diagnosing conditions along with treatment, "management" or cure and eradication of conditions (Dewar, Claus, Tucker, & Johnston, 2017; Falk-Rafael, 2005; Scullion, 2010). This means that the focus of health services for people with disability still tends to be on the assessment and treatment of body function and structure rather than on factors limiting engagement and participation (Dewar et al., 2017). This medical focus remains deeply entrenched in health professional education and flows on to the philosophies underpinning health care professional practice and research (Boyles, Bailey, & Mossey, 2008; Curtin, Adams, & Egan, 2017). When the social model of disability is adopted in practice, health professionals expand on their knowledge by examining not only the biology, but also the social and environmental factors that arise as part of the experience of disability.

The rest of this chapter explores health professionals' need to understand about the social determinants of health, discrimination and what constitutes a culture of *respect* when working with people with disability.

Social determinants of health and why these matter to people with disability

The social determinants of health include a range of factors that shape the conditions of daily life and contribute or impede people's experiences of health and wellbeing (World Health Organisation, 2011). When one experiences disability, there is likely to be a range of related socioeconomic, cultural and political disadvantages. When considered together, it becomes apparent that prevalent issues of disability discrimination, harm, abuse, and neglect are significant policy issues significantly impacting wellbeing and leading to poorer health outcomes.

In the work we do as professionals, it is vital to take up the challenge of tackling *ableism*. Ableism refers to attitudes, stereotypes, ideas, practices and physical and social structures that presume all are able neurotypical people (Chouinard, 1997). In doing so, people with disability are excluded and seen as Other, marginalised and devalued. Ableism may not be intentional, but results in many aspects of society being exclusive and oppressive to anyone who does not fit the "norm" of able and neurotypical (Campbell, 2009).

Ableism may be explicit or implied in everyday interactions (microaggressions), which communicate the message that people with disability are not worthy or equal. Take, for example, the many media stories that often use words that communicate the underlying message that people with disability are "dependent" and "a burden on society". Another example of implied and unintentional ableism lies in the design of buildings, spaces, places, events (and so on) that were often designed without consideration of the needs of people with disability. Often *accessibility* and inclusion are only considered as an afterthought.

Ableism may include the blanket assumption that the world would be better if people with disability did not exist—that it would be kinder for a person with disability to die. It may also include the belief that *all* people with disability are asexual, or adversely hypersexual. It may be seen as tragic or cruel should a person with disability have children.

When people are not aware of these implicit messages, such beliefs and attitudes relegate people with disability as "lesser" and "inferior". It is these negative beliefs and attitudes that impact relationships between health care professionals and people with disability.

Research demonstrates that there is a tendency for health professionals (reflective of broader society) to make assumptions about people's capability levels, which may come across as patronising, insulting and disrespectful (Kroll, Jones, Kehn, & Neri, 2006). Many studies looking at the experiences of people with physical and intellectual disability report similar themes of avoidance, fear and differential treatment by health professionals. The studies report a tendency for health professionals to assume the health complaint is part of the disability, overlooking secondary health conditions (Kroll et al., 2006; Morrison, George, & Mosqueda, 2008; Pelleboer-Gunnink, Van Oorsouw, Van Weeghel, & Embregts, 2017; Shabas & Weinreb, 2000). It is important to note that in many cases disadvantages may be further compounded by intersectional issues of discrimination, such as racism, sexism and ageism.

Box 10.3 Case study—Paula

Paula, a 28-year-old Aboriginal woman with intellectual disability, became increasingly distressed and was taken to emergency with two disability support workers from her home (a residential group home). She had been feeling sick, and the support workers decided it was serious. The paramedic asks questions about Paula's health and then asks whether she has been partying too hard or drinking too much alcohol. The paramedic does not investigate and instead casts the issue off as an alcoholism issue. Several hours later Paula dies. The coroner later finds that Paula had a twisted bowel. The coroner also found that the responding doctor had assumed that Paula was "playing up" and that the case was not urgent.

- What factors could have prevented Paula from receiving timely and appropriate care?
- Discuss how issues of gender, racism and ableism influenced the doctor's assumptions?
- What should have the doctor done to better support Paula?

https://www.sbs.com.au/nitv/nitv-news/article/2016/12/22/not-normal-allegations-aboriginal-woman-died-after-being-treated-differently

When people with disability are not considered as part of the planning, implementation and delivery of health services, this leads to misunderstanding and exclusion with many flow on effects for their health. If health care professionals fail to acknowledge and manage their own biases about disability, then this significantly impacts quality of the health care. Ableism is a significant social determinant of health, equal to racism, sexism and other forms of discrimination, but remains largely ignored in policy and organisational frameworks. It is more likely to see these organisations working on issues such as sexism, racism and LGBTIQA+. Ableism is particularly pertinent to consider here and significantly contributes to poor delivery of health services and in some cases adds to trauma, or physical harm. People with disability may have experienced physical and psychological harm by not being listened to within health care services (Jackson & Waters, 2015). Each experience of having their needs ignored creates distrust and contributes to experiences of trauma. It may also lead to experiences of physical harm when care is not provided appropriately with attention to individuals' support needs. Culturally safe health care practice needs to be attentive to individual care needs and also integrate an understanding of trauma-informed practice among health professionals (Jackson & Waters, 2015). Ableism should be prioritised in health care and tackled as a human rights issue equal to that of racism or sexism. It is vital to recognise ableism underlying the other social determinants of health. This will be discussed in the following pages, demonstrating the bi-directional influence between health and social factors in the environment.

> **Box 10.4 Case study—James (Hamam, 2011)**
>
> James, a 60-year-old man with expressive aphasia after stroke, experienced medication-induced sexual dysfunction that bothered him for four years. The health care providers had never addressed any of these concerns. The problem was easily resolved once uncovered and had most likely persisted due to assumptions made about him.
>
> - Consider the reasons why it has taken so long for James to receive appropriate support.
> - What are some of the assumptions and beliefs that could have prevented James and his health care provider from addressing this issue?
>
> https://www.ncbi.nlm.nih.gov/pmc/articles/PMC3562917/

Systemic and systematic disability discrimination

People with disability are more likely to be exposed to social, cultural and material disadvantage across the life course, and this has a significant influence on health, particularly such people with complex support needs or with intellectual disability (Ali et al., 2013; Durvalsula & Beange, 2001; Hatton & Emerson, 2015; Ouellette-Kuntz, 2005). People with disability are more likely to:

- Live on or below the poverty line
- Experience social exclusion and discrimination from the community
- Be exposed to harm, exploitation and neglect
- Face barriers to accessing education (across the life course)
- Face barriers to work participation
- Have insecure and unstable access to housing and especially specialist housing
- Lack access to health care
- Be over-represented in legal and criminal justice systems

It is also important to acknowledge that many people may experience multiple forms of disadvantage and discrimination, not just in terms of disability, but also due to community perceptions related to race, gender, class, sexuality and ability. Such experiences of adversity and disadvantage are further compounded for disabled people who embody multiple marginalised and intersecting identities. Examples include Aboriginal and Torres Strait Islander peoples with disability, children and young people with disability, LGBTIQA+ with disability, and ethnic and cultural minorities with disability. For example, the experience of an Aboriginal woman with disability would be different to that of a non-Indigenous man with disability. These social determinants intersect and shape how people with disability experience disadvantage (Lakhani, Cullen, & Townsen, 2017).

The report *Shut Out: Experiences of People with Disability and Their Families in Australia* by the National People with Disabilities and Carer Council (NDPCC) Australia (2009) highlighted how deeply entrenched ableism is in every layer of society. It is rooted in the structures and systems that form how we relate to people in our homes, schools, workplaces and broader community. The report drew on findings from 750 submissions and 2,500 consultations with people with disability and their carers and advocates. It painted a picture of a disability service system that is under resourced, leading to situations of discrimination, abuse and neglect of people with disability (National People with Disabilities and Carer Council, 2009). This is still the case today (for a more recent report with similar findings, please see the report by the Australian Institute of Health and Welfare (2019).

Disabled people are more likely to experience poverty compared to non-disabled people and earn significantly less (Australian Institute of Health and Welfare, 2019). According to the Australian Bureau of Statistics (2004), people with disability were earning $225 a week compared to $407 per week for people without disability. This was true even if education levels were the same for people with and without disability (Directorate for Employment, Community, Labour and Social Affairs, 2009). Young people with disability (ages 17–24) are 10 times more likely to experience discrimination related to their disability than older people (over 65).

Recent data from the Australian Human Rights Commission (2016–2017) noted that disability discrimination complaints accounted for the highest number of complaints dealt with annually. The vast majority of these human rights complaints related to the workplace and access to common goods, services and facilities (Australian Human Rights Commission 2017). People with high and complex support needs, or who have a psychiatric or intellectual disability, are most at risk of discrimination (Ali et al., 2013; Kavanagh et al., 2015). Krnjacki et al. (2018) analysed data from the Australian Bureau of Statistics and found that experiences of disability discrimination significantly contributed to poorer health outcomes. Exposure to stressful and adverse experiences of discrimination has a long-term effect on individual health and wellbeing. A high level of stress can of itself increase blood pressure and cortisol secretion, which impacts both psychologically and physiologically (Schmitt, Branscombe, Postmes, & Garcia, 2014). People with disability also report "high" or "very high" levels of stress (32%) compared to 8% without disability (Australian Institute of Health and Welfare, 2019).

People with disability are more likely to experience violence, abuse and harm, particularly for people with intellectual disability, sensory disability, or complex communication needs. Krnjacki, Emerson, Llewellyn, and Kavanagh (2016) disaggregated data from the 2012 Australian Bureau of Statistics *Personal Safety Survey* and found that people with disability were much more likely to experience all forms of violence, harm and neglect compared to people without disability. These results indicate that women with disability are more likely to experience intimate partner violence, whereas men are more likely to experience physical violence. Of late there has been increased political pressure to address these issues of violence in the disability community with the introduction of the Royal Commission into Violence, Abuse and Neglect of People with Disability in 2019 (Royal Commission into Violence, Abuse and Neglect of People with Disability, 2020). Australian disability and family violence activist Ms Nicole Lee (Hill, 2019) argues that simply demonstrating awareness of issues of violence is not enough. As Nicole further details, awareness is not simply "a ribbon" or "a colour" or "a hashtag" (Hill, 2019, p. 337). At the heart of these issues of violence exist deeper societal issues in terms of community attitudes around misogyny, sexism, racism and ableism that must be addressed.

The prevalence of exposure to violence in the disability community has implications for health professionals. It also demonstrates the need to include consideration of people with disability as part of mainstream violence prevention and health care initiatives (Krnjacki, Emerson, Llewellyn, & Kavanagh, 2016).

It is also worth noting that children and young people with disability also experience significant disadvantage compared to those without disability. They are more likely to experience poor health and nutrition, are at a particular risk of experiencing family and housing instability (Emerson & Spencer, 2015) and are at a much greater risk of violence, abuse and neglect. As Robinson (2012) noted in her paper about enabling and protecting children and young people with disability from harm and neglect, a child's disability does not inherently cause vulnerability by default. Rather, the social and environmental factors surrounding the individual contribute to vulnerability.

As Robinson (2012, p. 2) explains, "the presence of Down syndrome does not render a teenager vulnerable." Furthermore, "lack of social connections and networks, the absence of a trusted adult in their life, and caregivers who do not understand any individual communication methods they have would make them vulnerable" (Robinson, 2012). The relationship between vulnerability and harm becomes increasingly significant based on "interaction between the person and the relationships and support systems" that are needed to live contently (Robinson, 2012, p. 12).

A range of barriers makes it harder to report issues of harm and neglect in the case of a person with disability, and it is harder still for people with disability to access mainstream violence-response services, including sexual or domestic violence services, health care services or legal and police services (Baldry, 2014; Frohmader & Ricci, 2016; Fraser-Barbour, Crocker, & Walker, 2018; Robinson et al., 2019).

Barriers and facilitators to developing culturally safe health care

By now you should have an understanding of the "big picture" of social disadvantage in the lives of people with disability and the impact this has on health outcomes. This next section will focus specifically on some of the barriers and facilitators that impact the development of culturally safe health care for people with disability. Culturally safe health care means health services are accessible to all and that people with disability are supported in a way that does not devalue, demean or disempower (Taylor, 2019). The following section explores some the barriers and facilitators to culturally safe health care specific to people with disability (this is by no means an exhaustive list).

Barriers to respectful communication

The relationship between health professionals and people with disability is critical. Yet data from the World Health Organisation (2011) highlighted that many people with disability struggled to find health professionals who were knowledgeable about their needs. This same data also indicated that people with disability were three times more likely to be denied health care services and were four times more likely to have negative experiences with health care providers compared to people without disability. Given this strong evidence of disadvantage for people with disability in health care service settings, it is vital to consider the barriers to respectful communication.

Poor quality of information and documentation as a barrier

Studies consistently indicate that many health care professionals have insufficient knowledge of how to appropriately communicate and adapt to meet the needs of people with disability, including specific knowledge of supporting people's mobility, communication and/or cognitive impairment (Lewis et al., 2017; Merrifield, 2011; Morrison et al., 2008; Nicolaidis et al., 2013; O'Halloran, Hickson, & Worrall, 2008; Simmons-Mackie et al., 2007). Nor is there enough understanding of how disability impacts day-to-day functions and the overlap between disability and health issues such as autism, intellectual or physical disability (Warfield et al., 2015).

Access to information is critical to quality of health care. Another barrier hindering culturally safe practice lies in poor documentation and quality of information. Inadequate information may lead to misdiagnosis, diagnostic overshadowing, delays and mistreatment (Krahn, Hammon, & Turner, 2006; Lewis et al., 2002; Reichard et al., 2004; Sandberg et al., 2015). First, information provided by health care professionals to consumers with disability may not be accessible, with poor organisation of appropriate supports and adaption, and/or poor gathering of information and documentation (Hwang et al., 2009; Krahn et al., 2006; Witko, Boyles, Smiler, & McKee, 2017). A range of factors impacts quality of information-sharing between people with disability and health professionals. There are specific issues with sharing of information between health care professionals, social care services, educational services and other relevant services who are part of the formal supports a person with disability may have in their lives. A number of recent inquiries into disability services in Australia have revealed an alarming number of preventable deaths in disability care settings. Many of these inquiries indicated that people with disability who were living in supported care were more prone to health conditions that should be identified by regular and routine screenings, such as cancer. Often these illnesses were not adequately screened for or diagnosed. There were also issues with choking and respiratory issues that were improperly addressed and required ongoing care and management (Office of the Public Advocate, 2016; Ombudsman of NSW, 2018). Many of these incidents could have been prevented had there been active partnership, communication and information shared between health care professionals and wider disability services.

Limited time and heavy caseloads as a barrier

Many health care professionals are busy with heavy caseloads and have limited time. This is an issue for people both with and without disability. However, people with disability may need more time to negotiate their access needs, and/or may have complex issues that need to be addressed and taken into consideration (Ward, Nichols, & Freedman, 2010). The quality of care depends on the time provided. Time is especially important when meeting a patient for the first time.

A study by Kroll et al. (2006) interviewed people with physical disability and found that there was a tendency for health care professionals to assume that their disability would be too complex to manage in a short appointment time, creating negative experiences for those who felt competent and able to manage their disability. At other times people with disability felt that they needed longer appointment times and that the short slot allocated was not enough time for an adequate examination. There are diverse reasons people may need flexibility with consultation times including, but not limited to,

- Physical access needs
- Information access needs
- Communication access needs
- Involvement of interpreters or key support people
- Adequate investigation of complex medical histories—potential need to gather information from, or share information with other specialists or primary care providers
- Paperwork, referrals and government forms

It is also worth noting that people with disability may often be spending a great deal of time following up on paperwork, asking for referrals or collecting information and tracking medical records. This can often take considerable time when there are multiple health care and government services involved (Morrison et al., 2008).

Many people with disability may be negotiating relationships with a wide range of health care and social services in their lives. Robinson (2018) argues that multiple referrals to health care, social and educational professionals need to be carefully considered as they are not always helpful. Robinson explored this issue in relation to children and young people and found that those with multiple complex health issues have a wide range of health care, social and educational professionals coming in and out of their daily lives at home and at school. This may present particular challenges, including the de-personalisation and unfamiliarity with the health care or social care services, and also fatigue. Referral and transitions from paediatrics to adult health care services can also be a time of stress and anxiety for people with disability and their families, particularly when they are familiar and comfortable with existing health care professionals but have to be referred elsewhere once they are 18 years of age.

Facilitator to respectful communication

Ideally, health professionals should provide a valuable point of contact and information for people with disability seeking;

a) diagnosis and information about their health condition or disability and
b) treatment, health care planning, rehabilitation, therapy and capacity building, or
c) linkage and referral to appropriate services and supports.

People with disability who have communication support needs or an intellectual disability find it difficult to self-refer and seek assistance from health care services on their own terms. Often access to health care relies on referral by a family member, friend or social care service providers (Hogg, 2001). Agencies providing regular support with people's daily needs may not always have the knowledge or skills to recognise when health care services are needed. We need to make concerted efforts in disability services to ensure that potential health issues are identified early and responded to adequately with referral and linkage to appropriate health care services (Michael & Richardson, 2008). Data from the Australian Institute of Health and Welfare (2015) indicated that around 1.2 million people with disability who needed to see a general practice doctor delayed or did not go. One of the main reasons for not attending primary health care services was the long waiting times, or in some cases services simply not being available. The costs, insurance and finances also impact on referrals to health care services. One in 10 people with disability delay accessing health care due to the costs (Australian Institute of Health and Welfare, 2010). Whilst cost is a concern for many people regardless of disability, people with disability

Box 10.5 Case study—Meryl

Meryl, 39, has cerebral palsy. She asks about a pap smear, as she has heard her friends saying that they have all had theirs but she has never had one. Meryl is not offered screening or appropriate support. Her doctors instead say this is only for people who are sexually active and therefore would not concern her and is not necessary.

- What assumptions have the doctors made about Meryl?
- How have these assumptions prejudiced the doctor's decision making?
- Consider why pap smears, which are offered to most other women, are not being considered for Meryl.
- When doctors make assumptions like this what are the consequences for Meryl?

were more likely to report issues with costs, and younger people with disability are less likely to have access to health insurance compared to older people with disability (Cannell et al., 2011). More efforts must be made to prioritise outreach of health promotion and routine screening in the disability community. This may include active engagement and consideration of how resources and campaigns outreach people living with disability—particularly those living in supported accommodation with severe to profound disability. It is also important to consider how health care services can be co-designed and evaluated with partnership and leadership from people with lived experiences of disability. Following are some practical strategies that may facilitate accessible health care.

Flexible and non-judgemental communication as a facilitator

Good communication is key. This means reserving judgment and assuming that the person with disability has capabilities and can make, or be supported to make, their own decisions. Even if the person with disability has a support person with them, it is important that you speak directly to the individual rather than talking about them in third person as if they are not in the room. Often health professionals can adapt their communication styles that can significantly hinder or strengthen accessibility. Research highlights that complicated jargon and medical terminology is very disempowering (Hemsley & Balandin, 2014; Nicolaidis et al., 2015). Instead, it helps everyone (including those who don't have a disability) if information can be made simple and clear with shorter sentences and concepts broken down into chunks, or step by step.

The use of images, pictures, visual schedules, 3D models and body maps can be particularly useful ways of improving access to information by "showing" people (Finan, 2002; Osborne, 2006). Another strategy may be the use of video to demonstrate and share information visually. These practical strategies are useful to consider in all aspects of health care: in the health care clinician's meeting rooms, but also in terms of how health care promotional materials, websites and resources can be adapted to improve health literacy of people with learning difficulties or complex communication needs (Alborz, McNally, & Glendinning, 2005; Backer, Chapman, & Mitchell, 2009; Osborne, 2006).

It is essential that health professionals recognise the power they have and avoid projecting negative views of disability onto their clients, colleagues or others (Hammell, 2007).

Table 10.1 contrasts a few examples of disempowering and respectful practices around communication, so you can evaluate your own style.

Table 10.1 Disempowering and respectful practices around communication

Disempowering practices	*Respectful practices*
Making assumptions about the person's abilities based on their diagnosis or condition alone	Asking about the person's support needs and being open-minded about what they can and can't do, keeping in mind how the condition impacts most people
Being inflexible with the communication style and expecting the disabled person to adapt and understand complex jargon and information	Being flexible and accommodating different ways of communicating, for example, using pictures or visual props to communicate information; waiting extra time for responses to questions; booking AUSLAN interpreters as requested.
Using language that refers only to deficits and assumes no quality of life	Acknowledges prejudice and intentionally puts aside preconceptions. Considers the individual, their background and situation.

Supportive decision making as a facilitator

A key component of respectful communication lies in supporting people with disability to have a say in decisions. This is especially important in health care where it is likely that bodily autonomy has been overridden by service providers and paid professionals, and there is a high risk of acquiescence without really understanding or being engaged in making decisions or providing consent. It can be particularly useful to consider how you will balance your relationship with the individual who has a disability, along with their supports and families. You may like to know about various types of supportive decision making models: an emerging field of best practice now being adopted by many advocacy organisations and disability groups (Watson, 2016; Watson, Wilson, & Hagiliassis, 2017). Adopting supportive decision making as part of your practice means recognising that all of us, regardless of our level of ability, are interdependent and may benefit from support of others around us when making decisions at some point in our life. It is important that as individuals, we have the opportunity to have a say, especially when it is about our body, our lives and our futures. There are multiple approaches and ways of negotiating supportive decision making. One such way is for the individual to nominate key support people who know them well and intentionally form a community that may come together and assist with decision making and planning. The roles of people within this support circle, along with the formality and set-up varies depending on the individual needs (Brady, Burke, Landon, & Oertle, 2019; Burke, 2016; Watson, 2016). Such models are proving particularly useful when assisting people with cognitive impairment to make "big" decisions about their health, accommodation or life. There are creative ways to facilitate supportive decision making, and they vary, depending on the person and their needs (Arstein-Kerslake, Watson, Browning, Martinis, & Blanck, 2017).

Collaboration as a facilitator

As a health professional, you should always focus on working directly with the individual with disability, ensuring that their needs and decisions are central to your work. However, there may be times where a consumer has additional support people involved. In these cases, it is necessary to recognise the potential roles of key support people such as carers, or disability service staff (Backer et al., 2009). These key people can offer support in several ways:

- Modelling how communication systems work, and translating or transmitting information as needed to health professionals who are not familiar with how individuals communicate
- Informing and providing historical and current or emerging information that may be relevant and useful to health care decisions
- Supporting people with their health care needs in their daily lives outside of the consultation room.

Many of these key support people are informally involved; others have formal arrangements with guardians and advocates who must be part of the decision-making process. Health professionals may need to rely on support people's accounts of information in order to gather a picture of the health concerns and past history. This requires health professionals to be mindful of adapting the consultation to improve accessibility of communication (providing more time, adapting the way the information is delivered) and the potential need to gather information (Noonan Walsh, & McConkey, 2009) as well as appropriate accommodation to adapt the information. The health care needs of people with disability should not solely be the responsibility of disability service sectors. There is a strong need for mainstream and specialist health care services to consider outreaching and including people with disability as a priority population group.

Streamlining information using technology as a facilitator

A valuable area of development in recent years has been the use of technology as a way to screen for access requirements and improve information gathering prior to consultations. If all consumers were asked a series of questions and their access needs were identified early, this would enable administration and health professionals to better prepare for their consultations by booking extra time, or by organising access requirements such as equipment or AUSLAN interpreters (Backer et al., 2009; Bradbury-Jones, Rattray, Jones, & MacGillivray, 2013; Robertson, Hatton, Baines, & Emerson, 2015).

Technology has also seen the rise of resources and tools to streamline and increase access to historical health records and documentation. Such platforms have the potential to make documentation and information more accessible, a particularly useful consideration for people with disability who are often accessing multiple health and disability services.

Liaison and specialist team models as facilitators

Some health care services have developed specialists support teams or are nominating liaison specialists within their teams who can offer specialist knowledge, consultancy and advice specific to disability (Backer et al., 2009; MacArthur, Brown, McKechanie, Mack, Hayes, & Fletcher, 2015). Such models are shown to be effective, particularly among nurses and regarding people with learning difficulties (Backer et al., 2009). Adopting such a model may mean that people with disability and their families have a point of contact for consultancy and support to help with navigating complex health care systems. The addition of specialist positions may also provide a point of contact and information to health professionals who may need it.

Barriers to accessing services

The location of service and accessibility for people with disability who may not be able to drive, or who rely on public transport, determines who receives a services and who does not (de Vries McClintock et al., 2015). People with disability living in remote or regional areas are even less likely to find health care services available in their local area (Baumbusch, Moody, Hole, Jokinen, & Stainton, 2019; Gallego et al., 2017). The health care service may exist locally, but it may not be accessible enough to allow people with disability to use the service due to infrastructure and poor planning of buildings. This could include lack of ramps and wide automatic doors. Inside the buildings, there may not be space to manoeuvre a wheelchair or other mobility aids in waiting or clinical rooms. Some buildings may not have access to lifts, or appropriate changing places such as hospitals can be very large and difficult to navigate with poor planning around things like accessible signage or tactile directions for people who may be blind or vision impaired (Morrison et al., 2008). Environmental access may also be an issue for people with sensory issues (such as autism), who benefit from a calm and quieter environment with low or natural lighting (Nicolaidis et al., 2015; Zerbo et al., 2015). The environment and design of building and health care facilities weighs in heavily for many people with various types of disability. The scarcity of health care facilities that are adequately built and designed with appropriate equipment are likely to have long waiting lists and wait times involved. Studies indicate that people with disability are more likely to have to wait longer than other people to see clinicians, and there are often waiting lists (Australian Institute of Health and Welfare, 2010).

Universal design as a facilitator when planning accessible health care

In Australia, our building codes dictate that most buildings will have access to basic features such as lifts or ramps, but the truth is that meeting these standards does not actually meet the needs of many people with disability who require additional specialist equipment and supports. It is also important to consider access to transport, parking and the geographical location, as these factors can further limit choices of health care services, especially in small metropolitan, rural or remote areas.

Box 10.6 Reflection—Accessibility

Ask yourself, how many health professionals' rooms have hoists for people who need to be transferred?

For example, how many allied health therapy practices have changing rooms suitable or adults?

The concept of Universal Design gives you a useful framework from which to evaluate, assess and innovate accessible respectful health care services. There are seven Universal Design principles (Centre for Excellence in Universal Design, 2014).

1. Equitable use (useful to people regardless of ability)
2. Flexibility (tailored and able to meet a wide range of preferences)

Table 10.2 Barriers and facilitators underlying culturally safe health care for people with disability

Barriers	*Facilitators*
Health care facilities/services being inaccessible in their location, building design and equipment, opening hours or waitlist systems	Consultation with disabled people and groups when designing health care facilities would improve access to health services for all people
Inaccessible information about what services exist, how relevant they are and how to access them	Adhering to universal design and standards of building and design to improve physical and environmental access
No attempts made to include people with disabilities in health promotion campaigns, standard health screenings like pap screens and prostate exams and mental health plans	Building health literacy and the capacity of people to self-refer or refer their family member
Health professionals are under skilled with how to obtain informed consent for medical treatments from people	Developing health promotion campaigns that specifically prioritise people with disability (designed collaboratively with disabled people)
Health professionals value building relationships with their clients but are under time pressures that prohibit planning for peoples' individual needs in terms of physical equipment or communication supports	Developing practical communication resources to facilitate relationship building and health care service delivery. For example 3D props, picture cards, video demonstrations, podcasts or audio descriptions, visual schedules and Easy-English health information
Information about people is fragmented, meaning people with disability have to repeat things, and key information is sometimes missed or not asked for due to the health professional's misconceptions and assumptions	Improving undergraduate health professional curriculum in relation to disability-specific knowledge for students. Developing disability-specific continuing professional education programs

3. Simple (uncomplicated and easy to understand, not dependent on expert knowledge or language)
4. Perceptible information (communication information is clear and in multiple accessible formats)
5. Tolerance for error (minimises consequences of accident or unintended actions)
6. Low physical effort (able to use the design efficiently and comfortably with minimal fatigue)
7. Size and space (appropriate space and design to comfortably use regardless of body, size, mobility or posture)

These principles can be applied not only when thinking about the physical design of buildings, hospitals and clinics, but also when considering the design and practicality of service systems, online platforms, and health care products. By adopting Universal Design as a model to work from, we can develop health care services that suit all people—not just those with disability—but also people who are sick, injured, young or elderly. The key to good universal design in health care settings lies in considering accessibility and inclusion of people with disability at the outset of health care planning, and not as an afterthought. This should always include consultation and ongoing dialogue with people with disability at all stages of design, implementation and evaluation of health care services (Table 10.2).

Conclusion

This chapter has described the barriers people with disability experience regarding access to health care, and has offered a range of strategies to improve and develop culturally safe health care. It is vital for all health professionals to recognise people with disability as a group deserving of explicit reference and consideration in health service delivery.

Whatever field of health you are working towards, it is also important to consider how your future practice will:

- Build the capacity of people with disability by developing accessible and informative health promotional resources and campaigns that effectively reach all people, including people who live in supported accommodation settings who have complex support needs and/or learning difficulties.
- Recognise and call out abuse, neglect or harm when you see it by providing access to services and reporting to appropriate statutory bodies.
- Respond and interact with people with disability in flexible and practical ways that demonstrates a willingness to work with individual communication, access needs and learning styles.
- Improve platforms and streamline access to information and case notes.
- Invest in inclusive health care systems that are culturally respectful of the needs of people with disability and make this a key priority for professional development and innovation.

Commitment to education and professional development

Health professionals to educate themselves on disability and update regularly. It is important that this includes evidence-based practice, but also exposure to real-life stories. This is key to addressing knowledge deficit barriers as well as the biases that lead to discrimination and disrespect (Backer et al., 2009; O'Halloran et al., 2008; Tracy & McDonald, 2015).

Box 10.7 Reflection—Ideas regarding disability

Consider where and how your ideas about disability develop.

- Are they mostly from beliefs and stories you have heard growing up, or are they gathered from media exposure, or from people you know?
- How many of these stories are constructed and written from the view of non-disabled journalists or writers?
- How many are authentically shared by people with lived experience of disability?
- How diverse are these experiences?

Keep in mind that one person with disability cannot represent all people with disability. It is important for all of us in health and medicine to make a commitment to increasing evidence-based practice and upskilling our knowledge, not just in terms of evidence-based knowledge, but seeking out, hearing and valuing the lived experiences and stories of people with disability. It is important that these lived experiences and stories from people with disability are given space to speak honestly without judgement. This will enhance our cultural sensitivity and respect to people with disability.

References

Alborz, A., McNally, R., & Glendinning, C. (2005). Access to health care for people with learning disabilities in the UK: Mapping the issues and reviewing the evidence. *Journal of Health Services Research and Policy*, *10*(3), 173–182. https://doi.org/10.1258/1355819054338997.

Ali, A., Scior, K., Ratti, V., Strydom, A., King, M., & Hassiotis, A. (2013). Discrimination and other barriers to accessing health care: Perspectives of patients with mild and moderate intellectual disability and their carers. *PLoS One*, *8*(8), 1–13. https://doi.org/10.1371/journal.pone.0070855.

Arstein-Kerslake, A., Watson, J., Browning, M., Martinis, J., & Blanck, P. (2017). Future direction in supported decision-making. *Disability Studies Quarterly*, *37*(1). https://doi.org/10.18061/dsq.v37i1.5070.

Aston, M., Breau, L., & MacLeod, E. (2014). Diagnoses, labels and stereotypes: Supporting children with intellectual disabilities in the hospital. *Journal of Intellectual Disabilities*, *18*(4), 291–304. https://doi.org/10.1177/1744629514552151.

Australian Bureau of Statistics. (2004). *Disability, ageing and carers, Australia* (no. 4430.0). https://www.abs.gov.au/AUSSTATS/abs@.nsf/Lookup/4430.0Main+Features12003?OpenDocument.

Australian Bureau of Statistics. (2015). *Disability, ageing and carers, Australia: Summary of findings, 2015* (no. 4430.0.). https://www.abs.gov.au/ausstats/abs@.nsf/Lookup/4430.0main+features202015.

Australian Bureau of Statistics. (2018). *Disability, ageing and carers, Australia: Summary of findings, 2018* (no. 4430.0.). https://www.abs.gov.au/ausstats/abs@.nsf/mf/4430.0.

Australian Human Rights Commission. (2017). *2016–2017 complaint statistics*. https://humanrights.gov.au/sites/default/files/AHRC_Complaints_AR_Stats_Tables%202016-2017.pdf.

Australian Institute of Health and Welfare. (2010). *Health of Australians with disability: Health status and risk factors*. https://www.aihw.gov.au/getmedia/070c288b-8603-4438-86a3-bac43f1845c3/11608.pdf.aspx?inline=true.

Australian Institute of Health and Welfare. (2015). *Access to health services by Australians with disability 2012*. https://www.aihw.gov.au/getmedia/eb1e8f89-2d0d-429a-be05-c31211812184/19001.pdf.aspx?inline=true.

Australian Institute of Health and Welfare. (2018). *Australia's health 2018*. https://www.aihw.gov.au/getmedia/7c42913d-295f-4bc9-9c24-4e44eff4a04a/aihw-aus-221.pdf.

Australian Institute of Health and Welfare. (2019). *People with disability in Australia 2019: In brief.* https://www.aihw.gov.au/getmedia/3bc5f549-216e-4199-9a82-fba1bba9208f/aihw-dis-74.pdf.aspx?inline=true -

Backer, C., Chapman, M., & Mitchell, D. (2009). Access to secondary healthcare for people with intellectual disabilities: A review of the literature. *Journal of Applied Research in Intellectual Disabilities, 22*(6), 514–525. https://doi.org/10.1111/j.1468-3148.2009.00505.x.

Baldry, E. (2014). Disability at the margins: Limits of the law. *Griffith Law Review, 23*(3), 370–388. https://doi.org/10.1080/10383441.2014.1000218.

Baumbusch, J., Moody, E., Hole, R., Jokinen, N., & Stainton, T. (2019). Using healthcare services: Perspectives of community-dwelling aging adults with intellectual disabilities and family members. *Journal of Policy and Practice in Intellectual Disabilities, 16*(1), 4–12. https://doi.org/10.1111/jppi.12264.

Boyles, C. M., Bailey, P. H., & Mossey, S. (2008). Representations of disability in nursing and healthcare literature: An integrative review. *Journal of Advanced Nursing, 62*(4), 428–437. https://doi.org/10.1111/j.1365-2648.2008.04623.x.

Bradbury-Jones, C., Rattray, J., Jones, M., & MacGillivray, S. (2013). Promoting the health, safety and welfare of adults with learning disabilities in acute care settings: A structured literature review. *Journal of Clinical Nursing, 22*(11–12), 1497–1509. https://doi.org/10.1111/jocn.12109.

Brady, A. M., Burke, M. M., Landon, T., & Oertle, K. (2019). Siblings of adults with intellectual and developmental disabilities: Their knowledge and perspectives on guardianship and its alternatives. *Journal of Applied Research in Intellectual Disabilities, 32*(5), 1078–1087. https://doi.org/10.1111/jar.12597.

Burke, S. (2016). Person-centered guardianship: How the rise of supported decision-making and person-centered services can help Olmstead's promise get here faster. *Mitchell Hamline Law Review, 42*(3), 873–896.

Cadwallader, J. R., Spivakovsky, C., Steele, L., & Wadiwel, D. (2018). Institutional violence against people with disability: Recent legal and political developments. *Current Issues in Criminal Justice, 29*(3), 259–272. https://doi.org/10.1080/10345329.2018.12036101.

Campbell, F. (2009). *Contours of ableism: The production of disability and abledness.* Springer.

Cannell, M. B., Brumback, B. A., Bouldin, E. D., Hess, J., Wood, D. L., Sloyer, P. J., Reiss, J. G., & Andresen, E. M. (2011). Age group differences in healthcare access for people with disabilities: Are young adults at increased risk? *Journal of Adolescent Health, 49*(2), 219–221. https://doi.org/10.1016/j.jadohealth.2010.11.251.

Centre for Excellence in Universal Design. (2014). *What is Universal Design? The 7 Principles.* http://universaldesign.ie/What-is-Universal-Design/The-7-Principles/The-7-Principles.html.

Chouinard, V. (1997). Making space for disabling difference: Challenges ableist geographies. *Environment and Planning D: Society and Space, 15*(4), 379–387. https://doi.org/10.1068/d150379.

Civil Society CRPD Report Working Group. (2019). Disability rights now 2019: Australian civil society shadow report to the United Nations Committee on the Rights of Persons with Disabilities: UN CRPD Review 2019. https://dpoa.org.au/wp-content/uploads/2019/08/CRPD-Shadow-Report-2019-English-PDF.pdf.

Curtin, M., Adams, J., & Egan, M. (2017) Evolution of occupational therapy within the health care context. In M. Curtin, M. Egan, & J. Adams (Eds.), *Occupational therapy for people experiencing illness, injury or impairment: Promoting occupation and participation* (7th ed., pp. 116–121). Elsevier.

de Vries McClintock, H. F., Barg, F. K., Katz, S. P., Stineman, M. G., Krueger, A., Colletti, P. M., Boellstorff, T., Bogner, H. R. (2015). Health care experiences and perceptions among people with and without disabilities. *Disability and Health Journal, 9*(1), 74–82. https://doi.org/10.1016/j.dhjo.2015.08.007.

Dewar, R., Claus, A. P., Tucker, K., & Johnston, L. M. (2017). Perspectives on postural control dysfunction to inform future research: A delphi study for children with cerebral palsy. *Archives of Physical Medicine and Rehabilitation, 98*(3), 463–479. https://doi.org/10.1016/j.apmr.2016.07.021.

Directorate for Employment, Labour and Social Affairs. (2009). *Sickness, disability and work: Keeping on track in the economic downturn.* Organisation for Economic Co-operation and Development. http://www.oecd.org/employment/emp/42699911.pdf.

Durell, S. (2014). How the social model of disability evolved. *Nursing Times, 110*(50), 20–22.

Durvalsula, S., & Beange, H. (2001). Health inequalities in people with intellectual disability: Strategies for improvement. *Health Promotion Journal of Australia, 11*(1), 27–31.

Emerson, E., & Spencer, N. (2015). Health inequity and children with intellectual disabilities. In C. Hatton & E. Emerson (Eds.), *International review of research in developmental disabilities* (Vol. *48*, pp. 11–42). Academic Press. https://doi.org/10.1016/bs.irrdd.2015.03.001.

Falk-Rafael, A. (2005). Advancing nursing theory through theory-guided practice: The emergence of a critical caring perspective. *Advances in Nursing Science*, *28*(1), 38–49.

Finan, N. (2002). Visual literacy in images used for medical education and health promotion. *Journal of Audiovisual Media in Medicine*, *25*(1), 16–23. https://doi.org/10.1080/014051102201l837X

FitzGerald, C., & Hurst, S. (2017). Implicit bias in healthcare professionals: A systematic review. *BMC Medical Ethics*, *18*(1), 1–18. https://doi.org/10.1186/s12910-017-0179-8.

Fraser-Barbour, E. F., Crocker, R., & Walker, R. (2018). Barriers and facilitators in supporting people with intellectual disability to report sexual violence: Perspectives of Australian disability and mainstream support providers. *The Journal of Adult Protection*, *20*(1), 5–16. https://doi.org/10.1108/JAP-08-2017-0031.

Frohmader, C., & Ricci, C. (2016). *Improving service responses for women with disability experiencing violence: 1800RESPECT: Final report*. Women with Disabilities Australia. http://wwda.org.au/wp-content/uploads/2016/09/1800RESPECT_Report_FINAL.pdf.

Gallego, G., Dew, A., Lincoln, M., Bundy, A., Chedid, R. J., Bulkeley, K., Brentnall, J., & Veitch, C. (2017). Access to therapy services for people with disability in rural Australia: A carers' perspective. *Health and Social Care in the Community*, *25*(3), 1000–1010. https://doi.org/10.1111/hsc.12399.

Garden, R. (2010). Disability and narrative: New directions for medicine and the medical humanities. *Medical Humanities*, *36*(2), 70–74. https://doi.org/10.1136/jmh.2010.004143.

Goering, S. (2015). Rethinking disability: The social model of disability and chronic disease. *Current Reviews in Musculoskeletal Medicine*, *8*(2), 134–138. https://doi.org/10.1007/s12178-015-9273-z.

Guy-Coichard, C., Nguyen, D. T., Delorme, T., & Boureau, F. (2008). Pain in hereditary neuromuscular disorders and myasthenia gravis: A national survey of frequency, characteristics, and impact. *Journal of Pain and Symptom Management*, *35*(1), 40–50. https://doi.org/10.1016/j.jpainsymman.2007.02.041.

Hadden, K. L., & von Baeyer, C. L. (2005). Global and specific behavioural measures of pain in children with cerebral palsy. *The Clinical Journal of Pain*, *21*(2), 140–146. https://doi.org/10.1097/00002508-200503000-00005.

Haegele, J. A., & Hodge, S. (2016). Disability discourse: Overview and critiques of the medical and social models. *Quest*, *68*(2), 193–206. https://doi.org/10.1080/00336297.2016.1143849.

Hallahan, L. (2010). Inside Kew Cottages. *History Australia*, 7(3), 63.1–63.3. https://doi.org/10.2104/ha100063.

Hamam, N. (2011). Sex, drugs and the medical role: A case report of a man prescribed Alprazolam following stroke. *The Australasian Medical Journal*, *4*(11), 608–609. https://doi.org/10.4066/AMJ.2011.1045.

Hammell, K. W. (2007). Experience of rehabilitation following spinal cord injury: A meta-synthesis of qualitative findings. *Spinal Cord*, *45*(4), 260–274. https://doi.org/10.1038/sj.sc.3102034.

Hatton, C., & Emerson, E. (2015). Introduction: Health disparities, health inequity, and people with intellectual disabilities. *International Review of Research in Developmental Disabilities*, *48*, 1–9. https://doi.org/10.1016/bs.irrdd.2015.04.001.

Hemsley, B., & Balandin, S. (2014). A metasynthesis of patient-provider communication in hospital for patients with severe communication disabilities: Informing new translational research. *Augmentative and Alternative Communication*, *30*(4), 329–343. https://doi.org/10.3109/07434618.2014.955614.

Heslop, P., Blair, P. S., Fleming, P., Hoghton, M., Marriott, A., & Russ, L. (2013). The confidential inquiry into premature deaths of people with learning disabilities: A population-based study. *The Lancet*, *383*(9920), 889–895. https://doi.org/10.1016/S0140-6736(13)62026-7ht.

Hill, J. (2019). Fixing it. In J. Hill (Ed.), *See what you made me do: Power, control and domestic abuse*. Black Inc.

Hogg, J. (2001). Essential healthcare for people with learning disabilities: Barriers and opportunities. *Journal of the Royal Society of Medicine*, *94*(7), 333–336. https://doi.org/10.1177/014107680109400704.

Hwang, K., Johnston, M., Tulsky, D., Wood, K., Dyson-Hudson, T., & Komaroff, E. (2009). Access and coordination of health care service for people with disabilities. *Journal of Disability Policy Studies*, *20*(1), 28–34. https://doi.org/10.1177/1044207308315564.

Jackson, A. L., & Waters, S. E. (2015). Taking Time: Framework: A trauma-informed framework for supporting people with intellectual disability. *Berry Street*. https://learning.berrystreet.org.au/sites/default/files/2018-05/Taking-Time-Framework.pdf.

James, T. A. (2018). Setting the stage: Why health care needs a culture of respect. *Harvard Medical School Lean Forward*. https://leanforward.hms.harvard.edu/2018/07/31/setting-the-stage-why-health-care-needs-a-culture-of-respect

Kavanagh, A. M., Krnjacki, L, Aitken, Z, LaMontagne, A. D., Beer, A., Baker, E., & Bentley, R. (2015) Intersections between disability, type of impairment, gender and socio-economic disadvantage in a nationally representative sample of 33,101 working-aged Australians. *Disability and Health Journal*, *8*(2), 191–199. https://doi.org/10.1016/j.dhjo.2014.08.008.

Krahn, G. L., Hammond, L., & Turner, A. (2006). A cascade of disparities: Health and health care access for people with intellectual disabilities. *Mental Retardation and Developmental Disabilities Research Reviews*, *12*(1), 70–82. https://doi.org/10.1002/mrdd.20098.

Krnjacki, L., Emerson, E., Llewellyn, G., & Kavanagh, A. (2016). Prevalence and risk of violence against people with and without disabilities: Findings from an Australian population-based study. *Australian and New Zealand Journal of Public Health*, *40*(1), 16–21.

Krnjacki, L., Priest, N., Aitken, Z., Emerson, E., Llewellyn, G., King, T., & Kavanagh, A. (2018), Disability-based discrimination and health: Findings from an Australian-based population study. *Australian and New Zealand Journal of Public Health*, *42*(2), 172–174. https://doi.org/10.1111/1753-6405.12735.

Kroll, T., Jones, G. C., Kehn, M., & Neri, M. T. (2006). Barriers and strategies affecting the utilisation of primary preventive services for people with physical disabilities: A qualitative inquiry. *Health and Social Care in the Community*, *14*(4), 284–293. https://doi.org/10.1111/j.1365-2524.2006.00613.x.

Lakhani, A., Cullen, J., & Townsend, C. (2017). The cost of disability for Indigenous people: A systematic review. *Journal of Social Inclusion*, *8*(1), 34–45. https://doi.org/10.36251/josi.116.

Lewis, M. A., Lewis, C. E., Leaker, B., King, B. H., & Lindemann, R. (2002). The quality of health care of adults with developmental disabilities. *Public Health Reports*, *117*(2), 174–184. https://doi.org/10.1016/S0033-3549(04)50124-3.

Lewis, P., Gaffney, R. J., & Wilson, N. J. (2017). A narrative review of acute care nurses' experiences nursing patients with intellectual disability: Underprepared, communication barriers and ambiguity about the role of caregivers. *Journal of Clinical Nursing*, *26*(11–12), 1473–1484. https://doi.org/10.1111/jocn.13512.

Linton, K. F., Krcek, T. E., Sensui, L. M., & Spillers, J. L. H. (2014). Opinions of people who self-identify with autism and Asperger's on DSM-5 criteria. *Research on Social Work Practice*, *24*(1), 67–77. https://doi.org/10.1177/1049731513495457.

MacArthur, J., Brown, M., McKechanie, A., Mack, S., Hayes, M., & Fletcher, J. (2015). Making reasonable and achievable adjustments: The contributions of learning disability liaison nurses in getting it right for people with learning disabilities receiving general hospitals care. *Journal of Advanced Nursing*, *71*(7), 1552–1563. https://doi.org/10.1111/jan.12629.

Manning, C. (2009). Imprisoned in state care? Life inside Kew Cottages 1925–2008. *Health and History*, *11*(1), 149–171.

Marks, D. (1997). Models of disability. *Disability and Rehabilitation*, *19*(3), 85–91. https://doi.org/10.3109/09638289709166831ht.

Merrifield, J. (2011). Meeting the needs of people with a learning disability in the emergency department. *International Emergency Nursing*, *19*(3), 146–151. https://doi.org/10.1016/j.ienj.2010.07.004.

Michael, J., & Richardson, A. (2008). Healthcare for all: The independent inquiry into access to healthcare for people with learning disabilities. *Tizard Learning Disability Review*, *13*(4), 28–34. https://doi.org/10.1108/13595474200800036.

Monk, L. A. (2010). Exploiting patient labour at Kew Cottages, Australia, 1887–1950. *British Journal of Learning Disabilities*, *38*(2), 86–94. https://doi.org/10.1111/j.1468-3156.2010.00634.x.

Morrison, E. H., George, V., & Mosqueda, L. (2008). Primary care for adults with physical disabilities: Perceptions from consumer and provider focus groups. *Clinical Research and Methods*, *40*(9), 645–651.

National People with Disabilities and Carer Council. (2009). *Shut out: The experiences of people with disabilities and their families in Australia: National disability strategy consultation report*. https://www.dss.gov.au/sites/default/files/documents/05_2012/nds_report.pdf.

Nicolaidis, C., Raymaker, D., McDonald, K., Dern, S., Boisclair, W. C., Ashkenazy, E., & Baggs, A. (2013). Comparison of healthcare experiences in autistic and non-autistic adults: A cross-sectional online survey facilitated by an academic-community partnership. *Journal of General Internal Medicine*, *28*(6), 761–769. https://doi.org/10.1007/s11606-012-2262-7.

Nicolaidis, C., Raymaker, D. M., Ashkenazy, E., McDonald, K. E., Dern, S., Baggs, A. E., Kapp, S. K., Weiner, M., & Boisclair, W. C. (2015). Respect the way I need to communicate with you: Healthcare experiences of adults on the autism spectrum. *Autism, 19*(7), 824–831. https://doi.org/10.1177/1362361315576221.

Noonan Walsh, P., & McConkey, R. (2009). Inclusive health and people with intellectual disabilities. In R. M. Hodapp (Ed.), *International review of research in mental retardation, Volume 38* (pp. 33–67). Academic Press.

Oddson, B. E., Clancy, C. A., & McGrath, P. J. (2006). The role of pain in reduced quality of life and depressive symptomology in children with spina bifida. *The Clinical Journal of Pain, 22*(9), 784–789. https://doi.org/10.1097/01.ajp.0000210929.43192.5d.

Office of the Public Advocate. (2016). *Upholding the right to life and health: A review of the deaths in care of people with disability in Queensland.* Queensland Government. https://www.justice.qld.gov.au/__data/assets/pdf_file/0008/460088/final-systemic-advocacy-report-deaths-in-care-of-people-with-disability-in-Queensland-February-2016.pdf.

O'Halloran, R., Hickson, L., & Worrall, L. (2008). Environmental factors that influence communication between people with communication disability and their healthcare providers in hospital: A review of the literature within the International Classification of Functioning, Disability and Health (ICF) framework. *International Journal of Language and Communication Disorders, 43*(6), 601–632. https://doi.org/10.1080/13682820701861832.

Oliver, M. (1983). *Social work with disabled people.* Macmillan.

Oliver, M. (2013). The social model of disability: Thirty years on. *Disability & Society, 28*(7), 1024–1026. https://doi.org/10.1080/09687599.2013.818773.

Ombudsman of New South Wales. (2018). *Report of reviewable deaths of people in 2014–2017: Deaths of people with disability in residential care.* https://www.ombo.nsw.gov.au/news-and-publications/publications/annual-reports/reviewable-deaths/report-of-reviewable-deaths-of-people-in-2014-2017-deaths-of-people-with-disability-in-residential-care.

Osborne, H. (2006). Health literacy: How visuals can help tell the healthcare story. *Journal of Visual Communication in Medicine, 29*(1), 28–32. https://doi.org/10.1080/01405110600772830.

Ouellette-Kuntz, H. (2005). Understanding health disparities and inequalities faced by individuals with intellectual disabilities. *Journal of Applied Research in Intellectual Disabilities, 18*(2), 113–121. https://doi.org/10.1111/j.1468-3148.2005.00240.x.

Pelleboer-Gunnink, H., Van Oorsouw, W. M. W. J., Van Weeghel, J., & Embregts, P. J. C. M. (2017). Mainstream health professionals' stigmatising attitudes towards people with intellectual disabilities: A systematic review. *Journal of Intellectual Disability Research, 61*(5), 411–434. https://doi.org/10.1111/jir.12353.

Reichard, A., Sacco, T. M., & Turnbull, H. R. III. (2004). Access to health care for individuals with developmental disabilities from minority backgrounds. *Mental Retardation, 42*(6), 459–470. https://doi.org/10.1352/0047-6765(2004)42<459:ATHCFI>2.0.CO2.

Robertson, J., Hatton, C., Baines, S., & Emerson, E. (2015). Systematic reviews of the health or health care of people with intellectual disabilities: A systematic review to identify gaps in the evidence base. *Journal of Applied Research in Intellectual Disabilities, 28*(6), 455–523. https://doi.org/10.1111/jar.12149.

Robinson, S. (2012). *Enabling and protecting: Proactive approaches to addressing the abuse and neglect of children and young people with disability.* Children with Disability Australia. http://a4.org.au/sites/default/files/CDA%20Enabling%20and%20Protecting%20Issues%20nPaper.pdf.

Robinson, S. (2018). Safety and harm in school: Promoting the perspectives of students with intellectual disability. *Journal of Research in Special Educational Needs, 18*(S1), 48–58. https://doi.org/10.1111/1471-3802.12417.

Robinson, S., Oakes, P., Murphy, M., Ferguson, P., Lee, F., Ward-Boas, W., Codognotto, M., Nicks, J., & Theodoropoulos, D. (2019). *Building safe and respectful cultures in disability services for people with disability.* Disability Services Commissioner. https://www.odsc.vic.gov.au/wp-content/uploads/BSRC-Report-June-2019-WEB.pdf.

Royal Commission into Violence, Abuse and Neglect of People with Disability. (2020). *Interim report.* Commonwealth of Australia. https://disability.royalcommission.gov.au/system/files/2020-10/Interim%20Report.pdf.

Sandberg, M., Ahlström, G., & Kristensson, J. (2015). Access to healthcare for people with intellectual disability. *BMC Nursing*, *14*(Suppl 1), 1. https://doi.org/10.1186/1472-6955-14-S1-S1.

Schmitt, M. T., Branscombe, N. R., Postmes, T., & Garcia, A. (2014). The consequences of perceived discrimination for psychological well-being: A meta-analytic review. *Psychological Bulletin*, *140*(4), 921–948. https://doi.org/10.1037/a0035754.

Scullion, P.A. (2010). Models of disability: Their influence in nursing and potential role in challenging discrimination. *Journal of Advanced Nursing*, *66*(3), 697–707. https://doi.org/10.1111/j.1365-2648.2009.05211.x.

Shabas, D., & Weinreb, H. (2000). Preventive healthcare in women with multiple sclerosis. *Journal of Women's Health & Gender-Based Medicine*, *9*(4), 389–395. https://doi.org/10.1089/15246090050020709.

Shakespeare, T. (2006). The social model of disability. *The Disability Studies Reader*, *2*, 197–204.

Simmons-Mackie, N. N., Kagan, A., O'Neill Christie, C., Huijbregts, M., McEwen, S., & Willems, J. (2007). Communicative access and decision making for people with aphasia: Implementing sustainable healthcare systems change. *Aphasiology*, *21*(1), 39–66. https://doi.org/10.1080/02687030600798287.

Straetmans, J. M., van Schrojenstein Lantman-de Valk, H. M., Schellevis, F. G., & Dinant, G. J. (2007). Health problems of people with intellectual disabilities: The impact for general practice. *The British Journal of General Practice*, *57*(534), 64–66.

Taylor, K. (2019). *Health care and Indigenous Australians: Cultural safety in practice* (3rd ed.). Red Globe Press.

Tracy, J., & McDonald, R. (2015). Health and disability: Partnerships in health care. *Journal of Applied Research in Intellectual Disabilities*, *28*(1), 22–32. https://doi.org/10.1111/jar.12135.

United Nations. (2006). *Convention on the rights of persons with disabilities and optional Protocol*. https://www.un.org/disabilities/documents/convention/convoptprot-e.pdf.

Ward, R. L., Nichols, A. D., & Freedman, R. I. (2010). Uncovering health care inequalities among adults with intellectual and developmental disabilities. *Health and Social Work*, *35*(4), 280–290. https://doi.org/10.1093/hsw/35.4.280.

Warfield, M. E., Crossman, J. D., Delahaye, J., Der Weerd, E., & Kuhlthau, K. A. (2015). Physician perspectives on providing primary medical care to adults with autism spectrum disorders. *Journal of Autism and Developmental Disorders*, *45*(7), 2209–2217. https://doi.org/10.1007/s10803-015-2386-9.

Watson, J. (2016). Assumptions of decision-making capacity: The role supporter attitudes play in the realisation of Article 12 for people with severe or profound intellectual disability. *Laws*, *5*(1), 1–9. https://doi.org/10.3390/laws5010006.

Watson, J., Wilson, E., & Hagiliassis, N. (2017). Supporting end of life decision making: Case studies of relational closeness in supported decision making for people with severe or profound intellectual disability. *Journal of Applied Research in Intellectual Disabilities*, *30*(6), 1022–1034.

Witko, J., Boyles, P., Smiler, K., & McKee, R. (2017). Deaf New Zealand sign language users' access to healthcare. *The New Zealand Medical Journal*, *130*(1466), 53–61. https://assets-global.website-files.com/5e332a62c703f653182faf47/5e332a62c703f685cc2fd42e_Witko-FINAL.pdf.

World Health Organisation. (2002). Towards a common language for functioning, health and disability: ICF, International classification of functioning, health and disability. https://www.who.int/classifications/icf/icfbeginnersguide.pdf.

World Health Organisation. (2011). *World report on disability*. https://www.who.int/disabilities/world_report/2011/report.pdf.

Zerbo, O., Massolo, M. L., Qian, Y., & Croen, L. A. (2015). A study of physician knowledge and experience with autism in adults in a large integrated health system. *Journal of Autism and Developmental Disorders*, *45*(12), 4002–4014. https://doi.org/10.1007/s10803-015-2579-2

11 Gender and health

Alexander Workman, Rocco Cavaleri, Elias Mambo Machina, Stewart Alford and Tinashe Dune

Learning outcomes

After working through this chapter, students should be able to:

1. Understand that gender is a social construction and therefore a social determinant of health.
2. Explain how constructions of gender influence health outcomes.
3. Identify Australian policies and systems regarding gender and health.
4. Discuss the ways in which health policies and systems may influence the health and wellbeing of people of different genders.
5. Reflect upon how gender-based health programs can support cultural safety in Australia.
6. Explore the role that health professionals play in reinforcing and/or challenging social constructions of gender.

Key terms

Cisgender: A term used to describe individuals whose gender identity and expression matches the biological sex with which they were presumed at birth.
Femininity: A socially constructed set of attributes, behaviours and characteristics considered "typical" or "appropriate" for girls and women.
Gender diverse: A term used to describe individuals whose gender identity does not necessarily align with their presumed sex.
Gender sensitivity: An iterative process by which people demonstrate awareness and responsiveness to the influence of gender on behaviour and wellbeing. A gender-sensitive clinician appreciates and positively responds to the differences, inequalities, and varying needs of individuals of differing gender identifies.
Gender: A socially constructed characterisation of people based on their roles, attitudes, behaviours, attributes and opportunities. There are many ways in which an individual may choose to define their gender, including those who identify as being agendered or non-binary (neither a man nor a woman).
Hegemony: The social dominance of one group over another, supported by legitimising norms and the subordination of other social groups or identities.
LGBTIQA+: An evolving acronym that stands for lesbian, gay, bisexual, transgender, intersex, queer/questioning, asexual and other terms (such as non-binary and pansexual) that people use to describe experiences of their gender, sexuality and physiological sex characteristics.
Masculinity: A socially constructed set of attributes, behaviours and characteristics considered "typical" or "appropriate" for boys and men.
Sex: The term sex can have different meanings in different contexts. Sex can refer to a person's physical characteristics, including their genitals and reproductive organs, or to their assigned or legal status. Sex can also refer to engaging in sexual activities.

Chapter summary

In this chapter, students will explore the ways in which constructions of gender influence health outcomes throughout Australia. Students will analyse this impact through the lens of social determinants, reflecting upon activities that demonstrate how men and women experience health. A discussion of health policies and systems introduces students to the influence of gender on treatment avenues and practitioner engagement. This chapter also provides students with discussions on evidence-based programs that encourage gender-sensitive and culturally safe practices. At its closing, this chapter invites students to challenge their constructions of gender and explore their role in supporting major health issues faced by people of differing genders.

Introduction

As early as a few weeks past conception, family, friends, and strangers begin to ask, "Is it a boy or a girl?" It is often from this time that our gender is decided and others begin surrounding us with expectations. Pink clothing may be bought for girls and blue clothing for boys. However, an important distinction is needed when discussing the impact of these labels and behaviours on health and wellbeing. *Sex* refers to biological characteristics, distinguishing individuals based upon a combination of their gametes (sex cells), hormonal balances, and chromosomal makeup, while *gender* represents a social construct (Butler, 2004). Accordingly, there are many ways in which an individual may choose to define their gender, including those who identify as being agendered or non-binary (neither a man nor a woman). As you will be aware from reading previous chapters, and as will be expanded in the following chapter, our understanding of gender has significant repercussions on how we experience health and wellbeing.

The way we navigate health systems or are perceived by health practitioners is often based on a binary system of being male or female. While rapidly changing, there persists the belief that males will perform "masculine" roles, adopting the familial role of provider, performing yard work, watching or playing sport, and suppressing outward expressions of their emotions (Connell, 2011; Javaid, 2017; Jewkes et al., 2015; Messerschmidt, 1993; White et al., 2017). Conversely, females are expected to be empathetic caregivers, performing household chores and actively displaying a broad spectrum of emotions (Budgeon, 2014; Carmody, 2015).

Although it is acknowledged that males and females have different health needs and priorities, there exist inequalities in how these needs are met in a variety of contexts. These inequalities often reinforce stereotypical beliefs that men and women ought to be treated differently, promoting differences in health service access, delivery and utilisation (Annandale & Hunt, 2000; Butler, 2004; Workman & Dune, 2019). For context, students are introduced to the concepts of *masculinity* and *femininity* and how the health care system responds to people according to this binary. However, it remains important to emphasise the great variance that exists in terms of gender and its expressions.

Box 11.1 Reflection—Gender and society

How does society define a boy/man or girl/woman? Consider the following:

- Hairstyle, clothing/fashion
- Occupation, leisure activities, sporting pursuits

Has there ever been a time where you were unsure about someone's gender identity? How did you come to identify their gender?

Social constructions of gender

Constructions of masculinity

Through media and popular culture, we are often exposed to images reinforcing the ways in which men and women "should" perform their masculine and feminine roles, respectively. These images have been shown to reinforce societal barriers, depicting men as absent fathers, violent football fans, or underachieving students (Mac an Ghaill, & Haywood, 2007). Men are stereotypically characterised as inherently aggressive, with this trait manifesting itself in the form of "taking charge", exhibiting dominating behaviours or violence (Connell, 2011; Javaid, 2017; Jewkes et al., 2015; Messerschmidt, 1993; White et al., 2017). *Hegemonic masculinity* describes practices that legitimise the "dominant" position of heterosexual white men in society and justify subordination of other gender identities or sexual orientations (Connell, 2011; Treadwell & Garland, 2011). The hegemonic male must be successful, athletic, competitive and stoic, taking risks and engaging in aggressive or thrill-seeking behaviours. Physical fitness may be prioritised along with work success, and mental or emotional difficulties are kept hidden from all but the most intimate of female partners (Johansson & Ottemo, 2015; Tolman et al., 2016). In some cases, these traits may be exaggerated and reflect *hyper-masculinity,* which is characterised by callous sexual attitudes towards women, the belief that violence is acceptable or "manly" and the perception of danger as exciting (Bengtsson, 2016). Such individuals are more likely to drink alcohol to excess, be involved in fatal car accidents and commit acts of violence, online bullying or sexual harassment (Courtenay, 2000; Mahalik et al., 2007). Hyper-masculine males, in particular, are less likely to engage with health professionals for fear of being considered "weak" and consequently demonstrate poorer health outcomes (Courtenay, 2000; Levant et al., 2009; Mahalik et al., 2007).

Pressure to conform to hegemonic masculine "norms" may create a false sense of self, leading individuals to question their "manhood" or alter their outward persona (Courtenay, 2000; Levant et al., 2009; Mahalik et al., 2007). Anxiety and depression are common amongst men who believe they do not possess hegemonic masculine qualities (Courtenay, 2000; Levant et al., 2009; Mahalik et al., 2007). The societal advantages seen amongst hegemonic males may also cause resentment or frustration amongst those who do not receive such advantage. This frustration may elicit *protest masculinity*, whereby males actively protest the "ideal" of hegemonic masculinity (Anderson & McGuire, 2010; Elliott, 2020; Noble et al., 1998). This form of masculinity is most often observed among ethnic minorities or individuals of low socioeconomic status (Anderson & McGuire, 2010; Elliott, 2020; Noble et al., 1998). Protest masculinity can be "anomic", where men exert their masculinity by suppressing health- and help-seeking behaviours, engaging in criminal activities and pursuing multiple female sexual partners, or "disciplined", where men institute social controls and behaviours (e.g., de-emphasising sexual prowess) to increase solidarity amongst others in similar positions (Walker, 2006).

Constructions of femininity

Although there has been considerable investigation regarding constructions of masculinity and the relationships between them, femininity remains relatively under-conceptualised. Most research into gender relations has not included specific consideration of femininity as a concept, instead only referring to this construct in terms of its interplay with, or subordination to, masculinity (Paechter, 2018). Indeed, many traditional feminine "characteristics" are those that appear to serve men, such as being slim and attractive, wearing makeup, exhibiting submissiveness and fulfilling one's "duty" as a caring mother. The same qualities that characterise depression and low social rank, including subordination, lack of autonomy, and wishing to escape a scenario but remaining "trapped" due to fear or obligation, are often regarded as normal and even desirable qualities of femininity (World Health Organisation, n.d.). Pressure to portray feminine characteristics has indeed been associated with increased rates of mental health disorders among women (World Health Organisation, n.d.). This pressure may also manifest itself in the form of intensive bodily surveillance and unhealthy relationships with food or exercise (Cosgrove & Riddle, 2003; Martz et al., 1995). At its extreme, *hyper-femininity* is characterised by the belief that success is determined by maintaining one's romantic relationship with a man, and that sexuality can be used to maintain this relationship (Matschiner & Murnen, 1999; Murnen & Byrne, 1991). Women in this category are less likely to report instances of domestic violence or advocate for severe punishment following sexual abuse, reinforcing their institutionalised view of themselves as "objects" (Sailors et al., 2016; Tolman et al., 2016). Such damaging portrayals of femininity are not uncommon throughout popular culture (Warsh, 2011).

While traditional gender constructions accord *hegemony* (social dominance) exclusively to men, modern conceptualisations of *hegemonic femininity* have begun to emerge. Paechter (2018) contends that in some contexts, hegemonic femininity may share characteristics with hegemonic masculinity, rather than simply being subordinate to it. Although both uphold traditional gender binaries and preserve a gender order dominated by men, they can operate socially in distinct ways. Under this framework, hegemonic females are not subservient or male-focused, instead positioning themselves as strong, independent, and mobilising power in relation to other females and non-hegemonic males (Paechter, 2018). Interestingly, findings by Schippers (2007) suggest that, even amongst different ethnicities, white women are perceived as the hegemonic feminine group. In this study, Korean and Vietnamese second-generation migrant women described white females as self-confident, successful and assertive, embodying the modern notion of hegemonic femininity (Schippers, 2007).

Box 11.2 Reflection—The constructions of masculinity and femininity

Do you identify with the constructions of masculinity and femininity presented here? Have you ever felt pressure (subtle or overt) to conform to gender stereotypes? Consider:

- The sports in which you were encouraged to participate
- The set-up (colour, toy selection, wall posters) throughout your childhood bedroom
- The nicknames or terms by which you have been addressed

Have societal expectations ever shaped your approach towards your health and wellbeing? Are there certain gender stereotypes with which you do not conform?

The relationship between gender constructions and health outcomes

Sex and gender are being increasingly recognised as important determinants of health. Biological differences notwithstanding, gender roles and societal expectations influence the ways in which people access and experience health services. Gender-based differences in health care may emanate from sociocultural and political processes that exacerbate biological susceptibilities or generate inequalities of their own accord (Afifi, 2007). Gender-sensitive and culturally safe practitioners must appreciate the varying needs of individuals across all gender identifies and understand the interrelationship between these identifies and health outcomes.

Despite the importance of taking a broad sociocultural approach, most research into the relationship between gender and health adheres to "traditional" binary perspectives. Gender biases have also been shown to influence research and health policy discourse. For example, the relationship between women's reproductive functioning and their mental health has received ongoing analysis over many years, while other areas of women's health have been neglected (World Health Organisation, n.d.). While it is true that certain health experiences are exclusive to females, such as endometriosis, menopause or pregnancy, the mental health consequences of many of these factors has been shown to be strongly mediated by psychosocial factors, rather than biological or hormonal differences (Dennerstein, 1996; World Health Organisation, n.d.). By contrast, the contribution of male reproductive functioning to mental health has been largely ignored. The small amount of research that has been conducted suggests that men respond similarly to women in a number of contexts, including a relatively common occurrence of depression following the birth of a child (Soliday et al., 1999).

Box 11.3 Reflection—Perceptions of health

Open a new web page, and search for images of "men's health" and "women's health". Consider the following when you do:

1. What is presented in these images?
2. Do the representations of health differ between males and females? If yes, how so?
3. What are the commonalities between the images?
4. Do the images focus on a singular aspect of health, or are they broader?
5. Do the images create healthy or unhealthy perceptions of what men or women "should" look like?
6. What was the race/ethnicity of those portrayed in the images? Did one group dominate the portrayals? What does this tell us regarding images of health?

Australian men, on average, die four years younger than Australian women (Australian Institute of Health and Welfare, 2019a). Males account for over 60% of premature deaths, and the majority of these deaths are potentially avoidable (Australian Institute of Health and Welfare, 2019a). Death rates by heart disease and lung cancer are nearly twice as high among Australian men, and men are more likely to experience severe chronic conditions from an earlier age (Australian Institute of Health and Welfare, 2019a). Evidence suggests that men of all ages are more likely than women to engage in over 30 behaviours that increase risk of disease, injury and death (Courtenay, 2000). Indeed, men are more likely than women to drive while intoxicated and smoke cigarettes, and less likely to use safety belts or attend health screenings (Courtenay, 2000; Mahalik et al., 2007). Many of the practices that undermine men's health reflect societal pressures to embody hegemonic masculinity. When a man boasts, "I haven't been to a doctor in years", he is not only describing a health practice, but also positioning himself in a masculine arena as someone who does not need to "fuss" about his body or welfare (Mahalik et al., 2007). Likewise, the fact that men are less likely to see health practitioners reflects adherence to the stereotype that men should deny vulnerability and not acknowledge their pain or suffering (Johansson & Ottemo, 2015; Tolman et al., 2016). Men may also construct their gender identities by refusing to take sick leave from work, taking on high workloads and sacrificing sleep for productivity (Mahalik et al., 2007). Driving dangerously or engaging in contact sports may also be a form of expressing masculinity and "fearlessness". Such factors likely contribute to men accounting for over 70% of all road fatalities throughout Australia and being more than twice as likely as women to be hospitalised with traumatic brain injuries (Australian Institute of

Health and Welfare, 2007; Department of Infrastructure, Transport, Regional Development and Communication, 2020).

Gender constructions and expectations are also often detrimental to health outcomes amongst women. Depression and anxiety represent two of the most significant contributors to the global burden of disease and occur approximately twice as often in women as in men (Afifi, 2007; World Health Organisation, n.d.). While completed suicide rates are higher among men, women demonstrate higher rates for suicide attempts (Weissman et al., 1999). Gender-based violence is a significant predictor of depression and suicidal tendencies amongst women, with over 20% of women who have experienced violence attempting suicide (Stark & Flitcraft, 1995). Approximately one in four Australian women has experienced physical or sexual violence from an intimate partner (Australian Bureau of Statistics, 2017). Such experiences have been associated with elevated rates of post-traumatic stress disorder, phobias, and affective disorders amongst women worldwide (World Health Organisation, n.d.). Accumulating evidence indicates that the increased prevalence of many psychological conditions amongst women reflects greater exposure to domestic violence, familial responsibilities and other stressors, as opposed to any kind of biological predisposition (World Health Organisation, n.d.). Men have been shown to develop alternate disorders in response to such stressors, such as antisocial behaviour and alcohol dependency (Kessler et al., 1994; Linzer et al., 1996). Physical expectations regarding femininity have also been shown to contribute to health disparities, with women representing the majority of people diagnosed with anorexia nervosa and bulimia worldwide (Burns, 2004).

Box 11.4 Reflection—Sexual harassment

Some statistics that may surprise you (Australian Bureau of Statistics, 2017; Australian Institute of Criminology, 2017):

- 1 in 4 young Australians believe that it is normal for a man to pressure a woman into sex.
- 85% of Australian women have been sexually harassed, with 25% experiencing sexual harassment in the workplace.
- In 70% of workplace-based sexual harassment cases, witnesses make no attempt to intervene.
- 53% of women experienced sexual harassment by a male or female perpetrator across their lifetime.
- 1 in 7 men have experienced emotional abuse within a relationship.
- 1 in 19 men have experienced physical or sexual violence from a partner.
- There are no male-specific services available for victims of abuse in New South Wales, and when services are available, male victims rarely utilise them.

Questions for reflection:

- What factors do you think contribute to these statistics?
- Do you think that gender constructions or expectations influence the behaviours of those witnessing sexual harassment?
- Why may men be reluctant to utilise victim support services?

Gender-based biases and stereotypes extend to the provision and utilisation of health care services themselves. Medical professionals are more likely to prescribe psychotropic drugs to women than men, even when they present with identical symptoms or scores on standardised depression assessment measures (World Health Organisation, n.d.). Women are more likely to disclose mental health problems to general practitioners, while men tend to see specialist mental health care (Allen et al., 1998; World Health Organisation, n.d.). Men are also more likely to discuss alcohol-related health issues (Allen et al., 1998). Gender-based expectations regarding women's mental health and alcohol dependency among men, as well as a reluctance to discuss symptoms of depression among men, reinforce social stigma and may contribute to these patterns of health care access (Allen et al., 1998). Certain diagnoses, such as osteoporosis, may be underdiagnosed in men due to the perception that they are "female diseases" (Regitz-Zagrosek, 2012). Conversely, expectations regarding gender and cardiovascular health have seen women with myocardial infarction, heart failure and atrial fibrillation receive less evidence-based assessment and treatment than men, who are thought to reflect the "typical" patient with cardiovascular issues (Regitz-Zagrosek, 2012).

Limitations of existing research

Though imperative to our understanding of gender as a social determinant of health, research into the relationship between gender constructions and health outcomes are by no means representative. Australia is one of the most ethnoculturally diverse populations in the world, with over 25% of inhabitants being born overseas (Australian Bureau of Statistics, 2014). Additionally, in the 2016 Australian census, approximately 600,000 Australians identified with a sexual orientation other than heterosexual, and more than 10,000 people reported identifying with a gender other than male or female (Australian Bureau of Statistics, 2018). Despite these figures, research into the influence of gender on health has largely been conducted on heterosexual Caucasian individuals. A gender binary predominates in Australian research, with a lack of comprehensive data being available regarding the gender diverse population. The term *gender diverse* is used to refer to people whose gender identity does not necessarily align with their presumed sex (Riggs et al., 2014). Current research largely neglects this potentially vulnerable population. Indeed, the small amount of research that has been conducted in this area suggests that gender diverse and non-heterosexual individuals are more likely to experience violence, self-harm, and psychological distress than heterosexual, cisgender people (National LGBTI Health Alliance, 2016; Riggs et al., 2014). The term *cisgender* is used to describe individuals whose gender identity and expression matches the sex with which they were presumed at birth. A high prevalence of depression, anxiety and suicidality has also been identified among non-binary individuals and those who do not adhere to gender stereotypes (National LGBTI Health Alliance, 2016). These sequelae may manifest as a result of leading marginalised lives, experiencing a lack of acceptance, facing pressure to hide one's sexuality or abuse from intolerant communities (Riggs et al., 2014).

More culturally diverse investigations regarding the relationship between health and gender are required. Research suggests that Western terminology is often inadequate or inappropriate when discussing gender across a range of contexts. For example, referring to Indigenous Australian *sistergirls* or *brotherboys* as transgender has been shown not to adequately capture the distinct and sovereign relationship to country that these individuals hold (Riggs & Toone, 2017). Given the rich and diverse nature of the Australian population, it is imperative that research and policy discourse strives to reflect such diversity. Where research is not yet available, clinicians must consistently reflect upon their own experiences and their patient's values in order to achieve the best possible health care practices (Cavaleri et al., 2018).

Australian health policies and systems

Australia has demonstrated ongoing commitment to its policies regarding gender and culturally safe practice. The *Sex Discrimination Act 1984* prohibits discrimination on the basis of sex, relationship status, sexual orientation, or gender identity. The *Workplace Gender Equality Act 2012,* administered by the Australian Workplace Gender Equality Agency, aims to promote gender equality and remove gender-based barriers in the Australian workforce. Despite these positive steps, institutional gender disparities do exist. For example, women in Australia currently earn, on average, $244.80 per week less than men (Workplace Gender Equality Agency, 2018). This difference represents a full-time "gender pay gap" of approximately 15%, contributing to a socioeconomic disadvantage that has been associated with poorer mental health outcomes amongst women (Afifi, 2007). This is compounded by the significant degree of unpaid work performed by women, who represent approximately 70% of the primary carers in Australia (Workplace Gender Equality Agency, 2018). Although many theories regarding the gender pay gap exist, at least some portion of it has been attributed to direct gender discrimination (Workplace Gender Equality Agency, 2018). The average Australian woman has $113,660 less superannuation for retirement than the average Australian man (Association of Superannuation Funds of Australia, 2017). As a result, women are more likely to experience financial hardships and poverty following retirement and are more likely to be dependent upon the Age Pension when compared to men of a similar age (Tanton et al., 2009).

Gender bias has also been identified within Australian policies themselves. Until January 2019, tampons, sanitary pads, and other feminine hygiene products were sold with a 10% goods and services tax included because they were regarded as "non-essential" items (Cook & Ayoub, 2018; Hunter, 2016). This tax was successfully removed following an 18-year campaign highlighting that the policy constituted discrimination, as items like condoms, lubricant, and male sexual enhancement medications were exempt from the tax and considered *essential.* Interestingly, other policies regarding *gender and health* have been synonymous with *women's health*, and funding for male reproductive health initiatives is substantially lower than initiatives for women. An Australian senate committee highlighted that breast and ovarian cancer research receives nearly double the funding dedicated to prostate and testicular cancer research, despite the conditions demonstrating similar mortality rates (Australian Parliament, 2009). Such policies and practices may reinforce institutionalised beliefs that men should downplay the significance of their health care problems, or that reproductive health concerns are exclusive to women.

Systems providing medical professionals with the means of supporting gender-diverse populations have also been shown to be inadequate. Studies have consistently demonstrated misgendering and discriminatory language from health care providers when treating gender-diverse populations (Ansara, 2012; Sperber et al., 2005). Recent evidence suggests that at least 50% of transgender individuals have had to educate their health care provider regarding transgender health issues (Grant et al., 2011). Practitioners have also been found to discount the knowledge held by gender-diverse clients, opting for prescriptive, binary treatment options regardless of a patient's gender identity (Poteat et al., 2013). These studies highlight an ongoing need for improving systems and policies regarding gender as a social determinant of health.

Box 11.5 Reflection—Gender and health professions

Consider the following data:

- Men make up just 12% of the registered nursing workforce in Australia.
- The vast majority of orthopaedic (94%) and cardiothoracic (88%) surgeons are men.
- The only medical specialists with more women practicing than men are endocrinologists (59%), pathologists (58%), and paediatricians (53%).

Questions for reflection:

- What social factors do you believe may contribute to these statistics?
- What do you picture when you think of a "typical" nurse or doctor? Do these images differ? If so, why do you think this may be the case?
- How could we start to address potential biases in the health care workforce?

Gender-based health programs and cultural safety

The ongoing need to strive for gender-sensitive and culturally safe practice has prompted the development of Australian initiatives dedicated towards mitigating gender-based health disparities. These initiatives have a particular focus on identifying gender stereotypes and the ways in which they undermine health, as well as offering support to marginalised or disadvantaged individuals.

Men's Sheds

Men's Sheds represent a growing movement within Australia in the form of community locations where men engage in a variety of activities and socialise with peers. These "Sheds" seek to address issues of social isolation and promote emotional wellbeing among men. Sheds offer a "safe space", where the focus is often not exclusively on discussing mental health, but instead seeking to instil a sense of mutual support that fosters acceptance and openness over time (Wilson et al., 2015). An intrinsic mateship is thought to promote discussions regarding health in a more organic manner, helping to overcome many men's reluctance to discuss such issues in more traditional, clinically focussed environments (Wilson et al., 2015). Many also include health promotion work, providing support to marginalised populations including disengaged youth, Indigenous men, and men with disabilities. Among men with disabilities, Sheds are considered to be enabling environments that reject deficit views of masculinity and focus on what men can do rather than what they cannot (Hansji et al., 2015). Men's Sheds have been particularly successful in attracting older men that are traditionally difficult to engage through conventional health, employment, and training initiatives (Cordier & Wilson, 2014). Sheds have been shown to normalise many experiences, reducing anxiety associated with aging, unemployment, disability, isolation, and gender-based expectations (Wilson et al., 2015). The initiative has yielded positive mental health outcomes amongst participants, also translating to increased reported levels of wellbeing amongst partners and families (Cordier & Wilson, 2014; Hansji et al., 2015; Wilson et al., 2015). Such benefits have been recognised by the Australian National Male Health Policy, which allocated AU$3 million over four years to develop an infrastructure for ensuring the growth and sustainability of Men's Sheds (Wilson et al., 2015).

A particularly successful example of a Shed has been the collaboration between the Men's Health Information and Resource Centre (MHIRC) and the Holy Family Church at Mount Druitt, New South Wales. This Shed is funded by the Commonwealth Department of Health and Ageing and provides support to men at risk of mental health issues and suicide, often due to cumulative stress associated with disadvantaged situations (Macdonald & Welsh, 2012). Most of these men are of Aboriginal and Torres Strait Islander origin, and the Shed places a particular emphasis on culturally safe support networks (Macdonald & Welsh, 2012). The Shed's appreciation of the socioeconomic, cultural, and gender-based determinants of health has elicited widespread benefits. Community leaders and Indigenous Australian Elders are actively involved in directing participants towards resources, public housing providers, legal services, or financial counsellors. Employment and mental health service providers also engage with activities through the Shed, offering support once appropriate rapport has been established (Macdonald & Welsh, 2012).

Box 11.6 Reflection—Suicide

Consider the following data:

- In Australia, there are over 3000 deaths by suicide each year, with this rate steadily increasing.
- Three out of every four suicides are males.
- Aboriginal people, Torres Strait Islanders, and individuals living in remote communities experience higher rates of suicide than the national average (Australian Institute of Health and Welfare, 2015).

Questions for reflection:

- Why do you think these populations may be over-represented in terms of mental health issues and suicide? Consider the influence of historical context, gender expectations, and broader sociocultural factors.
- What role would your profession and others have in the prevention, reparation, or support of communities facing this health issue in Australia?
- What cultural safety principles would health professionals need to demonstrate to effectively engage with diverse groups of people with mental health issues?

African Women Australia Inc.

African Women Australia Inc. (AWAU) is a non-profit organisation focused on the holistic development of African women in Australia in terms of social, health, economic and civic participation (African Women Australia Inc., 2020). The organisation represents a hub for the most comprehensive and up-to-date resources regarding African women in Australia. AWAU operates within a strengths-based human rights framework, recognising and centralising diversity. The work of AWAU is guided by African women themselves through extensive consultations with African communities (African Women Australia Inc., 2020). In 2014, AWAU developed a Charter promoting a human rights approach regarding female genital mutilation and providing a guide to culturally safe engagement with diverse groups (African Women Australia Inc., 2014). The organisation has represented African Australian women at the United Nations Commission on the Status of Women, which is the principal global intergovernmental body dedicated to gender equality. AWAU provides cultural safety and human rights training, offering mechanisms by which to simultaneously promote mutual respect and raise the profile of African women throughout Australia. The organisation is also a conduit for the dissemination of evidence regarding the experiences of African women, having conducted research on sexual health, education, and the use of health services among this population. Their work has brought to light African migrant women's unique understanding and construction of health in Australia, encouraging reflection of the appropriateness of current policies, service delivery and health promotion throughout multicultural Australia.

Box 11.7 Reflection—Female genital mutilation (FGM)

Female genital mutilation (FGM) and/or cutting has no health benefits. Rather, the act is performed for complex social and cultural reasons that vary across ethnicity and region. It is estimated that FGM impacts over 200 million women and girls worldwide. In Australia, FGM is Illegal in all States and Territories (Australian Institute of Health and Welfare, 2019b).

Consider the role of health care providers in the prevention and management of female genital mutilation:

- Which health professions may be involved?
- What cultural safety principles would health professionals need to demonstrate to effectively engage with the diverse groups of women who have experienced or are at risk of FGM?
- What role would your profession or others have in the prevention, reparation or support of women and communities facing this health issue in Australia?

The role of the health professional

Gender-sensitive and culturally safe practice requires a concerted effort not only across governmental and organisational levels, but also at the level of the health professional. A gender-sensitive approach involves understanding and appreciating gender as a social determinant of health. For individual practitioners, this may involve reflection upon one's own identify and experience throughout the health care system. Health professionals should recognise gender as a spectrum, striving to educate themselves regarding individual patient needs rather than developing assumptions based upon certain observable characteristics. This may involve seeking ongoing professional development opportunities in this area. Gender-sensitive practice acknowledges the influence of gender in all interactions and appreciates the different experiences, expectations, pressures and inequalities faced by men, women and gender-diverse populations (Mental Health, Drugs and Regions Division, Department of Health, 2011). The European Institute for Gender Equality (2019) provides an extensive toolkit on gender-sensitive communication, including recommendations regarding appropriate use of preferred pronouns and avoidance of stereotyping or gender binary language. The toolkit also offers opportunities to test and reflect upon one's own biases and knowledge of gender-sensitive practice. Indeed, health care providers have the responsibility to adapt their practice to ensure gender-sensitive and culturally safe health care delivery for all Australians, irrespective of their individual gender identities.

Conclusion

This chapter has introduced gender as a significant social determinant of health. Students should now have an appreciation for social constructions of masculinity and femininity, as well as the ways in which these constructions influence health and wellbeing. Limitations of existing research have been presented, and the intersection of health and gender has been explored across socio-political, organisational and individual levels of health care provision. Students are encouraged to challenge preconceived notions and expectations regarding gender and to strive to promote equality throughout our increasingly diverse nation. The next step in this process is developing a multidimensional understanding of gender as socially constructed and the implications this may have on sexuality and gender-diverse people. The following chapter will expand on these concepts and provide evidence to help students explore cultural safety in the context of LGBTIQA+ populations.

References

Afifi, M. (2007). Gender differences in mental health. *Singapore Medical Journal, 48*(5), 385–391.

African Women Australia Inc. (2014). *Charter of Ethical practice.* https://netfa.com.au/wp-content/uploads/2019/10/AMA-CHARTER-2014.pdf.

African Women Australia Inc. (2020). *African Women Australia Inc.: Raising the voices and profile of African women in Australia.* https://awau.org.au/.

Allen, L. M., Nelson, C. J., Rouhbakhsh, P., Scifres, S. L., Greene, R. L., Kordinak, S. T., Davis Jr, L. J., & Morse, R. M. (1998). Gender differences in factor structure of the self-administered alcoholism screening test. *Journal of Clinical Psychology, 54*(4), 439–445. https://doi.org/10.1002/(sici)1097-4679(199806)54:4<439::aid-jclp6>3.0.co;2-i.

Anderson, E., & McGuire, R. (2010). Inclusive masculinity theory and the gendered politics of men's rugby. *Journal of Gender Studies, 19*(3), 249–261. https://doi.org/10.1080/09589236.2010.494341.

Annandale, E., & Hunt, K. (2000). *Gender inequalities in health.* Open University Press.

Ansara, Y. G. (2012). Cisgenderism in medical settings: How collaborative partnerships can challenge structural violence. In I. Rivers & R. Ward (Eds.), *Out of the ordinary: LGBT lives* (pp. 102–122). Cambridge Scholars Publishing.

Association of Superannuation Funds of Australia. (2017). *Superannuation account balances by age and gender.* https://www.superannuation.asn.au/ArticleDocuments/359/1710_Superannuation_account_balances_by_age_and_gender.pdf.aspx.

Australian Bureau of Statistics. (2014). *Foundation for a national data collection and reporting framework for family, domestic and sexual violence, 2014* (no. 4529.0.00.003). https://www.abs.gov.au/ausstats/abs@.nsf/Lookup/by Subject/4529.0.00.003~2014~Main Features~Cultural and Linguistic Diversity (CALD) Characteristics~13 - :~:text=DESCRIPTION%3A,person's origins and cultural diversity.

Australian Bureau of Statistics. (2017). *Personal safety, Australia* (no. 4906.0). https://www.abs.gov.au/ausstats/abs@.nsf/mf/4906.0.

Australian Bureau of Statistics. (2018). *Sex and gender diversity in the 2016 census* (no. 2071.0). https://www.abs.gov.au/ausstats/abs@.nsf/Lookup/by Subject/2071.0~2016~Main Features~Sex and Gender Diversity in the 2016 Census~100.

Australian Institute of Criminology. (2017). *Barriers to male victims accessing formal support services.* https://www.aic.gov.au/publications/rpp/rpp126

Australian Institute of Health and Welfare. (2007). *Disability in Australia: Acquired brain injury.* https://www.aihw.gov.au/reports/disability-services/disability-australia-acquired-brain-injury/contents/table-of-contents.

Australian Institute of Health and Welfare. (2015). *Leading cause of premature mortality in Australia fact sheet: Suicide.* https://www.aihw.gov.au/getmedia/de29fe77-427e-451c-8f71-c7d55118c5c7/phe193-suicide.pdf.aspx.

Australian Institute of Health and Welfare. (2019a). *The health of Australia's males.* https://www.aihw.gov.au/reports/men-women/male-health/contents/who-are.

Australian Institute of Health and Welfare. (2019b). *Towards estimating the prevalence of female genital mutilation cutting in Australia.* https://www.aihw.gov.au/reports/men-women/female-genital-mutilation-cutting-australia/notes.

Australian Parliament. (2009). *Select committee on men's health.* https://www.aph.gov.au/Parliamentary_Business/Committees/Senate/Former_Committees/menshealth/report/index.

Bengtsson, T. T. (2016). Performing hypermasculinity: Experiences with confined young offenders. *Men and Masculinities, 19*(4), 410–428. https://doi.org/10.1177/1097184X15595083.

Budgeon, S. (2014). The dynamics of gender hegemony: Femininities, masculinities and social change. *Sociology, 48*(2), 317–334. https://doi.org/10.1177/0038038513490358.

Burns, M. (2004). Eating like an ox: Femininity and dualistic constructions of bulimia and anorexia. *Feminism and Psychology, 14*(2), 269–295. https://doi.org/10.1177/0959353504042182.

Butler, J. (2004). *Undoing gender.* Routledge.

Carmody, M. (2015). *Sex and ethics in young people.* Palgrave Macmillan.

Cavaleri R., Bhole S., & Arora A. (2018). Critical appraisal of quantitative research. In P. Liamputtong (Ed.), *Handbook of research methods in health social sciences.* Springer. https://doi.org/10.1007/978-981-10-2779-6_120-2.

Connell, R. (2011). *Masculinities.* Allen & Unwin.

Cook, L., & Ayoub, J. (2018). *Removing GST on feminine hygiene products.* Parliament of Australia. https://tinyurl.com/yb3o7clz.

Cordier, R., & Wilson, N. J. (2014). Community-based men's sheds: Promoting male health, wellbeing and social inclusion in an international context. *Health Promotion International, 29*(3), 483–493. https://doi.org/10.1093/heapro/dat033.

Cosgrove, L., & Riddle, B. (2003). Constructions of femininity and experiences of menstrual distress. *Women and Health, 38*(3), 37–58. doi:10.1300/J013v38n03_04.

Courtenay, W. H. (2000). Constructions of masculinity and their influence on men's well-being: A theory of gender and health. *Social Science and Medicine, 50*(10), 1385–1401. https://doi.org/10.1016/s0277-9536(99)00390-1.

Dennerstein, L. (1996). Well-being, symptoms and the menopausal transition. *Maturitas, 23*(2), 147–157. https://doi.org/10.1016/0378-5122(95)00970-1.

Department of Infrastructure, Transport, Regional Development and Communication. (2020). *Road deaths Australia.* https://www.bitre.gov.au/publications/ongoing/road_deaths_australia_monthly_bulletins.

Elliott, K. (2020). Bringing in margin and centre: Open and closed as concepts for considering men and masculinities. *Gender, Place and Culture,* 1–22. https://doi.org/10.1080/0966369X.2020.1715348.

European Institute for Gender Equality. (2019). *Toolkit on gender-sensitive communication.* https://eige.europa.eu/publications/toolkit-gender-sensitive-communication.

Grant, J. M., Motter, L. A., & Tanis, J. (2011). *Injustice at every turn: A report of the national transgender discrimination survey.* https://dataspace.princeton.edu/jspui/handle/88435/dsp014j03d232p.

Hansji, N. L., Wilson, N. J., & Cordier, R. (2015). Men's sheds: Enabling environments for Australian men living with and without long-term disabilities. *Health and Social Care in the Community, 23*(3), 272–281. https://doi.org/10.1111/hsc.12140.

Hunter, L. (2016). The tampon tax: Public discourse of policies concerning menstrual taboo. *Hinckley Journal of Politics, 17,* 11–12.

Javaid, A. (2017). The unknown victims: Hegemonic masculinity, masculinities, and male sexual victimisation. *Sociological Research Online, 22*(1), 28–47. https://doi.org/10.5153/sro.4155.

Jewkes, R., Morrell, R., Hearn, J., Lundqvist, E., Blackbeard, D., Lindegger, G., Quayle, M., Sikweyiya, Y., & Gottzén, L. (2015). Hegemonic masculinity: Combining theory and practice in gender interventions. *Culture, Health & Sexuality, 17*(sup2), 112–127. https://doi.org/10.1080/13691058.2015.1085094.

Johansson, T., & Ottemo, A. (2015). Ruptures in hegemonic masculinity: The dialectic between ideology and utopia. *Journal of Gender Studies, 24*(2), 192–206. https://doi.org/10.1080/09589236.2013.812514.

Kessler, R. C., McGonagle, K. A., Zhao, S., Nelson, C. B., Hughes, M., Eshleman, S., … Kendler, K. S. (1994). Lifetime and 12-month prevalence of DSM-III-R psychiatric disorders in the United States: Results from the National Comorbidity Survey. *Archives of General Psychiatry, 51*(1), 8–19. https://doi.org/10.1001/archpsyc.1994.03950010008002.

Levant, R. F., Wimer, D. J., Williams, C. M., Smalley, K. B., & Noronha, D. (2009). The relationships between masculinity variables, health risk behaviors and attitudes toward seeking psychological help. *International Journal of Men's Health, 8*(1), 3–21. https://doi.org/10.3149/jmh.0801.3.

Linzer, M., Spitzer, R., Kroenke, K., Williams, J. B., Hahn, S., Brody, D., & DeGruy, F. (1996). Gender, quality of life, and mental disorders in primary care: Results from the PRIME-MD 1000 study. *The American Journal of Medicine, 101*(5), 526–533. https://doi.org/10.1016/S0002-9343(96)00275-6.

Mac an Ghaill, M., & Haywood, C. (2007). *Gender, culture and society, contemporary femininities and masculinities.* Palgrave Macmillan.

Macdonald, J., & Welsh, R. (2012). *The shed in Mount Druit. Addressing the social determinants of male health and illness.* https://www.westernsydney.edu.au/__data/assets/pdf_file/0003/1308234/MHIC0437_TheShedMtDruitt_FA_LR.pdf.

Mahalik, J. R., Levi-Minzi, M., & Walker, G. (2007). Masculinity and health behaviors in Australian men. *Psychology of Men and Masculinity, 8*(4), 240–249. https://doi.org/10.1037/1524-9220.8.4.240.

Martz, D. M., Handley, K. B., & Eisler, R. M. (1995). The relationship between feminine gender role stress, body image, and eating disorders. *Psychology of Women Quarterly, 19*(4), 493–508. https://doi.org/10.1111/j.1471-6402.1995.tb00088.x.

Matschiner, M., & Murnen, S. K. (1999). Hyperfemininity and influence. *Psychology of Women Quarterly, 23*(3), 631–642. https://doi.org/10.1111/j.1471-6402.1999.tb00385.x.

Mental Health, Drugs and Regions Division, Department of Health. (2011). *Service guideline on gender sensitivity and safety.* https://www2.health.vic.gov.au/about/publications/policiesandguidelines/service-guideline-for-gender-sensitivity-and-safety.

Messerschmidt, J. (1993). *Masculinities and crime, critique and reconceptualization of theory.* Rowman & Littlefield Publishers.

Murnen, S. K., & Byrne, D. (1991). Hyperfemininity: Measurement and initial validation of the construct. *Journal of Sex Research, 28*(3), 479–489. https://doi.org/10.1080/00224499109551620.

National LGBTI Health Alliance. (2016). *Snapshot of mental health and suicide prevention statistics for LGBTI people.* https://lgbtihealth.org.au/resources/snapshot-mental-health-suicide-prevention-statistics-lgbti-people/.

Noble, G., Tabar, P., & Poynting, S. (1998). If anyone called me a wog, they wouldn't be speaking to me alone: Protest masculinity and Lebanese youth in Western Sydney. *Journal of Interdisciplinary Gender Studies, 3*(2), 76.

Paechter, C. (2018). Rethinking the possibilities for hegemonic femininity: Exploring a Gramscian framework. *Women's Studies International Forum, 68*, 121–128. https://doi.org/10.1016/j.wsif.2018.03.005.

Poteat, T., German, D., & Kerrigan, D. (2013). Managing uncertainty: A grounded theory of stigma in transgender health care encounters. *Social Science and Medicine, 84*, 22–29. https://doi.org/10.1016/j.socscimed.2013.02.019.

Regitz-Zagrosek, V. (2012). Sex and gender differences in health: Science and society series on sex and science. *EMBO Reports, 13*(7), 596–603. https://doi.org/10.1038/embor.2012.87.

Riggs, D.W., Coleman, K., & Due, C. (2014). Healthcare experiences of gender diverse Australians: A mixed-methods, self-report survey. *BMC Public Health, 14*(1), 1–5. https://doi.org/10.1186/1471-2458-14-230.

Riggs, D. W., & Toone, K. (2017). Indigenous sistergirls' experiences of family and community. *Australian Social Work, 70*(2), 229–240. https://doi.org/10.1080/0312407X.2016.1165267.

Sailors, P. R., Teetzel, S., & Weaving, C. (2016). Core workout: A feminist critique of definitions, hyperfemininity, and the medicalization of fitness. *International Journal of Feminist Approaches to Bioethics, 9*(2), 46–66.

Schippers, M. (2007). Recovering the feminine other: Masculinity, femininity, and gender hegemony. *Theory and Society, 36*(1), 85–102. https://doi.org/10.1007/s11186-007-9022-4.

Soliday, E., McCluskey-Fawcett, K., & O'Brien, M. (1999). Postpartum affect and depressive symptoms in mothers and fathers. *American Journal of Orthopsychiatry, 69*(1), 30–38. https://doi.org/10.1037/h0080379.

Sperber, J., Landers, S., & Lawrence, S. (2005). Access to health care for transgendered persons: Results of a needs assessment in Boston. *International Journal of Transgenderism, 8*(2–3), 75–91. https://doi.org/10.1300/J485v08n02_08.

Stark, E., & Flitcraft, A. (1995). Killing the beast within: Woman battering and female suicidality. *International Journal of Health Services, 25*(1), 43–64. https://doi.org/10.2190/H6V6-YP3K-QWK1-MK5D

Tanton, R., Vidyattama, Y., McNamara, J., Vu, Q. N., & Harding, A. (2009). Old, single and poor: Using microsimulation and microdata to analyse poverty and the impact of policy change among older Australians. *Economic Papers: A Journal of Applied Economics and Policy, 28*(2), 102–120. https://doi.org/10.1111/j.1759-3441.2009.00022.x.

Tolman, D. L., Davis, B. R., & Bowman, C. P. (2016). That's just how it is: A gendered analysis of masculinity and femininity ideologies in adolescent girls' and boys' heterosexual relationships. *Journal of Adolescent Research, 31*(1), 3–31. https://doi.org/10.1177/0743558415587325.

Treadwell, J., & Garland, J. (2011). Masculinity, marginalization and violence: A case study of the English Defence League. *The British Journal of Criminology, 51*(4), 621–634. https://doi.org/10.1093/bjc/azr027.

Walker, G. W. (2006). Disciplining protest masculinity. *Men and Masculinities, 9*(1), 5–22. https://doi.org/10.1177/1097184X05284217.

Warsh, C. K. (2011). *Gender, health, and popular culture: Historical perspectives*. Wilfrid Laurier University Press.

Weissman, M. M., Bland, R. C., Canino, G. J., Greenwald, S., Hwu, H. G., Joyce, P. R., Karam, E. G., Lee, C. K., Lellouch, J., Lepine, J.-P., & Newman, S. C. (1999). Prevalence of suicide ideation and suicide attempts in nine countries. *Psychological Medicine, 29*(1), 9–17. https://doi.org/10.1017/S0033291798007867.

White, R., Haines, F., & Asquith, N. (2017). *Crime and Criminology* (7th ed.). Oxford University Press.

Wilson, N. J., Cordier, R., Doma, K., Misan, G., & Vaz, S. (2015). Men's sheds function and philosophy: Towards a framework for future research and men's health promotion. *Health Promotion Journal of Australia, 26*(2), 133–141. https://doi.org/10.1071/HE14052.

Workman, A., & Dune, T. M. (2019). A systematic review on LGBTIQ intimate partner violence from a Western perspective. *Journal of Community Safety and Well-Being, 4*(2), 22–31. https://doi.org/10.35502/jcswb.96.

Workplace Gender Equality Agency. (2018). *Australia's gender pay gap statistics*. Australian Government. https://www.wgea.gov.au/sites/default/files/documents/gender-pay-gap-statistic_0_1.pdf.

World Health Organisation. (n.d.). *Gender disparities in mental health*. https://www.who.int/mental_health/media/en/242.pdf?ua=1

12 Australians of diverse sexual orientations and gender identities

Cristyn Davies, Kerry H. Robinson, Atari Metcalf, Kimberley Ivory, Julie Mooney-Somers, Kane Race and S. Rachel Skinner

Learning outcomes

After working through this chapter, students should be able to:

1. Define the differences between the terms *sex*, *sexuality* and *gender*.
2. Discuss the role of intersectionality in understanding identity, sexuality and gender diversity.
3. Identify facilitators and barriers to health care for sexuality and gender diverse people.
4. Demonstrate an understanding of the impact of stigma and discrimination on health outcomes for people of diverse sexual orientation and gender identity.
5. Acknowledge the impact of health professionals' knowledge and attitudes about sexuality and gender diversity on patient/client outcomes.
6. Demonstrate awareness of culturally safe models of health care for people of diverse sexual orientations and gender identities.

Key terms

Cultural safety: An environment that is spiritually, socially and emotionally safe, as well as physically safe for people; where there is no assault challenge or denial of their identity, of who they are and what they need.
Culturally sensitive care: Care that reflects the ability to be appropriately responsive to the attitudes, feelings or circumstances of groups of people that share a common and distinctive racial, national, religious, linguistic or cultural heritage.
Discrimination: Occurs when a person is excluded from benefits generally available to other members of a society because of a perceived difference or a stigmatised identity.
Gender binary: A classification system consisting of two genders, male and female, and underpins the social foundations of Australian society and many other societies globally.
Gender diversity: An umbrella term that is used to describe gender identities that demonstrate a diversity of expression beyond the binary framework.
Gender dysphoria: In medical discourse, gender dysphoria refers to distress arising from incongruence between one's internal sense of gender, the sex they were presumed at birth and/or their body.
Gender expression: Outward gender presentation and behaviour that may communicate gender to others.
Gender fluidity: A spectrum of gender identities that are not exclusively masculine or feminine—identities that are outside the gender binary.
Gender identity: A person's internal view of their gender—that is, one's innermost sense of themselves as a gendered person. A person's gender identity may or may not correspond with their sex presumed at birth. Gender identity often influences the name and pronouns people use.

Heteronormativity: Everyday interactions, practices and policies that construct individuals as heterosexual.

Homophobia and biphobia: Negative beliefs, prejudices and stereotypes that exist about people who are not heterosexual.

Intersectionality: The interconnected nature of social categorisations such as race, class and gender as they apply to a given individual or group, regarded as creating overlapping and interdependent systems of discrimination or disadvantage.

LGBTIQA+: An evolving acronym that stands for lesbian, gay, bisexual, transgender, intersex, queer/questioning, asexual and other terms (such as non-binary and pansexual) that people use to describe experiences of their gender, sexuality and physiological sex characteristics.

Non-binary: When a person's gender identity does not align with binary gender, male/female. Non-binary people may identify as gender fluid, trans masculine, trans feminine, agender, bigender, gender queer and a multitude of other such terms.

Sex: The term *sex* can have different meanings in different contexts. Sex can refer to a person's physical characteristics, including their genitals and reproductive organs, or to their assigned or legal status. Sex can also refer to engaging in sexual activities.

Sexuality: Encompasses who a person may be attracted to romantically and sexually.

Social and medical gender affirmation: Social affirmation is when a person makes changes in appearance and social situations to reflect their gender. This may include changes to hairstyle and clothing, name and pronoun changes, and use of different bathrooms/gendered facilities. They may choose to do this all at once, or only in specific social circles such as with close family and friends. Medical affirmation could include hormone therapy to help develop secondary physical characteristics of gender (such as voice deepening or development of breast tissue) or gender affirmation surgery so that genitalia reflects the person's gender.

Stigma: Defined as the co-occurrence of labeling, stereotyping, separation, status loss and discrimination in a context in which power is exercised.

Transgender: People whose gender is not aligned with the gender presumed for them at birth.

Transphobia: Negative beliefs, prejudices and stereotypes that exist about transgender/trans and gender diverse people.

Chapter summary

In this chapter diverse sexual orientations and gender identities in Australia are introduced, and differences and intersections between gender, sex and sexuality are explored. A brief history of Australian gender and sexuality diverse communities, relevant legislation and human rights issues are provided. Changing language used to describe people of diverse sexual orientations and gender identities is addressed, with particular reference to the areas of medicine, health and human rights. The impact of stigma, discrimination and minority stress on people of diverse sexual orientations and gender identities in the Australian health care system is explored by showing how these experiences are key social determinants of health. Students are asked to consider their personal and professional roles in relation to cultural safety. Case studies are provided to assist students to understand the power imbalance between health providers and those accessing a health service, and to identify strategies to minimise it. This chapter also outlines ways that health professionals' knowledge and attitudes about sexuality and gender diversity, and their conscious and unconscious bias, aids in the creation and reduction of stigma and discrimination. By the end of the chapter, students will have developed an understanding of current key principles for inclusive and respectful practices in health care settings for working with people of diverse sexual orientation and gender identity.

Introduction

This chapter focuses on the cultural safety of gender and sexuality diverse people when accessing health care in Australia. Research demonstrates that gender and sexuality diverse people experience barriers to health care, despite universal health coverage (UHC) in Australia (Byron, Rasmussen, Wright Toussaint, Lobo, Robinson, & Paradise, 2017; Kang et al., 2018; Koh, Kang, & Usherwood, 2014; Mooney-Somers, Deacon, Scott, Price, & Parkhill, 2018; Robinson, Bansel, Denson, Ovenden, & Davies, 2014; Smith, Jones, Ward, Dixon, Mitchell, & Hillier, 2014; Strauss, Cook, Winter, Watson, Wright Toussaint, & Lin, 2017). According to the Organisation (WHO), universal health coverage has three objectives: equity in access to health services, good quality health services and protection against financial risk as a result of accessing health services.

It is critical to understand the differences and intersections between gender, sex and sexuality and the changing use of language and discourses, including those within health, medicine, and human rights. Understanding these differences, intersections and discourses will better equip you to identify and address stigma and discrimination in health care policy, practice and provision for people of diverse sexual orientation and gender identity. The importance of intersectionality of identity is also highlighted in this chapter. As Ruth McNair (2017) argues, "negotiating multiple identities influences health outcomes" (pp. 444–445).

The chapter explores how health professionals' knowledge and attitudes about sexuality and gender diversity may also impact on the stigma and discrimination experienced by gender and sexuality diverse communities. You will be invited to consider the role of conscious and unconscious bias and your personal and professional roles in improving health outcomes for gender and sexuality diverse people through an introduction to the cultural safety framework. Case studies will be used as instructive examples to assist your knowledge and understanding and to promote methods and practices to address the patient–health professional power imbalance. This chapter provides a definition of intersex and highlights key resources for further information, but does not provide detailed discussion of the complex issues faced by people with intersex variations.

Key principles for inclusive and respectful work practice that can be applied across a range of health contexts are outlined in this chapter.

Relevant terms

This section offers a guide of key terms that health professionals and policy makers will need when addressing the needs of people who are gender and/or sexuality diverse. Language and terminology can change quickly as communities create discourses that best describe their gender, sexuality and sexual and romantic relationships or interactions. Having an understanding of this language and terminology can help ensure that health care settings and organisations are inclusive and respectful. It is important to use the terms that patients or clients use and to check whether the term applies to them.[1]

In use since the 1990s, the LGBT acronym was considered to be a more inclusive descriptor than the general term in usage, "gay community". LGBT is an umbrella term pertaining to gender and sexuality diversity. In more recent years, "I" for Intersex and "Q" for Queer or Questioning, have sometimes been added to the acronym, as have the "A" for asexual, and "+" to indicate other communities that may fall outside gender and sexual norms. The acronym originated to promote political and social solidarity and visibility regarding human rights across these heterogeneous identities and experiences. However, there are critiques of this acronym, including the lack of focus of the specific and diverse issues experienced by each of these identities or labels included under the umbrella term.

Gender

The terms *sex* and *gender* are often used interchangeably in health policy and practice, but they have distinctly different meanings. The term **sex** can have different meanings in different contexts. For example, **sex** can refer to a person's physical characteristics, including their genitals and reproductive organs, or to their assigned or legal status. **Sex** can also refer to engaging in sexual activities. **Gender** refers to the range of characteristics that a culture identifies as masculine or feminine. **Gender** is constructed through relationships, expectations and practices that are institutionalised, for example, through the family, education, religion, cultural practices and rituals and health care systems and settings. These expectations and practices can change across time, culture and location. In many cultures, binary gender has been established as the social norm. **Gender binary** refers to a classification system consisting of two genders, male and female, and underpins the social foundations of Australian society and many other societies globally. Queer theorists have argued against the idea of binary gender as normative, pointing out the multiplicity of gender, its complexities and fluidity (Butler, 1990; Jagose, 1996). **Gender norms** determine what is expected, allowed and valued of girls and women, boys and men, and transgender, gender diverse and non-binary people. In most societies, including Australia, many differences and inequalities exist between people who identify as women, men, transgender, gender diverse or non-binary people.

Gender identity refers to a person's internal view of their gender—that is, one's innermost sense of themselves as a gendered person. A person's gender identity may or may not correspond with their sex presumed at birth. Gender identity often influences the name and pronouns people use. **Gender expression** refers to outward gender presentation and behaviour that may communicate gender to others. Some people identify as **non-binary**, which is when a person's gender identity does not align with binary gender, male/female. **Non-binary** people may identify as gender fluid, trans masculine, trans feminine, agender, bigender, gender queer and a multitude of other such terms.

Transgender refers to people whose gender is not aligned with the gender presumed for them at birth. It is not a diagnostic descriptor and does not imply a medical or psychological condition. In June 2018, the World Health Organisation, released the 11th version of the *International Classification of Diseases* (ICD-11) removing trans-related categories from the mental health chapter (World Health Organisation, 2018). Being transgender or gender diverse is part of the natural spectrum of human diversity. Not all people whose gender identity differs from their sex presumed at birth identify as transgender or use this term to describe themselves. In Australia, **sistergirls** and **brotherboys** are terms used in some Aboriginal and Torres Strait Islander communities to describe being trans in a way specific to First Nations people. **Sistergirls** are First Nations women presumed male at birth, and **brotherboys** are First Nations men presumed female at birth. In some regions, sistergirls (sometimes Yimpininni in the Tiwi Islands) and brotherboys have distinct cultural identities and roles (LGBTIQ+ Health Australia, 2013). **Cisgender** refers to a person whose gender identity and gender expression matches the sex they were presumed at birth. Inequalities and disadvantages are prevalent between cisgendered and trans, gender diverse and non-binary people with regard to accessing social, economic, health and education opportunities and resources.

Gender affirmation refers to processes that a person undertakes to align their internal sense of gender with their gender expression (ACON, 2019). These processes may involve social and/or medical steps. Examples of social steps include changing one's name and pronouns, wearing clothing and/or participating in social activities and behaviours that align with their gender. For example, as part of a process of gender affirmation, a person may change their pronouns to she/her, he/him and/or they/them rather than pronouns that signify male or female. There are also medical interventions available to assist individuals to affirm their gender; however, not all transgender or gender diverse people necessarily undertake all or any medical steps (Coleman et al., 2012; Telfer, Tollit, Pace, & Pang, 2018). These include hormone replacement therapy (or in the case of adolescents, hormone blockers such as gonadotropin-releasing hormone agonists to prevent irreversible bodily changes during puberty) and surgeries (e.g., masculinising chest surgery (mastectomy) or breast augmentation, gonadectomy, genital reconstruction, thyrocondroplasty, among others) or speech therapy later in life. Distress arising from incongruence with one's internal sense of gender, the sex they were presumed at birth and/or their body, referred to in medical discourse as "gender dysphoria", can start very early in life around three years of age, or may present in adolescence or adulthood (Riley, Sitharthan, Clemson, & Diamond, 2011; Strauss et al., 2017). Many transgender or gender diverse people can experience significant and persistent emotional distress, underscoring the importance of accessible and culturally safe health care and support (Callander et al., 2018; Coleman et al., 2012; Telfer et al., 2018).

Intersex

While intersex is often included in the Lesbian, Gay, Bisexual, Trans*/Transgender— LGBTI acronym, health concerns faced by people with intersex variations are unique and require different frameworks to address issues encountered within the Australian health care system. However, like non-intersex people, some people with intersex variations may also be gender and/or sexuality diverse. Intersex is distinct from sex, sexual orientation and gender identity (Intersex Human Rights Australia, 2019). **Intersex** people are born with physical sex characteristics that do not fit medical norms for female or male bodies (including genitals, gonads and chromosome patterns) (Carpenter, 2016). **Intersex traits** vary across individuals, with some visible at birth, or for others, these traits are not evident until puberty (Carpenter, 2016; Intersex Human Rights Australia, 2019). For other people, intersex variations may not be visible at all (Carpenter, 2016). In clinical settings, the terms "disorders of sex development" or "differences of sex development", and individual diagnostic terms, may be used. Some people with intersex variations old enough to have agency to express an identity may identify as gender or sexuality diverse (Carpenter, 2018), while many identify as heterosexual (Intersex Human Rights Australia, 2019; Jones, Hart, Carpenter, Ansara, Leonard, & Lucke, 2016). People who do not have intersex variations are referred to as **endosex**.

Sexuality

Sexuality encompasses who a person may be attracted to romantically and sexually. It is produced in complex ways and is "the intricate and multiple ways in which our emotions, desires and relationships are shaped by the society" in which we live (Cartledge & Ryan, 1983, p. 1). **Sexual orientation** refers to the set of meanings through which people describe their sexual attractions. Sexual orientation includes attraction, behaviour and sexual identity. **Attraction** can be sexual, emotional, spiritual, psychological and/or political. **Sexual behaviour** refers to what a person does sexually and/or with whom. **Sexual identity** refers to the language and terms a person uses to refer to their sexual orientation, which may be influenced by attraction, behaviour, family, culture and community. Together, sexual attraction, behaviour and identity form what is known as the **sexuality triad** (Fairley, Russell, & Bradford, 2005). While there is generally congruence between sexual attraction, behaviour and identity, a person's sexual behaviour does not necessarily indicate their attraction or identity. For example, a bisexual person may be in a long-term monogamous relationship with a person of one gender while feeling attraction for people of other genders; the gender of their partner does not indicate their sexual identity. Sexual attraction, behaviour and identity are not static, and each can shift over a person's lifetime. The acronym **MSM** is frequently used, especially in health research, to refer to men who have sex with men, but who may not identify as gay or bisexual (Fairley, Russell, & Bradford, 2005; Perez-Brumer, Parker, & Aggleton, 2017). Trans and gender diverse people experience the same spectrum of sexual orientations as cisgender people (Callander et al., 2018; Robinson et al., 2014; Smith et al., 2014).

Gender and sexuality diversity

In this chapter, we use the terms **gender and sexuality diversity**, which incorporates identity, sexual attraction and gender identity and expression. **Lesbian** refers to a cisgender, trans or gender diverse woman or non-binary person who is emotionally and physically attracted to other women. **Gay** is the term used for someone who is emotionally and physically attracted to people of the same gender. It is often used to refer to cisgender, trans or gender diverse men or non-binary people who are emotionally and physically attracted to men. **Bisexual** refers to people whose sexual, romantic or physical attraction is to people of more than one gender. **Pansexual** refers to a person whose sexual, romantic or physical attraction is not limited by sex, gender or gender identity. **Asexual** refers to people who do not experience sexual attraction. Asexual people can experience platonic attraction but may have no sexual desire or need within relationships. Historically, **queer** was a pejorative term used against those who were sexuality diverse in the late 19th century. The term was re-signified in the late 1980s by queer theorists and activists and was used as a politically radical alternative challenging labels and categories, such as lesbian, gay, bisexual, or transgender (Butler, 1990; Jagose, 1996). For many people, *queer* is an inclusive term for diverse sexual and gender identities. However, it can still be used pejoratively as slur or insult.

Heteronormativity

Within the Australian health care system, **heteronormativity** prevails, and this refers to the way that everyday interactions, practices and policies construct individuals as heterosexual. This process of "compulsory heterosexuality", as coined by Adrienne Rich (1980), is integral to the way that heterosexuality is normalised and holds priority, and non-heterosexual relationships can be characterised as deviant from the norm. Through heteronormativity, a culture of power is institutionalised through structures, systems and everyday practices that reinforce heterosexuality as normative (Robinson & Díaz, 2016). This process often silences and renders invisible the ways in which economic, social, health and educational institutions organise class, race, sexuality, gender, ability and other differences. This silencing is a root cause of the inequity we see in health and inclusion. **Cisnormative** refers to the assumption that all people are cisgender (have a gender identity that matches the sex they were presumed at birth). The assumptions of heteronormativity and cisnormativity in most institutions means there is often no designated space for inclusion of transgender, gender and sexuality diverse people in health care settings.

Minority stress

Gender and sexuality diverse people can experience **minority stress** (Meyer, 2003). This refers to the impact of internal and external stressors, such as stigma and discrimination, or the distress experienced as a result of having to conceal one's sexual orientation and/or gender identity due to fear or discrimination, rejection or violence. These systemic issues have both physical and psychological impacts on those who experience them. Notably, experiencing or internalising discrimination causes physiological arousal of the hypothalamic–pituitary–adrenal (HPA) axis and triggers the release of cortisol. This causes metabolic changes, affects the immune system and produces mood changes and cognitive impairment (Kaholokula, Grandinetti, Keller, Nacapoy, Kingi, & Mau, 2012). Sustained elevation of cortisol over time leads to glucocorticoid-driven structural changes and abnormal afferent neurotransmitter inputs that may contribute to the development of adverse mental and physical health consequences. Even experimental lowering of perceived social status has negative effects on affect and stress-related physiological systems. Within the minority stress model, there are proximal stressors, including:

- **Internalised homophobia or transphobia**, refers to internalised negative beliefs and attitudes about one's own sexuality, or gender identity;
- **Concealment**, refers to stress associated with concealing sexual orientation and/or gender identity for fear of harm; and
- **Stigma consciousness**, refers to the increased vigilance and expectations or rejection in social interactions based on sexuality or gender identity (Morandini, Blaszczynski, Dar-Nimrod, & Ross, 2015).

Introduction to stigma and discrimination

Social determinants of health

There is substantial evidence that stigma and discrimination are important social determinants of health (Hatzenbuehler, Bellatorre, & Muennig, 2014; Rosenstreich, Comfort, & Martin, 2011). The social determinants of health framework is used by the World Health Organisation (WHO) to identify a range of social factors that influence the health of populations (Commission on Social Determinants of Health, 2008, World Health Organisation, 2011). Social exclusion, which is an outcome of stigma and discrimination, is one of the factors that negatively impacts on people's health.

As a social determinant of health, stigma can negatively impact many life chances at the same time. Michael Marmot et al. (1991) demonstrated that the less autonomy one has in life, the more likely one is to have poorer health outcomes. Socio-economic status, individual power and social supports can determine health outcomes. The more support you have, the better connected you are, and the more social capital you have in any setting, the more you benefit from your society and the more positive your health outcomes are likely to be.

Stigma

Mark Hatzenbuehler et al. (2013) state, "stigma is defined as the co-occurrence of labeling, stereotyping, separation, status loss, and discrimination in a context *in which power is exercised*" (p. 813). They argue that discrimination is a "constitutive feature of stigma", and stigma cannot exist without discrimination, but stigma is broader than discrimination alone. Stigmatisation occurs in situations when social, economic or political power allows for and supports the identification of difference leading to disapproval or rejection.

Stigma impacts in three main ways (Quinn & Chaudoir, 2009). **Internalised stigma** refers to negative stereotypes about a person's identity that they believe applies to them (e.g., others say people with mental illness are weak therefore I am weak). A high degree of internalized stigma is consistently related to lower psychological wellbeing. **Enacted stigma** is discrimination as a direct result of a disclosed stigmatised identity (e.g., the local baker refuses to make the cake for a gay wedding). **Anticipated stigma** refers to the negative treatment people with a concealed stigmatised identity believe they might receive if their identity was known (e.g., an employee has not told their boss about having a history of depression due to a fear of not being promoted).

Some of our identities are externally apparent, but others may be concealed in some settings but not in others. For example, your professional identity may not be apparent when you are playing sport on the weekend but would be apparent in your work setting. Sexuality and gender minority identities are often concealable because some people can choose when, where and to whom they reveal this identity. In most societies, minority sexuality or gender identities are stigmatised. Stigma results in lowered power and status and can lead to discriminatory outcomes.

There are a range of impacts a concealable stigmatised identity (CSI) may have on an individual depending on the *valence* of the CSI, i.e., whether the CSI makes the person feel better or worse about themselves, and the *magnitude* of the CSI, i.e., the size of the CSI as part of the sense of self. There is a great deal of variation within stigmatised groups in the valence and magnitude of the CSI. For example, a transgender man who has had positive acknowledgement and support from family and friends throughout his gender affirmation may feel more positive about his identity than someone who did not. For some people, their sexuality is a large part of their sense of self, but for others it is less so, and is merely one small part of how they view their identity.

As health professionals, our aim is to improve health outcomes for all. Reducing stigma and discrimination for people seeking our care is essential to health promotion and provision of effective health care.

Discrimination

Discrimination occurs when a person is excluded from benefits generally available to other members of a society because of a perceived difference or a stigmatised identity. This definition from social epidemiologist Nancy Krieger (2001) is a helpful starting point when considering the impact of discrimination on health:

> [Discrimination is] the process by which a member, or members, of a socially defined group is, or are, treated differently (especially unfairly) because of their membership of that group … this unfair treatment arises from socially derived beliefs each group holds about the other, and patterns of dominance and oppression, viewed as expressions of a struggle for power and privilege.
>
> (p. 693)

Some gender and sexuality diverse people can experience many forms of discrimination as they hold multiple disadvantaged identities. This can result in poorer health outcomes than groups with a single marginalised identity. **Intersectionality** recognises that people have multiple identities, shaped by socio-cultural and political power and privilege. Coined by Kimberlé Crenshaw (1989), the term is useful to understand multiple identity categories that may marginalise people. For example, a person who is an Aboriginal or Torres Strait Islander and gender and/or sexuality diverse is more likely to experience greater marginalisation and disadvantage than someone who is gender and/or sexuality diverse and benefits from privileges associated with being White.

Discrimination can also be enacted towards certain groups by institutions (often termed "structural discrimination" or "institutional discrimination"). Examples of this type of discrimination include:

- Under-representation of minority group members in the media;
- Reinforcement of negative stereotypes, or misinformation, in media reporting involving minority groups; and

- Limitations on or exclusions from access to education, health care or social services and employment for minority group members.

The relationship between gender and sexuality diverse people and health care settings has a troubled history and people who are gender and/or sexuality diverse have frequently been criminalised, pathologised and excluded. Until 1973, homosexuality was classified as a mental illness in the *Diagnostic and Statistical Manual of Mental Disorders* (DSM II), and the diagnosis of "gender dysphoria" still persists in the *Diagnostic and Statistical Manual of Mental Disorders*, Fifth Edition (DSM V) (American Psychiatric Association, 2013).

Institutional discrimination may occur in overt and subtle ways. Examples of subtle discrimination are not recognising a sexuality diverse partner as the next of kin (or referring to a partner as "a friend"); the use of non-inclusive options on intake forms, such as, sex: male or female, or father or mother rather than parent 1 and parent 2; or failing to provide gender neutral bathrooms. Examples of overt discrimination include requiring transgender and gender diverse people to undergo surgeries or divorce their partners before allowing them to change legal identity documents such as birth certificates to reflect their gender, a lack of inclusive and non-discriminatory policies, and limited education in the culturally appropriate care of gender and sexuality diverse people.

Many gender and sexuality diverse people experience poorer health and social outcomes compared with their heterosexual and cisgender peers (Leonard et al., 2012). Clinical care is also affected by a health care professional's own experiences, social positioning and values (gender and sexual identity, cultural background, socio-economic class, ability and so on) and structural features, including funding and resources, clinical protocols, health policies, guidelines and practice of the health care setting.

Barriers and facilitators to culturally safe health care for gender and sexuality diverse Australians

Doctors and allied health professionals often lack appropriate skills in providing best practice health care to gender and sexuality diverse people (Aggleton, Bhana, Clarke, Crewe, Race, & Yankah, 2018; Knight, Shoveller, Carson, & Contreras-Whitney, 2014; Newman, Kidd, Kippax, Reynolds, Canavan, & de Wit, 2013), either implicitly (by relying on assumed heteronormative practices) or explicitly (through lack of appropriate training). For example, health professionals have commented that they are not adequately equipped with a clinical skill set to effectively provide care for gender and sexuality diverse youth about issues related to their sexual health (Brooks et al., 2018; Knight et al., 2014).

Compared to the general population, gender and sexuality diverse people experience higher rates of illness and morbidity. This is primarily related to the interplay of social factors, exposures and risks and failures of the health system. Institutional norms and values (heteronormative and cis-normative assumptions, stigma and social exclusion) result in gender and sexuality diverse people's exposure to social determinants that influence their health-related outcomes (Mooney-Somers et al., 2018; Robinson et al., 2014; Strauss et al., 2017).

Young gender and sexuality diverse people experience specific barriers to accessing quality health care, which is further impacted by their age and other intersectional aspects of their identities. In *Growing up Queer* (Robinson et al., 2014), a national study about issues faced by gender and sexuality diverse young Australians (ages 16–27 years), 55.7% of young people who identified as gender and/or sexuality diverse had *not* disclosed their sexuality and/or gender identity to a doctor: 37.6% told their doctor who *was* supportive, and 6.7% told their doctor, who was *not* supportive. In "You learn from each other" (Byron et al., 2017), a study about sexuality and gender diverse young people's (ages 16–25 years) access to mental health support, most people (76%), surveyed felt it was necessary to discuss gender or sexuality diversity with health professionals, yet only 46% reported good experiences in doing so, and 41% said they had not discussed these matters with health professionals. Therefore, there is a discrepancy between what participants wanted to disclose and their practices about gender and/or sexuality diversity disclosure with health professionals. In *Access 3* (Kang et al., 2018), which examined health care access and health system navigation for young people (ages 12–24 years) in NSW with a focus on several marginalised groups, gender and/or sexuality diverse people experienced higher levels of psychological distress and significant structural barriers to accessing health care compared to the rest of the sample.

In these studies, barriers to accessing health care reported by participants included fears of homophobia, transphobia and other discriminations, judgmental responses, gendered assumptions, concerns regarding confidentiality, prohibitive cost of the service, difficulty getting to the service, and young people not having their own Medicare card.

Fear of disclosing and non-disclosure of sexuality and/or gender diversity to health professionals can be major barriers to preventive health practices, including screening, and have been associated with lower mental health outcomes (Durso & Meyer 2012). Not being aware of a patient's gender or sexuality means patients may not be informed of relevant and clinically important health issues, such as a higher likelihood of mental ill-health or smoking (Deacon & Mooney-Somers, 2017), or a heightened risk of HIV for men who have sex with men. Many general practitioners (GPs) do not ask about sexuality because they assume patients are heterosexual, prefer patients to disclose, or think sexuality is irrelevant (McNair, Hegarty, & Taft, 2015). They may also not appreciate that disclosure is important for developing a productive doctor–patient relationship. However, many patients do not disclose as they fear practitioner reaction and subsequent treatment, do not believe it is clinically relevant or they wait for the health provider to ask. For these reasons, patients prefer practitioners to ask about their sexuality.

Disclosure may also be particularly fraught for people with intersectional identities. Research demonstrates that there are lower rates of disclosure among people of colour and who had been born overseas, those who report lower educational attainment or income or those people living in rural areas (Durso & Meyer, 2012). Generally, intake forms should acknowledge the full range of human identity and sexual expression, including gender identity, sexual orientation and a range of sexual behaviours. McNair and colleagues provide excellent guidance for health practitioners on how to ask sensitively about sexuality (McNair et al., 2015).

It is important to take a sexual and social history from all patients, not just those who identify themselves as LGBTQ+, in a way that normalises the discussion of sexual health by emphasising that such a discussion is routine with all patients. When taking a sexual history, it is important to understand that sexual identity, orientation and behaviour may not align. For example, a man who identifies as heterosexual may engage in sex with men (Newman et al., 2018). Sexuality and gender diverse populations are known to be more at risk for certain health issues, such as substance use (including tobacco), certain cancers and sexually transmitted infections (STIs), depression, suicide and violence (including intimate partner violence) (Ovenden et al., 2019). Therefore, health professionals should ask pertinent, non-judgmental questions about these issues in the interests of providing culturally safe care (McGarry, Hebert, Kelleher, & Potter, 2008).

Creating inclusive health settings

Health services can demonstrate inclusivity by making visible the rainbow symbol in health care settings, inclusive use of language on service intake forms, websites, administrative systems and in policies, and offering staff professional development and training in the diversity of experiences across the spectrum of gender and sexuality. In addition, respectful communication, visible user-friendly opening hours and notification of free or subsidised services can help to create an inclusive environment. Partnerships between mainstream health services and LGBT community organisations, accreditation by programs such as *"Rainbow Tick"*,[2] or participation in workplace inclusivity programs like *"Pride in Health + Wellbeing"*, demonstrate a genuine, sustained and high-level commitment to ensure safe and inclusive service provision.

Digital health interventions

Digital health interventions aimed at gender and sexuality diverse young people should offer diverse and comprehensive sexual health information that links mental and sexual health, that is not risk focused, but rather focuses on the strengths of these communities (Byron et al., 2017; Robinson et al., 2014). Online interventions should complement rather than stand in for sexual health education strategies delivered in face-to-face environments through a variety of settings: schools, at home, clinical settings, and youth support service settings (Davies et al., 2017). These strategies may be particularly useful for young people as they are generally very engaged online (Davies, Skinner, Odgers, Khut, & Morrow, 2018; Guse et al., 2012), and digital interventions may assist in overcoming some of the barriers to accessing health services. Gender and sexuality diverse people are heterogeneous (despite being grouped together) with distinct health concerns. Gender diverse and transgender young people are often marginalised in public health and educational interventions and have fewer digital tools to meet their sexual health and reproductive needs. Research collaboration and community consultation with gender and sexuality diverse communities regarding their sexual health needs and care should be part of all health interventions and strategies.

Box 12.1 Brief overview of legislations and human rights impacting gender and sexuality diverse Australians

Decriminalisation of sex between men: South Australia was the first state to decriminalise male homosexuality in 1975. Most other jurisdictions decriminalised in the 1980s (Tasmania decriminalised in 1997). Legislation to allow men to apply to have their record expunged because they were convicted when homosexual acts were a crime were only passed recently (2014: NSW, Victoria; 2017: Queensland; 2018: Tasmania, WA); this meant men would no longer have to declare convictions when applying for a job or a travel visa, nor could they be discriminated against for the now expunged conviction.

A common age of consent: Age of consent was set by jurisdictions once sex between men was decriminalised. While some jurisdictions immediately made a common age of consent (e.g. 1980/81: Victoria), others set the age of consent two to five years higher for sex between men (1983: NT; 1984: NSW; 1990: Western Australia), or higher for anal sex (1990: Queensland). In 1994 the United Nations Human Rights Council found Australia in breach of its International Covenant on Civil and Political Rights regarding anti-sodomy laws and differing ages of consent for homosexuals and heterosexuals. The same year the Commonwealth government passed the *Human Rights (Sexual Conduct) Act* to override all state and territory legislation pertaining to sexual conduct for consenting adults 18 years of age and over. All jurisdictions now have an age of consent of 16 or 17 years of age.

Anti-discrimination laws: Although sex between men was still illegal, in 1982, NSW became the first jurisdiction to include homosexuality in anti-discrimination laws. However, the *Commonwealth Sex Discrimination Act* was not amended until 2013, making it unlawful to discriminate against people on the basis of sexual orientation, gender identity and intersex status. The act contained exemptions about sexual orientation and gender identity that allowed faith-based schools to discriminate against students (e.g., exclude them, not take action on bullying on the basis of sexuality or gender diversity) and teachers (e.g., dismiss them), and faith-based hospitals and welfare services (e.g., family counselling services, family violence services), to discriminate against patients, families and staff were exempted.

Gay panic defence: In 1992, the so-called gay panic defence was successfully used to downgrade a charge of murder to manslaughter. This defence is where a defendant claims they acted against a victim in response to an unwanted sexual advance. Its use was upheld by the High Court of Australia in 1997. Many jurisdictions abolished this defence in the 2000s (beginning with Tasmania). However, it was not abolished in NSW until 2014 and in Queensland until 2017 (although a clause allows a magistrate to rule in exceptional circumstances).

Marriage equality: In 2004 the government amended the *Commonwealth Marriage Act* to add to the definition of marriage to restrict it to a union between a man and a woman to the exclusion of others; this explicitly excluded sexuality diverse couples. In 2013, the ACT passed marriage equality, legislation that was subsequently quashed by the High Court of Australia. In 2017, the Australian Marriage Law Postal Survey results showed 61% of those who responded supported marriage equality, and 38.4% did not. The federal government legislated marriage equality the same year.

Legal inequity in employment, superannuation laws and adoption: In 1992 the government removed the ban on sexuality diverse people serving in the military but did not extend equal benefits to sexuality diverse couples, e.g., equal access to veteran's pension for sexuality diverse partners, until 2005. In 2009, the government passed legislation to remove discrimination against sexuality diverse couples from 85 federal laws relating to areas such as tax, veterans' affairs, social security and health. In the same year, de facto couples (heterosexual or homosexual) were given similar rights to those who were legally married (at the time only heterosexual couples could marry). Legislative changes to allow sexuality diverse couples to adopt are relatively recent (2004: ACT; 2010: NSW; 2013: Tasmania; 2016: Victoria, Queensland, SA; 2018: NT).

Gender recognition, forced divorce/surgery, and hormones: Legal advances for trans and gender diverse people are very recent. In 2011, the government passed passport legislation allowing for an "x" gender option and the ability for trans people to select their gender without medical intervention. Several jurisdictions subsequently changed legislation to allow trans and gender diverse people to change the sex on their birth certificate without gender-affirming surgery (2014: ACT; 2016 SA: 2019: Tasmania; Victoria). Tasmania is the only jurisdiction to make gender optional on birth certificates (2019). At the time of writing, trans and gender diverse people are still required to have gender-affirming surgery (including sterilisation) to change the sex on their birth certificate in NSW and Queensland. In 2018 most jurisdictions (NT, Victoria, Queensland, NSW) removed the "forced divorce" requirement, where married trans and gender-diverse people had to divorce a previously heterosexual marriage if they wanted legal recognition of their gender (e.g., on birth certificates). Tasmania and WA passed similar legislation in 2019. In 2017, the Family Court of Australia ruled that transgender young people diagnosed with gender dysphoria no longer needed to seek court approval to access gender affirming hormones (unless there is disagreement between parents or between treating doctors and parents). This overturned a 2013 decision that even if parents consented, court approval was required (Australia was the only country in the world to require this).[3] In 2018, the Family Court of Australia ruled that transgender young people diagnosed with gender dysphoria are no longer required to seek court authorisation for gender affirming surgery where they are *Gillick* competent (unless there is disagreement between parents or between treating doctors and parents).[4]

We acknowledge Winsor (2017) for much of the preceding content.

Cultural safety: Addressing stigma and discrimination in health care

The principles that underpin cultural safety, which is a term that came into prominence in the late 1980s and early 1990s that draws on the work of Maori nurses in New Zealand (Ramsden, 2002), can also be considered within the context of health care provision for people of diverse gender and sexuality. Cultural safety promotes a health care:

> environment that is safe for people: where there is no assault, challenge or denial of their identity, of who they are and what they need. It is about shared respect, shared meaning, shared knowledge and experience of learning, living and working together with dignity and truly listening.
>
> (Williams, 1999)

Case studies

We have provided four case studies. The first three case studies require you to apply the knowledge and understanding you have developed by reading this chapter to the following cases by responding to the questions. In the fourth case study, we have provided responses that reflect best Australian allied health and clinical practice at the time of writing this chapter. For each case study, please consider the implications of cultural safety for gender and sexuality diverse people from different perspectives, including health policy and practice, health research, clinical considerations, and where relevant, multidisciplinary or interdisciplinary care, and social support services.

Box 12.2 Case study—Caring for a trans or gender diverse young person

Jack is a 13-year-old boy, who was presumed female at birth. Part of the way through his first year of high school at a co-educational school, he refuses to attend. Jack has been subjected to bullying from some of his peers during class, in the school grounds, on the way to and from school, and especially during PE and sport. Jack is particularly worried about going into the school toilets and dressing rooms, where most of the bullying is encountered. Some of his teachers do not intervene in this bullying. Jack also finds it very stressful when the school separates students by gender for activities, which happens nearly on a daily basis. Lillian, Jack's mother, is called to the school to discuss Jack's non-attendance with his year advisor, the school principal and the school counsellor. Lillian requests that Jack's social worker who is part of his multidisciplinary health care team at a children's hospital also attend the meeting.

1. What can the school do to address issues contributing to Jack's reluctance to attend?
2. What support organisations are available in your jurisdiction to help the school with strategies that promote inclusion of transgender and gender diverse young people in education settings? What role can they play in ensuring Jack's safe return to school?
3. What can the social worker and school counsellor do to support Jack's return to school?
4. What strategies can allied health professionals use to work collaboratively with schools to ensure culturally safe education settings for all young people?

Box 12.3 Case study—Caring for a sexuality diverse attracted woman

Molly is a 42-year-old woman who has been married to a cisgender man since her early twenties. She has three children from this relationship ages 14, 11 and 7 years. She recently told her husband that she has started a relationship with a woman she met online a few months ago. Molly's communication with her husband is tense, and they have not disclosed to the children what is happening. Molly is worried that her children will reject her, and that she will have to move out of the family home. She expresses shame about possibly "ruining" her children's lives and hurting her husband by pursuing this new relationship. Molly presents to her GP seeking psychosocial support for her relationship breakdown. She also discloses that she is drinking a bottle of wine most nights.

1. What are the important issues that you need to consider so that Molly can experience culturally safe health care provision?
2. What support is available for Molly around her drinking in your jurisdiction?
3. What psychosocial support is available for Molly and her family?
4. What resources and services are available in your jurisdiction to assist Molly with her sexual identity?

Box 12.4 Case study—Caring for a sexuality diverse attracted man

Mo is a 28-year-old gay man who is concerned about his continuing fatigue and difficulty motivating himself. He has lost his appetite and feels run down. Sen, his male partner of 6 years, has been complaining that this is affecting their life together and berates Mo for being lazy and not caring about their relationship. Sen has started to restrict Mo's Internet use and check his phone, saying he is spending too much time on social media and talking to other people. Mo presents to his GP regarding his depressive symptoms.

Sen is also Mo's manager, and Mo feels that he can't talk to his colleagues. Mo's family live overseas, and they do not know he is gay.

1. What are the important issues that you need to consider to enable Mo to access and experience culturally safe health care?
2. What psychosocial support is available for Mo in your jurisdiction?
3. Do you have any concerns about Mo's relationship? How might you raise these with Mo? How could you identify culturally safe referral options in your jurisdiction?
4. What other health issues might you need to rule out, and how would you approach this with Mo?

Box 12.5 Case study—Cervical screening case study for trans and gender diverse men

Ben is a 36-year-old transgender man who began testosterone replacement therapy 12 years ago. He has had chest surgery to affirm his gender but has not had any genital or reproductive surgeries. Ben presents to a primary health care setting that a friend has recommended to ask the practice nurse about screening for human papillomavirus (HPV test) and whether or not he needs it. He has never had a cervical screening test, and his usual doctor located at another setting has never raised the issue.

1. What factors might contribute to trans and gender diverse patients having low participation rates in cervical screening?
   - Perception by providers/and or clients that screening is not required for transgender men;
   - Testosterone causes vaginal atrophy, and internal examinations may be very uncomfortable;
   - Assumptions by providers about what surgery may have occurred;
   - Non-disclosure by client that he is transgender;
2. What are the important communication and cultural safety issues when providing sexual health care in trans and gender diverse patients?
   - Use of correct name and pronouns;
   - Use of non-judgmental language;
   - Discuss anatomical language with Ben regarding the words he would prefer his health care provider use to describe different body parts;
   - Sensitively discussing the history of medical and surgical treatments undertaken to affirm gender;
   - Important to broach the need for contraception with Ben as testosterone alone does not guarantee infertility.

By providing inclusive and informed care, the practice nurse was able to improve health outcomes for Ben, who agreed to participate in screening. Cervical cancer incidence and mortality have both decreased in Australia since the National Cervical Screening Program began in 1991, but in countries with well-developed cervical screening programs, such as Australia, being either never, or under-screened (Saville, Hawkes, Mclachlan, Anderson, & Arabena, 2018) is one of the most significant risk factors for developing cervical cancer.

Acknowledgements

Thank you to Morgan Carpenter, Co-Executive Director of Intersex Human Rights Australia, for his review of and contribution to content in this chapter related to intersex people.

Cristyn Davies is a researcher, Skinner is an investigator, and Julie Mooney-Somers is an associate investigator within the Wellbeing Health and Youth (WH&Y) NHMRC Centre of Research Excellence in Adolescent Health (APP 1134984).

Cristyn Davies is a Board Director at Twenty10 Inc. GLCS, NSW, Australia. Atari Metcalf and Julie Mooney-Somers are Directors at ACON, NSW, Australia.

Notes

1 Various terms are used across the health care sector to describe people accessing health care services including, but not limited to, patients, clients, service users and consumers. All of these terms can connote power-relations between those accessing a service and service provision and are influenced by context and institutional setting. Throughout this chapter we have tried to avoid use of these terms, but where necessary have referred to both patients and clients.

2 Rainbow tick information: https://www.qip.com.au/standards/rainbow-tick-standards/. Pride in Health + Wellbeing: https://www.prideinclusionprograms.com.au/health/.

3 *Re Kelvin* [2017] FamCA 78.

4 *Re: Matthew [2018] FamCA 161 (16 March 2018).*

References

ACON. (2019). *A blueprint for improving the health and wellbeing of the trans and gender diverse community in NSW.* https://www.acon.org.au/wp-content/uploads/2019/04/ACON-TGD-Health-Blueprint-Booklet.pdf.

Aggleton, P., Bhana, D., Clarke, D. J., Crewe, M., Race, K., & Yankah, E. (2018). HIV education: Reflections on the past, priorities for the future. *AIDS Education and Prevention, 30*(3), 254–266. https://doi.org/10.1521/aeap.2018.30.3.254.

American Psychiatric Association. (2013). *Diagnostic and statistical manual of mental disorders* (5th ed.). American Psychiatric Association. https://doi.org/10.1176/appi.books.9780890425596.

Brooks, H., Llewellyn, C. D., Nadarzynski, T., Pelloso, F. C., Guilherme, F. D. S., Pollard, A., & Jones, C. J. (2018). Sexual orientation disclosure in health care: A systematic review. *British Journal of General Practice, 68*(668), e187–e196. https://doi.org/10.3399/bjgp18X694841.

Butler, J. (1990). *Gender trouble: Feminism and the subversion of identity*. Routledge.

Byron, P., Rasmussen, S., Wright Toussaint, D., Lobo, R., Robinson, K. H., & Paradise, B. (2017). *You learn from each other: LGBTIQ young people's mental health help-seeking and the RAD Australia online directory.* Young and Well Cooperative Research Centre. https://doi.org/10.4225/35/58ae2dea65d12.

Callander, D., Wiggins, J., Rosenberg, S., Cornelisse, V. J., Duck-Chong, E., Holt, M., Pony, M., Vlahakis, E., MacGibbon, J., & Cook, T. (2018). *The 2018 Australian trans and gender diverse sexual health survey: Report of findings.* The Kirby Institute. https://kirby.unsw.edu.au/sites/default/files/kirby/report/ATGD-Sexual-Health-Survey-Report_2018.pdf.

Carpenter, M. (2016). The human rights of intersex people: Addressing harmful practices and rhetoric of change. *Reproductive Health Matters, 24*(47), 74–84. https://doi.org/10.1016/j.rhm.2016.06.003.

Carpenter, M. (2018). The normalisation of intersex bodies and othering of intersex identities. In J. M. Scherpe, A. Dutta, & T. Helms (Eds.), *The legal status of intersex persons* (pp. 445–514). Intersentia. https://doi.org/10.1017/9781780687704.

Cartledge, S., & Ryan, J. (1983). *Sex and love: New thoughts on old contradictions.* The Women's Press.

Coleman, E., Bockting, W., Botzer, M., Cohen-Kettenis, P., DeCuypere, G., Feldman, J., … Monstrey, S. (2012). Standards of care for the health of transsexual, transgender, and gender-nonconforming people, version 7. *International Journal of Transgenderism, 13*(4), 165–232. https://doi.org/10.1080/15532739.2011.700873.

Commission on Social Determinants of Health. (2008). *Closing the gap in a generation: Health equity through action on the social determinants of health.* World Health Organisation. https://www.who.int/social_determinants/final_report/csdh_finalreport_2008.pdf.

Crenshaw, K. (1989). Demarginalizing the intersection of race and sex: A black feminist critique of antidiscrimination doctrine, feminist theory and antiracist politics. *University of Chicago Legal Forum, 1*(8), 139–168.

Davies, C., Skinner, S. R., Odgers, H. L., Khut, G. P., & Morrow, A. (2018). The use of mobile and new media technologies in a health intervention about HPV and HPV vaccination in schools. In L. Grealy, C. Driscoll & A. Hickey-Moody (Eds.), *Youth, technology, governance, experience* (pp. 175–195). Routledge.

Davies, C., Skinner, S. R., Stoney, T., Marshall, H. S., Collins, J., Jones, J., Hutton, H., Parrella, A., Cooper, S., McGeechan, K., Zimet, G., & for the HPV.edu Study Group. (2017). Is it like one of those infectious kind of things? The importance of educating young people about HPV and HPV vaccination at school. *Sex Education, 17*(3), 256–275.

Deacon, R. M., & Mooney-Somers, J. (2017). Smoking prevalence among lesbian, bisexual and queer women in Sydney remains high: Analysis of trends and correlates. *Drug and Alcohol Review, 36*(4), 546–554. https://doi.org/10.1111/dar.12477.

Durso, L. E., & Meyer, I. H. (2012). Patterns and predictors of disclosure of sexual orientation to healthcare providers among lesbians, gay men, and bisexuals. *Sexuality Research and Social Policy, 10*(1), 35–42. https://doi.org/10.1007/s13178-012-0105-2.

Fairley, C., Russell, D. B., & Bradford, D. (Eds.). (2005). *Sexual health medicine.* IP Communications.

Guse, K., Levine, D., Martins, S., Lira, A., Gaarde, J., Westmorland, W., & Gilliam, M. (2012). Interventions using new digital media to improve adolescent sexual health: A systematic review. *Journal of Adolescent Health, 51*(6), 535–543. https://doi.org/10.1016/j.jadohealth.2012.03.014.

Hatzenbuehler, M. L., Bellatorre, A., & Muennig, P. (2014). Anti-gay prejudice and all-cause mortality among heterosexuals in the United States. *American Journal of Public Health, 104*(2), 332–337. https://doi.org/10.2105/AJPH.2013.301678.

Hatzenbuehler, M. L., Phelan, J. C., & Link, B. G. (2013). Stigma as a fundamental cause of population health inequalities. *American Journal of Public Health, 103*(5), 813–821. https://doi.org/10.2105/AJPH.2012.301069.

Intersex Human Rights Australia. (2019). Intersex for allies. https://ihra.org.au/allies/.

Jagose, A. (1996). *Queer theory: An introduction.* New York University Press.

Jones, T., Hart, B., Carpenter, M., Ansara, G., Leonard, W., & Lucke, J. (2016). *Intersex stories and statistics from Australia.* Open Book Publishers. https://doi.org/10.11647/OBP.0089.

Kaholokula, J. K. A., Grandinetti, A., Keller, S., Nacapoy, A. H., & Mau, M. K. (2012). Association between perceived racism and physiological stress indices in Native Hawaiians. *Journal of Behavioral Medicine, 35*(1), 27–37. https://doi.org/10.1007/s10865-011-9330-z.

Kang, M., Robards, F., Sanci, L., Steinbeck, K., Jan, S., Hawke, C., Luscombe, G., Kong, M., & Usherwood, T. (2018). *Access 3: Young people and the healthcare system in the digital age final research report.* Department of General Practice Westmead, the University of Sydney, & the Australian Centre for Public and Poulation Health Research, University of Technology. https://www.uts.edu.au/sites/default/files/2019-04/Access3_young people and the health system in the digital age.pdf.

Knight, R. E., Shoveller, J. A., Carson, A. M., & Contreras-Whitney, J. G. (2014). Examining clinicians' experiences providing sexual health services for LGBTQ youth: Considering social and structural determinants of health in clinical practice. *Health Education Research, 29*(4), 662–670. https://doi.org/10.1093/her/cyt116.

Koh, C. S., Kang, M., & Usherwood, T. (2014). I demand to be treated as the person I am: Experiences of accessing primary health care for Australian adults who identify as gay, lesbian, bisexual, transgender or queer. *Sexual Health, 11*(3), 258–264. https://doi.org/10.1071/SH14007.

Krieger, N. (2001). A glossary for social epidemiology. *Journal of Epidemiology & Community Health, 55*(10), 693–700. https://doi.org/10.1136/jech.55.10.693.

Leonard, W., Pitts, M., Mitchell, A., Lyons, A., Smith, A., Patel, A., Couch, M., & Barrett, A. (2012). *Private lives 2: The second national survey of the health and wellbeing of GLBT Australians.* Australian Research Centre in Sex, Health and Society. https://www.acon.org.au/wp-content/uploads/2015/04/PrivateLives2-report-2012.pdf.

LGBTIQ+ Health Australia. (2013). *Inclusive language guide: Respecting people of intersex, trans and gender diverse experience.* https://d3n8a8pro7vhmx.cloudfront.net/lgbtihealth/pages/160/attachments/original/1587966204/Alliance_Health_Information_Sheet_Inclusive_Language_Guide_on_Intersex__Trans_and_Gender_Diversity_0.pdf?1587966204.

Marmot, M. G., Stansfeld, S., Patel, C., North, F., Head, J., White, I., Brunner, E., Feeney, A., & Smith, G. D. (1991). Health inequalities among British civil servants: The Whitehall II study. *The Lancet*, *337*(8754), 1387–1393. https://doi.org/10.1016/0140-6736(91)93068-K

McGarry, K., Hebert, M. G., Kelleher, J., & Potter, J. (2008). Taking a comprehensive history and providing relevant risk-reduction counseling. In H. Makadon, K. H. Mayer, J. Potter, & H. Goldhammer (Eds.), *The Fenway guide to lesbian, gay, bisexual, and transgender health* (pp. 419–442). American College of Physicians.

McNair, R. P. (2017). Multiple identities and their intersections with queer health and wellbeing. *Journal of Intercultural Studies*, *38*(4), 443–452. https://doi.org/10.1080/07256868.2017.1341398.

McNair, R., Hegarty, K., & Taft, A. (2015). Disclosure for same-sex attracted women enhancing the quality of the patient–doctor relationship in general practice. *Australian Family Physician*, *44*(8), 573–578.

Meyer, I. H. (2003). Prejudice, social stress, and mental health in lesbian, gay, and bisexual populations: Conceptual issues and research evidence. *Psychological Bulletin*, *129*(5), 674–697. https://doi.org/10.1037/0033-2909.129.5.674.

Mooney-Somers, J., Deacon, R. M., Scott, P., Price, K., & Parkhill, N. (2018). Women in contact with the Sydney LGBTQ communities: Report of the SWASH lesbian, bisexual and queer women's health survey 2014, 2016, 2018. Sydney Health Ethics, University of Sydney. https://www.acon.org.au/wp-content/uploads/2020/01/Sydney-SWASH-Report-2018-FINAL.pdf.

Morandini, J. S., Blaszczynski, A., Dar-Nimrod, I., & Ross, M. W. (2015). Minority stress and community connectedness among gay, lesbian and bisexual Australians: A comparison of rural and metropolitan localities. *Australian and New Zealand Journal of Public Health*, *39*(3), 260–266. https://doi.org/10.1111/1753-6405.12364.

Newman, C. E., Kidd, M. R., Kippax, S. C., Reynolds, R. H., Canavan, P. G., & de Wit, J. B. (2013). Engaging nonHIV specialist general practitioners with new priorities in HIV prevention and treatment: Qualitative insights from those working in the field. *Sexual Health*, *10*(3), 193–198. https://doi.org/10.1071/SH12157.

Newman, C. E., Persson, A., Manolas, P., Schmidt, H. M. A., Ooi, C., Rutherford, A., & de Wit, J. B. (2018). So much is at stake: Professional views on engaging heterosexually identified men who have sex with men with sexual health care in Australia. *Sexuality Research and Social Policy*, *15*(3), 302–311. https://doi.org/10.1007/s13178-017-0291-z.

Ovenden, G., Salter, M., Ullman, J., Denson, N., Robinson, K., Noonan, K., Bansel, P., & Huppatz, K. (2019). Gay, bisexual, transgender, intersex and queer men's attitudes and experiences of intimate partner violence and sexual assault. Sexualities and Genders Research, Western Sydney University, & ACON. http://sayitoutloud.org.au/wp-content/uploads/2019/05/Sorting-It-Out_GBTIQ-Men-and-SDFV-ACON.pdf.

Perez-Brumer, A. G., Parker, R., & Aggleton, P. J. (2017). *Rethinking MSM, trans* and other categories in HIV Prevention*. Routledge.

Quinn, D. M., & Chaudoir, S. R. (2009). Living with a concealable stigmatized identity: The impact of anticipated stigma, centrality, salience, and cultural stigma on psychological distress and health. *Journal of Personality and Social Psychology*, *97*(4), 634–651.

Ramsden, I. (2002). Cultural safety and nursing education in Aotearoa and Te Waipounamu [Doctoral dissertation, Victoria University of Wellington]. https://croakey.org/wp-content/uploads/2017/08/RAMSDEN-I-Cultural-Safety_Full.pdf.

Rich, A. (1980). Compulsory heterosexuality and lesbian existence. *Signs: Journal of Women in Culture and Society*, *5*(4), 631–660.

Riley, E. A., Sitharthan, G., Clemson, L., & Diamond, M. (2011). The needs of gender-variant children and their parents: A parent survey. *International Journal of Sexual Health*, *23*(3), 181–195. https://doi.org/10.1080/19317611.2011.593932.

Robinson, K. H., Bansel, P., Denson, N., Ovenden, G., & Davies, C. (2014). *Growing up queer: Issues facing young Australians who are gender variant and sexuality diverse.* Young and Well Cooperative Research Centre. https://www.twenty10.org.au/wp-content/uploads/2016/04/Robinson-et-al.-2014-Growing-up-Queer.pdf.

Robinson, K. H., & Díaz, C. J. (2016). *Diversity and difference in early childhoods: Implication for theory and practice.* Open University Press.

Rosenstreich, G., Comfort, J., & Martin, P. (2011). Primary health care and equity: The case of lesbian, gay, bisexual, trans and intersex Australians. *Australian Journal of Primary Health, 17*(4), 302–308. https://doi.org/10.1071/PY11036.

Saville, M., Hawkes, D., Mclachlan, E., Anderson, S., & Arabena, K. (2018). Self-collection for under-screened women in a national cervical screening program: Pilot study. *Current Oncology, 25*(1), e27–e32. https://doi.org/10.3747/co.25.3915.

Smith, E., Jones, T., Ward, R., Dixon, J., Mitchell, A., & Hillier, L. (2014). *From blues to rainbows: The mental health and wellbeing of gender diverse and transgender young people in Australia.* Australian Research Centre in Sex Health and Society. https://www.beyondblue.org.au/docs/default-source/research-project-files/bw0268-from-blues-to-rainbows-report-final-report.pdf?sfvrsn=6f2e60ea_2.

Strauss, P., Cook, A., Winter, S., Watson, V., Wright Toussaint, D., & Lin, A. (2017). *Trans pathways: The mental health experiences and care pathways of trans young people.* Telethon Kids Institute. https://www.telethonkids.org.au/globalassets/media/documents/brain--behaviour/trans-pathways-report.pdf.

Telfer, M. M., Tollit, M. A., Pace, C. C., & Pang, K. C. (2018). *Australian standards of care and treatment guidelines for trans and gender diverse children and adolescents version 1.1.* The Royal Children's Hospital. https://www.shil.nsw.gov.au/NSWSexualHealthInfolink/media/SiteContent/Files/5-Australian-Standards-of-Care_TGD-children-and-adolescents.pdf.

Williams, R. (1999). Cultural safety—What does it mean for our work practice? *Australian and New Zealand Journal of Public Health, 32*(2), 213–214. https://doi.org/10.1111/j.1467-842x.1999.tb01240.x.

Winsor, B. (2017). *A definitive timeline of LGBT+ rights in Australia: A bittersweet look at where we've been, how far we've come, and how far we've got to go.* https://www.sbs.com.au/topics/sexuality/agenda/article/2016/08/12/definitive-timeline-lgbt-rights-australia.

World Health Organisation. (2011). *Rio political declaration on social determinants of health.* https://www.who.int/sdhconference/declaration/Rio_political_declaration.pdf?ua=1.

World Health Organisation. (2018). *International classification of diseases.* https://icd.who.int/browse11/l-m/en

13 Ageing Australians

Genevieve Z. Steiner, Emma S. George, Freya MacMillan and Kate A. McBride

Learning outcomes

After working through this chapter, students should be able to:

1. Discuss how individual factors, including geographic, cultural, social, ethnic, sexuality and gender diversity, influence our needs as we age.
2. Compare and contrast the range of physical and mental health and wellbeing complications that can emerge with advancing age.
3. Demonstrate an understanding of Australian legislation that protects the rights of older people.
4. Identify the health, wellbeing, social, and economic impacts of loneliness, social isolation, caregiver burden and health literacy in older people.
5. Identify the health care system challenges for an ageing population.
6. Discuss the roles and requirements for health care professionals working with older people, particularly in relation to the provision of cultural safety.

Key terms

Ageing: The process of growing old.
Ageism: Discrimination or prejudice based on age.
Caregiver burden: A multidimensional response to the psychological, emotional, physical, social and financial stress of caring for a family member who is elderly, disabled or ill.
Chronic conditions: Health conditions lasting 3 months or more.
Dementia: Cognitive impairment that interferes with everyday functioning.
Elder abuse: A single or repeated act, or lack of appropriate action, occurring within any relationship where there is an expectation of trust that causes harm or distress to an older person (World Health Organisation, 2020).
Health care system: The system in which the purpose of all the services and activities are to promote, restore or maintain health.
Health literacy: The ability to obtain, process, and understand basic health information and services in order to make appropriate health decisions.
Residential aged care: Care options and accommodation for older people who are unable to live independently in their own homes.
Social isolation: The state of lack of contact or minimal contact between an individual and society.

Chapter summary

The chapter will discuss the impact on Australia's population as a result of ageing and the implications that has for the health care system, and social determinants of health for Australians across the lifespan. Students will engage in reflexive activities where they will be asked to explore themselves across the lifespan. These activities will help students to describe the health, social and aged care services they would need and have access to, and what concerns they would have about their wellbeing and the health care system. From this, students will be introduced to ageism and the ways in which it can impact society at all levels, in addition to its impact on older Australians across all areas of social determinants (including housing, employment, etc.). Students will review national policies related to age discrimination and the role of health care professionals in supporting Australia's ageing population.

Introduction

Globally, the population is ageing. In the past 30 years, the number of people aged 60 years and over has more than doubled, and in the next 10 years, older people will outnumber children under the age of 10 (United Nations Department of Economic and Social Affairs, 2017). Australia is no exception, with more than one in every seven people aged 65 years and over in 2017. This chapter will introduce students to the contemporary health and wellbeing challenges of an ageing population in Australia. The multifactorial components of ageing will be discussed, including health complications, chronic conditions, and mental health changes as well as the social dynamics related to ageing and societal participation, including ageism, social exclusion, elder abuse, loneliness, caregiver burden and health literacy, in addition to the effects of ageing on the *health care system* and its workforce. This content will be supported by case studies, examples and activities relevant to national policies that highlight the diversity in Australia's ageing population. Students will also engage in reflective activities throughout where they will be asked to consider their health, independence, individual factors and place in society across the lifespan. The content and activities in this chapter will help students to develop a comprehensive understanding of the contemporary issues relevant to Australia's ageing population, including health, wellbeing, social dynamics, the health care system and its workforce.

Ageing in Australia

Ageing is a complex phenomenon resulting in a range of changes in mental, physical and social functioning that affects not only individuals' lives, but also their families and the wider community. Australia's ageing population is on the rise. From 1996 to 2016, the population aged 65 years and over increased from 12.0% to 15.3%, reaching 3.4 million (Australian Bureau of Statistics, 2015); this number is expected to double to 6.8 million by 2040, with the number of people aged 85 years and over expected to triple in the same timeframe (Australian Bureau of Statistics, 2013c). Most older Australians live in major cities (66%) and inner regional areas (32%) in NSW (33%) and Victoria (25%) (Australian Bureau of Statistics, 2017b).

There is a widespread perception that older Australians are "being taken care of" by society (Levy & Macdonald, 2016) and thereby limiting Australia's future prosperity. In reality, many older adults are healthy, independent and active contributors in our local communities. Most older Australians live in their own homes, 24% provide financial support to their adult children or relatives, 48% of older people aged 65–74 years donate their time to assist people within their community, 33% are active volunteers and 29% are involved with community organisations (Australian Institute of Health and Welfare, 2018c).

Australia's older population is culturally and linguistically diverse (CALD), with around one in every three Australians aged 65 years and older being overseas born (Australian Bureau of Statistics, 2017b). In 2016, 67% of these older Australians were born in Europe and 16% in Asia (Australian Bureau of Statistics, 2016), with 20% born in a non-English-speaking country (Australian Bureau of Statistics, 2017c). Due to the poorer health and lower life expectancy of Aboriginal and Torres Strait Islander Australians, aged care service planning takes place from 50 years and over, and in 2016, 23% of Australia's Aboriginal and Torres Strait Islander Peoples fell in this age group (Australian Institute of Health and Welfare, 2015a). Older Australians with CALD backgrounds can experience barriers to service access due to differing languages, norms and cultural practices and have lower socio-economic status compared to Anglo-Australians in the same age group (Federation of Ethnic Communities' Councils of Australia, 2015). Other diverse groups include veterans, those living in rural or remote areas, those who are homeless (16% of Australians age 55 and up) (Australian Bureau of Statistics, 2018a) and those who identify as lesbian, gay, bisexual, transgender, queer, intersex or asexual (LGBTIQA+); 5% of same-sex couple relationships are aged 65 years and over (Australian Bureau of Statistics, 2017b).

Box 13.1 Case study—Diversity and age

Mrs. L is a 69-year-old heterosexual, married woman of Filipino descent who was living at home alone prior to her admission into a *residential aged care* facility via hospital after being found at home by her son unconscious after a fall. Mrs. L speaks little English and was receiving community care services from support workers bilingual in Filipino and English languages prior to her admission to hospital. Mrs. L was diagnosed with vascular dementia, depression, diabetes, and post-traumatic stress disorder during her stay in hospital. Prior to Mrs. L's hospitalisation, she had expressed to the bilingual community health care workers that if anything major were to happen to her health, she wished to stay at home surrounded by family. Although Mrs. L's condition was stable when she was admitted to residential aged care, her condition worsened rapidly. She became subdued and withdrawn throughout the day, dozing mostly in her chair, and has not been sleeping in the evening, spending most of the night crying and calling out for her late husband in Filipino. The residential aged care facility is located closer to where her son lives, rather than where Mrs. L lived (due to both financial and convenience reasons), and bilingual support is limited. Her communication deteriorated to the extent that it has been assumed that she is now unable to communicate her wishes due to dementia.

Questions for reflection:

- Identify Mrs. L's geographic, cultural, social, ethnic, gender and sexuality factors.
- How do these social determinants of health shape Mrs. L's needs in older age?
- How have these social determinants of health affected Mrs. L's journey through the health care system and into residential aged care?

Ageing, health and wellbeing

Age-associated health complications

Older people face a range of physical and mental health challenges. As individuals age, they experience a range of age-associated complications, with the prevalence of many health conditions higher in older age groups. Excluding long and short sightedness, in Australia, the most common long-term health conditions experienced by older people include back pain, hearing loss, arthritis, diabetes, cardiovascular disease (CVD), chronic obstructive pulmonary disease (COPD), osteoporosis and cancer (Australian Institute of Health and Welfare, 2014a). Age-related vision problems are also common with cataracts, macular degeneration, blindness and glaucoma all affecting at least 2% of older individuals. Further, like Mrs. L in the preceding case study, many Australians have *dementia*, with an estimated 447,115 Australians diagnosed with the condition in 2018, 93% of whom are 65 years and older (Dementia Australia, 2018).

As people age, they are also likely to experience several of these *chronic conditions* at the same time (i.e., multimorbidity, defined as the coexistence of two or more chronic health conditions [Wang et al., 2017]), with older age characterised by complex health states, commonly termed geriatric syndromes. These syndromes invariably result as a consequence of multiple underlying factors such as frailty, urinary incontinence, falls, pressure ulcers and intellectual incapacity due to dementia and delirium (Noguchi et al., 2016; World Health Organisation, 2018). Geriatric syndromes are likely better predictors of mortality than the presence or number of specific diseases (Inouye et al., 2007).

Impacts on societal participation

This multimorbidity is often the norm, rather than the exception, in older people (Marengoni et al., 2011), with a recent study showing that the prevalence of multiple morbidities is likely to be higher than 80% among individuals older than 85 years (Salive, 2013). Multimorbidity has proven negative effects on wellbeing, function and mobility, which in turn can impact on societal participation activities (Galenkamp & Deeg, 2016; Marengoni et al., 2011), such as employment, volunteering, and informal caregiving, as well as participation in educational activities, social leisure activities and religious activities.

Chronic conditions

Specific chronic conditions, such as osteoporosis, and age-related health complications, including hearing and vision loss, are strongly associated with advancing age and already pose a significant challenge for the Australian health system. The next generation of older adults transitioning into the 65 years and over age group are also affected by a range of conditions driven by modifiable risk-factors (e.g., diabetes, CVD, cancer) and pose a two-fold challenge to health care providers.

As with all population age groups, chronic conditions are increasing among older Australians. Prevalence of these conditions is growing due to a complex interaction between non-modifiable risk factors such as genetics and ageing, social determinants of health and modifiable risk factors across the life-course, including consumption of low levels of fruits and vegetables, high levels of processed foods, alcohol and tobacco, as well as low levels of physical activity and high rates of sedentary behaviour (Australian Institute of Health and Welfare, 2015b). Tobacco consumption has particular impacts on the older population as it is highest among older age groups and is the leading risk factor for the burden of disease among Australians aged 65–80 years (Australian

Institute of Health and Welfare, 2018a). Smoking habits acquired earlier in life greatly increase the risk for CVD and COPD in old age, along with cancers and many other chronic diseases. Individuals in their 60s are also increasingly the most likely to exceed single-occasion risky drinking guidelines on at least 5 days per week: 5.7% in 2013 versus 7.0% in 2016 (Australian Institute of Health and Welfare, 2018a). These unhealthy behaviours, as well as the high prevalence of overweight and obesity, have contributed to the significant and continuing increase in the chronic disease burden in Australia (Australian Institute of Health and Welfare, 2014c). Dementia, for which obesity is now recognised as a significant risk factor, is also rapidly increasing, with the number of Australians affected by the disease estimated to reach ~1.1 million by 2058 (Australian Institute of Health and Welfare, 2012; Dementia Australia, 2018). Cancers associated with modifiable risk factors (e.g., excess body mass) such as bowel cancer, postmenopausal breast cancer, pancreatic cancer and prostate cancer (advanced) are also increasing, with an estimated 150,000 cancers in 2020—an increase of almost 40% from 2007 (Australia Institute of Health and Welfare, 2012). Prostate cancer for men, breast cancer for women, and bowel cancer for all present the biggest burden of cancer in Australia (Australia Institute of Health and Welfare, 2012).

Box 13.2 Reflection—Spotlight on the chronic conditions crisis in Western Sydney, Australia

Chronic conditions with high prevalence rates in older people including dementia, cancer, diabetes and cardiovascular disease pose a significant challenge for the Australian health system. This is a major problem for Western Sydney, as in comparison to the NSW average, the region faces a range of poorer health outcomes for older people (South Western Sydney Local Health District, 2016), including the following:

- The highest expected increase in the prevalence of dementia in all of NSW by 2050 (Alzheimer's Australia NSW & Deloitte Access Economics, 2014; Steiner et al., 2020)
- Higher prevalence of thyroid, kidney, liver, gastro-intestinal and lung cancer (South Western Sydney Local Health District, 2016)
- Higher rates of diabetes, with the National Diabetes Services Scheme implicating Blacktown, Mt Druitt, and Westmead amongst areas with the highest registered cases of diabetes in Australia (Essue et al., 2007)
- Higher standardised mortality rates from CVD (South Western Sydney Local Health District, 2016)
- Increased prevalence of health risk factors, including smoking, obesity and overweight, and inadequate vegetable intake and physical activity (South Western Sydney Local Health District, 2016)

The reasons for the disproportionately poorer health outcomes in Western Sydney are multifactorial and include population ageing (more >65- than <16-year-olds), lower levels of educational attainment (the second biggest risk factor for dementia), economic disadvantage, and high rates of vascular risk factors, including obesity and overweight, diabetes and hypertension (Australian Tax Office, 2015; Centre for Western Sydney, 2019b; South Western Sydney Local Health District and Medicare Local, 2014; South Western Sydney Local Health District, 2017).

Western Sydney is also the most diverse large urban region in Australia. Residents are from over 170 countries that speak over 100 different languages, with 38% of residents speaking a language other than English, the most common including India, China, Iraq, the Philippines and Vietnam (Centre for Western Sydney, 2019a). The diversity of the region in conjunction with the disadvantage faced by the Western Sydney community emphasises the multiple layers and complexity of the social determinants of health in relation to ageing.

Box 13.3 Case study—Cancer screening

Cancer risk increases with age, but other modifiable risk factors like obesity also increase the risk of cancers, including breast cancer among postmenopausal women. Obesity can also worsen breast cancer outcomes among older women, which is concerning given that obesity rates in Australia are rising rapidly. Despite these issues, breast screening participation rates in the free biennial Breast Screen Australia program offered to women ages 50–74 years are suboptimal, and even lower in higher risk, obese women (Ferrante et al., 2007; McBride et al., 2019). Exploratory Australian data shows that one of the reasons for this lower participation in screening may in part be due to social determinants of health, cultural competency, and lower perceived risk of postmenopausal breast cancer among overweight and obese women (McBride et al., 2019). Amongst these women, limited desire to prioritise personal health needs, reluctance to screen due to poor body image and prior negative mammographic experiences due to issues with weight were all reported by the women who took part in this study. Radiographers reported cultural barriers, a lack of education, and low levels of health literacy as barriers to breast screening participation amongst overweight and obese women from diverse backgrounds. These are all issues that are exacerbated by other age-related contextual factors such as comorbidities and mobility issues.

Questions for reflection:

- How might older age impact on taking part in preventative health programs like cancer screening?
- For someone like Mrs. L, how could these issues be exacerbated by cultural factors?
- Given these issues, how might we encourage older individuals to participate in cancer screening programs, such as Breast Screen Australia?
- How could screening programs focused on disease prevention and health promotion be culturally safe?

Mental health of older Australians

While dementia is a significant public health issue among older individuals, poor mental health is also highly prevalent. There is increasing recognition that good mental health is a key factor associated with healthy ageing (Cosco et al., 2017; Kane, 2005). Depression, for example, is a significant problem in older cohorts and may contribute to lower levels of independent functioning, increased perceptions of poor health, and use of health services (Bunce et al., 2012). Depression is also linked to risk of stroke, hip fracture, heart failure, and dementia risk (Birkenshaw, 1988; Bunce et al., 2012). Conversely, the mental health of older people can be affected by losing the ability to live independently, declining functional ability, bereavement (particularly through the death of a life partner), and an income drop following retirement (Phongsavan et al., 2013). Together, these factors can lead to *social isolation* and loneliness as well as increased psychological distress (World Health Organisation, 2017). Depression is often underdiagnosed among older adults, as the symptoms may be overlooked and untreated due to the co-occurrence with other health issues.

Box 13.4 Reflection—Reducing chronic conditions risk in older Australians

In 2018, academics at Western Sydney University published an Ageing Research White Paper (Steiner et al., 2018), which outlined the multifactorial challenges that older Australians face as they age. One of the key issues they identified was the need to prevent chronic conditions so that individuals who are now living longer could do so as healthier people. The university's researchers working on ageing concluded that real impact and change for older adults could occur through engagement with a broad range of partners, in local, state and federal government; health; research; industry; non-government organisations; not-for-profits; consumer advocacy agencies; policymakers; and quintessentially older adults, their carers and their families.

Questions for reflection:

- If you were creating a population-level health-promotion program aimed at encouraging older adults to lose weight to reduce their chronic conditions risk, who might you engage with?
- What might be the benefit of engaging multiple stakeholders in an obesity-prevention program?

Social dynamics of ageing

Ageism and social exclusion

Given their rich and diverse life experiences, older adults have much to contribute to society. Unfortunately, negative attitudes towards ageing fail to recognise these strengths, and many older adults report being discriminated against because of their age (Australian Human Rights Commission, 2013)

Box 13.5 Reflection—Age Discrimination Act

To protect the rights of older adults and ensure employers, educators and those in power do not discriminate on the ground of age, the *Age Discrimination Act* was introduced in 2004. This Act makes it unlawful to discriminate, either directly or indirectly, against a person on the ground of age in respect to:

- Employment
- Education
- Access to premises

- Provision of goods, services and facilities
- Provision of accommodation
- Disposal of land
- Administration of Commonwealth laws and programs
- Requests for information on which age discrimination might be based (Australian Government, 2004; *Age Discrimination Act 2004 (Cth)*)

Ageism involves negative attitudes towards older people and is a significant social issue. According to the Australian Human Rights Commission, many Australians associate ageing with negative stereotypes and characteristics, including forgetfulness, inflexibility and difficulty adapting to new or complex skills (Australian Human Rights Commission, 2013); this can have serious implications for older adults' employment and education opportunities. As life expectancy continues to rise, so too will the age at which Australians are eligible for the age pension. In turn, older Australians will need to remain in the workforce for longer and often extend their working career beyond the point at which they would like to retire (Zhu, 2016). As of 1 July 2017, the age pension eligibility age increased to 65 years and 6 months. The age at which adults are eligible for the pension is set to increase by a further 6 months every 2 years, until 1 July 2023 (Department of Human Services, 2018). For those wishing or requiring to remain in or re-enter the workforce, however, ageism presents a significant barrier for older people.

The transition into retirement can influence health positively and negatively. A large-scale Australian study of adults aged 45 years and older (Ding et al., 2016) found that retirement was associated with a reduction in the odds of smoking (for women), more physical activity, less sitting time and healthier sleep patterns. Conversely, retirement can also lead to a reduced sense of purpose, reduction in regular social interactions and loneliness (Segel-Karpas et al., 2018). To maintain social connectedness and a sense of purpose, it is imperative that older adults are treated with respect and dignity, and that their valuable contribution to the community is recognised. Gender differences also contribute to diversity in ageing and the transition into retirement. Women are twice as likely as men to be informal caregivers in older age and also have less superannuation to support retirement due to mid-life caregiving responsibilities and salary disparities.

Elder abuse

Elder abuse is defined as "a single or repeated act, or lack of appropriate action, occurring within any relationship where there is an expectation of trust, which causes harm or distress to an older person" (World Health Organisation, 2020). Elder abuse can be intentional or unintentional and includes

- Physical abuse, including acts of violence, physical punishment or use of restraints
- Psychological or emotional abuse, including threats, intimidation or forced isolation
- Financial abuse or material exploitation, which can include illegal or improper use of a person's money, property or assets or coercing a person into signing documents
- Sexual abuse, which can include any unwanted sexual behaviour or touching
- Neglect, including failure to provide adequate care, or failure to fulfil obligations or duties of care

(Hall et al., 2016)

Findings from systematic reviews indicate that elder abuse is prevalent in both the community (Yon et al., 2017) and institutional settings (Yon et al., 2019). In the community, approximately one in six adults age 60 years and older had experienced some form of abuse (Yon et al., 2017).

Prevalence estimates based on self-reported data on institutional abuse (Yon et al., 2019) indicate that psychological and emotional abuse was most prevalent in institutional care settings (33.4%).

In 2017, the issue of elder abuse was brought to Australia's attention after shocking evidence of neglect and abuse at the Oakden campus of the South Australian Older Persons Mental Health Service was revealed (Maker & McSherry, 2018). In response to claims of abuse from residents' family members, South Australia's Independent Commissioner Against Corruption (ICAC) launched an investigation into the maladministration of the service in 2017. This was followed by the introduction of a Royal Commission into Aged Care Quality and Safety on 8 October 2018, established by the Governor-General of Australia. The findings of this Royal Commission are due in March 2021, and this will have serious implications for the future of aged care service provision in Australia. While it is acknowledged that many aged care facilities provide comprehensive and high-quality care, the Royal Commission will shine a light on the industry, highlighting best practice approaches and providing an opportunity to review and improve current practices. It is expected there will be a greater focus on quality of care and staff to resident ratios.

On 1 July 2019, the Aged Care Quality and Safety Commission's new Aged Care Quality Standards came into effect. All organisations providing aged care services subsidised by the Commonwealth are required to comply with the eight new standards, which focus on consumer outcomes (Aged Care Quality and Safety Commission, 2018) (Figure 13.1).

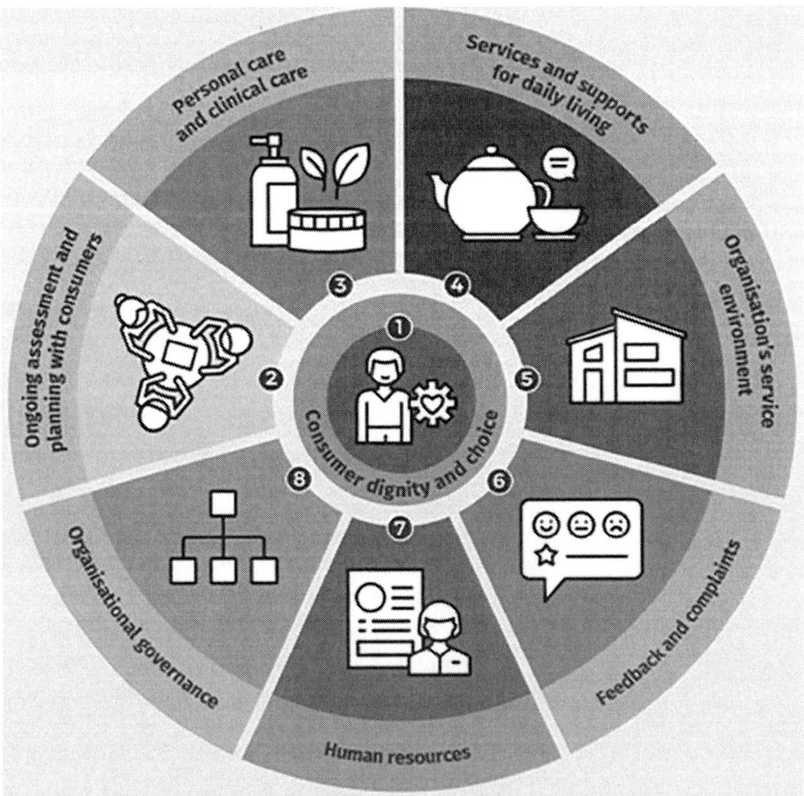

Figure 13.1 The Aged Care Quality Standards (Source: Australian Government Australian Aged Care Quality and Safety Commission. Guidance and Resources for Providers to support the new Aged Care Quality Standards, December 2019).

Box 13.6 Reflection—The Aged Care Quality Standards

The Aged Care Quality Standards stem from eight individual standards detailed in Figure 13.1.

Standard 1. Consumer dignity and choice
Standard 2. Ongoing assessment and planning with consumers
Standard 3. Personal care and clinical care
Standard 4. Services and supports for daily living (e.g., food services, domestic assistance, home maintenance, transport, recreational and social activities)
Standard 5. Organisation's service environment (i.e., the physical environment through which care and services are delivered)
Standard 6. Feedback and complaints
Standard 7. Human resources
Standard 8. Organisational governance

(Aged Care Quality and Safety Commission, 2018)

Loneliness

Loneliness is a negative feeling that can occur when social and emotional needs are not being met through existing relationships and interactions. Social isolation, while similar, is a distinct concept that is more objective and quantifiable. Social isolation can occur when an individual lives alone and has limited social network ties or irregular contact with friends, colleagues or family (Holt-Lunstad et al., 2015). The number of people one can rely on, the frequency of social interactions and the number of people a person lives with can be captured in a quantifiable way. A feeling of loneliness, however, is inherently subjective. While some people may feel lonely without frequent social contact and meaningful interactions, others may be content leading a solitary life. On the other hand, even when surrounded by friends, with regular social interactions and strong social networks, some may still feel a sense of loneliness as their social needs are not being fulfilled (Holt-Lunstad et al., 2015). Loneliness is common amongst older adults and is a public health concern. Loneliness stems from social isolation arising from multiple life changes such as age-related physical disability and illness, retirement, the death of a spouse or friends, and the feeling of being "pushed aside" as the role of being the hub of the family transitions to the next generation (Gerst-Emerson & Jayawardhana, 2015). Age-related changes, including a reduction in cognitive and physical functioning, onset of chronic health conditions and loss of friends and loved ones, can lead to increased social isolation and subsequent feelings of loneliness. Evidence suggests that loneliness, particularly in older adults, is associated with a range of health outcomes, including reduced physical activity, impaired cognitive performance, psychological distress and chronic conditions risk (Ong et al., 2016). It is therefore imperative that older adults continue to engage in meaningful social interactions to maintain a feeling of connectedness.

Box 13.7 Reflection—Physical activity and older people

Participation in moderate-to-vigorous physical activity can be difficult for older people, particularly those who have been inactive for long periods of time, but it is important for older adults to engage in some form of physical activity every day. Activities incorporating strength (e.g., light-intensity resistance training), fitness (e.g., walking) and balance and flexibility (e.g., yoga, tai chi, dancing) are ideal and should be included each week (Department of Health, 2017). Group-based activities, such as group fitness classes, dance classes and walking groups, may be particularly beneficial for older adults as they offer an opportunity for social interaction and mental stimulation. Learning a new skill or engaging in a new activity can also lead to a sense of belonging and accomplishment. Community centres, aged care facilities and health service providers should look for opportunities to keep older adults engaged in a variety of physical activities to promote physical and mental health and social connectedness.

- If you were to design a weekly physical activity program to be implemented in an aged care facility, what would you include? In your response, consider the characteristics of your participants (geographic, cultural, social and ethnic factors); the type, frequency and variety of activities; the skill and fitness levels required; and the health and social benefits associated with the activities.
- How would you tailor this program to encourage Mrs. L to be more physically active? Take into consideration Mrs. L's individual geographic, cultural, social, ethnic, gender and sexuality factors, in addition to her dementia symptoms.

Caregiver burden

Informal caregiving is characterised by the unpaid support and assistance provided by family members, friends or neighbours to those with chronic or disabling conditions (Lambert et al., 2017). As the number of older adults and rates of chronic conditions increase, informal caregiving is becoming more common, and providing ongoing care to an older person can have a substantial impact on the physical and mental health of caregivers (Colombo, Llena-Nozal, Mercier, & Tjadens, 2011). In Australia, 25.7% of informal caregivers in 2012 were born overseas (Australian Bureau of Statistics, 2012b). Yet, across all cultures, people who identify as women are most likely to be informal caregivers, with 71.8% of primary carers in 2018 (Australian Bureau of Statistics, 2018b).

Providing ongoing care can impact on a carer's personal life, social connectedness, employment, and education prospects (Garrido et al., 2018; Pinquart & Sörensen, 2003). A meta-analysis of psychological and physical health among caregivers and non-caregivers found that carers had higher rates of depression and stress, lower self-efficacy, and poorer physical health and general subjective wellbeing (Pinquart & Sörensen, 2003). A systematic review on caregiver burden for those caring for adults with dementia (Chiao et al., 2015) identified additional complex care factors, including a need to undertake increased responsibility as health and cognition deteriorate and a need to manage increasing dementia-related symptoms such as agitation, irritability, aggression, depression and withdrawal (Daly et al., 2015). As life expectancy and rates of chronic conditions continue to rise, it is likely that informal caregiving will become more common. To address caregiver burden, there is a need to provide informal caregivers with training and resources to support them and those they care for, particularly given that culturally diverse caregivers are less likely to use support services.

Box 13.8 Reflection—Caregiving

Caregiving is experienced differently across cultural contexts. Collectivistic cultures prioritise group and family (including extended family) needs over individual needs, whereas individualistic cultures preference individual needs and the immediate/nuclear family needs over the group and extended family. These differing cultural norms result in different expectations in relation to caregiving, caregiving behaviours and responses to caregiving demands (Willis, 2012). Collective cultural identification is linked with affection towards family members and willingness to provide informal care, whereas individualistic cultural identification provides informal care due to the feeling of necessity and lack willingness to provide care (Pyke & Bengtson, 1996). Cultural background also influences how particular causes of disability amongst older people are viewed. For example, some of the challenges faced by CALD dementia carers include (Vickrey et al., 2007):

- Language barriers to accessing resources and services
- Lack of culturally sensitive information, resources and services
- Stigma regarding open discussion of symptoms that can lead to stress and feelings of shame and limits support from family members
- Stigma, which creates a barrier to accessing resources and services
- Lack of awareness of programs, resources and services.

Health literacy in older adults

In Australia, it is estimated that only 40% of adults have a level of health literacy required to navigate the health system, understand and engage with health messages, make appropriate health decisions and function effectively in the health care environment (Australian Commission on Safety and Quality in Health Care, 2014). Adults over the age of 65 years tend to have lower rates of health literacy (Chesser et al., 2016), particularly mental health literacy (Farrer et al., 2008), than younger age groups. This means that older adults are often less adept at identifying depression and anxiety and may tend to hold misconceptions about depression, believing, for example, that it stems from weakness of character (Farrer et al., 2008). Reduced mental health literacy and pervasive misconceptions about depression and anxiety mean that—despite living in an information rich environment—older adults are also less likely to access resources or develop effective strategies for managing their symptoms. As few as 24% of older adults with depression actually seek treatment (Atkins et al., 2015), with the most recent available data from the 2007 Australian National Survey of Mental Health and Wellbeing finding that adults over 65 years of age are the least likely of all age groups to perceive a need for treatment for mental health issues (Forbes et al., 2017). In fact, many older people and their carers are often likely to attribute symptoms of depression to normal ageing, rather than viewing it as a treatable condition and are thus less likely to seek treatment (Sarkisian et al., 2003). When older people do seek treatment, they may express their mental health experiences in physical terms, making it more difficult for health practitioners to detect mental health issues (Sharpe et al., 2017).

Adults from CALD populations often experience additional barriers to effectively navigating the health care system and accessing required health care services (Jessup et al., 2017). Common barriers to health and mental health service utilisation include language and communication difficulties, lack of trust in health professionals, low perceived quality of care and limited knowledge of available services (Henderson & Kendall, 2011; Wohler & Dantas, 2017). Evidence also suggests that, for those from CALD backgrounds, dementia may be under-diagnosed and/or diagnosed at a later stage (Cooper, Tandy, Balamurali, & Livingston, 2010; Haralambous et al., 2014). This poses challenges for the treatment and management of dementia and associated symptoms and highlights a need for additional research into, and understanding of, the diversity of ways dementia is understood and experienced (Cox et al., 2019). It has been shown that positive outcomes for CALD populations are demonstrated when mainstream services for people with dementia and their caregivers work in partnership with cultural and ethnic specific services (Shanley et al., 2012) through the provision of culturally appropriate health information and services (Cooper et al., 2010).

Box 13.9 Reflection—Social isolation and loneliness

Shareefa is a 72-year-old woman with Muslim religious beliefs, who migrated to Australia 20 years ago from Pakistan. Her husband, Bisman, a man who is also of Pakistani descent with Muslim religiosity, was diagnosed with dementia three years ago, and he recently passed away. Shareefa dedicated all of her time to Bisman as his primary caregiver; the burden was extremely high as they did not have any family or close friends to assist and provide support. When Shareefa and Bisman first moved to Australia, the couple would frequently visit the local migrant community centre, where they formed friendships with other migrant families. When Bisman started to show signs of aggression and agitation, they stopped attending the centre, as they were too ashamed to socialise in case Bisman talked or behaved inappropriately. It was soon after that he was diagnosed with late-stage dementia. Shareefa now lives alone in a one-bedroom apartment in Sydney's western suburbs and lives on social welfare payments. Shareefa stopped going to the migrant community centre after Bisman's behaviour changed until after his passing—a total of nearly 5 years. Bisman was most fluent in spoken and written English as he worked when they arrived to Australia while Shareefa took care of the home and had fewer opportunities to practice her spoken English, although she is fluent in written English. She rarely ventures outside. On a few occasions when she was at the shops trying to buy groceries the clerks raised their voices, assuming Shareefa was hard of hearing when she struggled to communicate with them. Shareefa is nervous about interacting with people who do not speak her language and feels lonely and sad almost all of the time. She wants to reconnect with old friends, but she does not know where to start, and she is too ashamed to reach out to speak about the feelings of sadness and grief she has been experiencing since her husband's death.

Questions for reflection:

1. Can you identify the barriers Shareefa and Bisman faced in relation to health service access?
2. How may Shareefa's previous experiences have affected her willingness to connect with others?
3. What could your profession do to assist Shareefa to re-engage with her community?

Ageing and the health system

Australia's ageing population presents several challenges for the health care system due to an increased reliance on health care providers, increased rates of health-related complications, and greater diversity in the health needs of older adults. In the case of community-dwelling older adults living in households (as opposed to residential aged care), the 2011–2012 Australian Health Survey reported arthritis (49%), high-blood pressure (i.e., hypertension, 38%) and hearing loss (35%, complete or partial) as the most prevalent long-term health issues (apart from short- and long-sightedness) amongst people age 65 years and over (Australian Bureau of Statistics, 2012a).

Health system challenges faced in Australia include the following:

- **A declining workforce of suitably qualified health professionals.** This can be attributed to both reduced funding for health care providers and the ageing of its own workforce in some critical sectors, such as nursing (Health Workforce Australia, 2012; O'Loughlin et al., 2016). Increased capacity for health care services is required to deal with the growing ageing population and to combat the decreasing workforce.
- **Fragmented care between varying levels of health care services such as primary and secondary care, hospitals and community services.** For example, consider different patient health record systems between GPs and hospitals and difficulties in effective communication between health care workers in different settings (King et al., 2016). The introduction of MyAgedCare has added an additional level of complexity for health care professionals, older people and their families to navigate.
- **Barriers to accessing health services.** For example, navigating a complex aged-care system involving multiple layers of government departments including the introduction of MyAgedCare and the National Disability Insurance Scheme (NDIS), affordability, and delays, appropriate acknowledgement and sensitivity to the needs of LGBTQIA+ people (King et al., 2016) and a lack of access to specialists or GPs with specialist interests in aged care in rural locales. The diverse and unique needs of an ageing multicultural population, including Aboriginal and Torres Strait Islander peoples and people with CALD backgrounds, can also prove challenging when navigating the health system to access appropriate, culturally safe health care. There are further barriers due to the differing needs between genders (e.g., longer life expectancy of elderly women, compared to men, can result in additional psychological stress due to caregiver burden and loss of a life partner) (Zunzunegui et al., 2007).
- **Dementia and disability.** In Australia, dementia is the leading cause of disability for older Australians age 65 years and over (Australian Institute of Health and Welfare, 2012), and the leading cause of death in women (Australian Institute of Health and Welfare, 2018c). With this, comes pressure on health care providers such as residential aged care workers and home care providers (Steiner et al., 2019). The demand for high levels of care are increasing due to the additional health complications people with dementia often face, and this places a significant financial burden on the health system (Australian Institute of Health and Welfare, 2012).

Health care costs for older adults

The ageing population presents significant economic challenges for Australia's Health care System. Annually, the Australian Government spends ~$18 billion on aged care, with 67% ($12.4 billion) of this supporting residential aged care ($5.1 billion supports home care) (Australian Institute of Health and Welfare, 2019). An exploration of NSW inpatient hospital cost data found that care of individuals age 65 years and over accounted for 8.9% of all inpatient costs (Kardamanidis et al., 2007). It is expected that between now and 2050, health care expenditure for those over ages 65 and 85 years will rise approximately 7- and 12-fold, respectively (Private Health care Australia, 2019). It is predicted that total expenditure on health in older adults will rise from $166 billion to $320 billion between 2015 and 2035 (Harris and Sharma, 2018). Half of the total increase in public health care costs as a share of GDP between now and 2045 will be attributed to ageing (Banks, 2008). Pharmaceutical Benefit Scheme costs are over 20 times higher for those ages 65–74 compared to those ages 15–24 years (Australian Government The Treasury, 2007).

Increased health care demand and use with age

Residential aged care facilities and community services provide care for older adults within community settings funded through government, voluntary organisations, and individuals' contributions. In 2013, almost 169,000 older Australians were residents in residential aged care (Australian Institute of Health and Welfare, 2014b) facilities. Hospitalisation rates are over four times greater in adults aged 65 years and over compared to those under age 65 (McPake & Mahal, 2017). In 2016–2017, nearly one-third (38 million) of total Medicare claims for unreferred GP visits were by older adults aged 65+ (Australian Bureau of Statistics, 2017a), with over double the number of claims in older adults (10 claims) compared to those under age 65 (4 claims) (Department of Human Services, 2018). Private health insurance affiliation drops with age, with 59% of those ages 65–74 years having insurance, but this proportion reduces to 51% and 42% in those ages 75–84 and 85+ (Australian Institute of Health and Welfare, 2016), highlighting inequity in access to private health insurance with increasing age, particularly given that older people utilise health services more than their younger counterparts.

Diversity in health care needs and access for older adults

Challenges to accessing health care for older adults vary based on geographic location and transport access to health services, comorbidity (and particularly regarding increased costs to manage multiple conditions), as well as cultural background (van Gaans & Dent, 2018). Health service availability is not evenly distributed geographically or in terms of type of service offered, and this is particularly evident in services for older adults (van Gaans & Dent, 2018). For older adults living in remote and rural areas, a lack of services within their area or the requirement of long trips to access services may result in them having less interaction with health care professionals and longer duration to diagnosis and treatment. Health care needs thus may be greater and more complex than if they lived in a well-serviced area.

As highlighted earlier, older adults are more likely to present to health care services with multimorbidities and hence more complex needs than younger adults. Just under 50% of the older Australian population (65–74 years) reported having ≥5+ chronic conditions, and this increased to 70% for those aged 85 years and older (Australian Bureau of Statistics, 2010). The most common medical conditions recorded as first listed in older adults in residential care were circulatory disease (22%), musculoskeletal conditions (19%), and endocrine disorders (including diabetes; 8%) (Australian Institute of Health and Welfare, 2013). Over half of residents had dementia and depression (52% of the population for both conditions) (Australian Institute of Health and Welfare, 2013). Rates of disability are also greater in older adults compared to younger people, which presents issues around access to health services and support for activities of daily living. Approximately 53% of adults age 65 years and over reported having a disability in a national survey conducted in 2012 (Australian Bureau of Statistics, 2013b). The high rates of comorbidity in older adults highlights the need for screening and treatment of multiple conditions, both physical and mental, by health care services to ensure that their health needs are fully met. As mentioned in Part 1, great cultural diversity exists in older Australians. Older adults from CALD backgrounds are less likely than older Anglo-Australian adults to utilise health services (ELDAC, 2019) and have higher rates of chronic disease (Care, 2019; van Gaans & Dent, 2018). Culturally safe health care services are thus required to assist in the initial and ongoing engagement of older adults with services. The Australian Government's Aged Care Diversity Framework action plans and Aged Care Quality Standards provide a framework for health care organisations to guide the quality of their care for older people, taking into account essential diversity factors and optimising engagement (Aged Care Quality and Safety Commission, 2018; Australian Government Department of Health, 2020).

Social determinants of health and individual factors also impact on older adults' health and access and use of health care services, particularly for women, Aboriginal and Torres Strait Islander peoples, those from regional and rural locations, those from non-English-speaking backgrounds and those of low socio-economic status. For example, older women are more likely than men to require support for daily activities, with 49% of women age 65 years and older requiring support with ≥1 activity, compared to 34% of men the same age (Australian Bureau of Statistics, 2013b). Older adults of Aboriginal and Torres Strait Islander background have poorer health and greater disability rates than their peers of non-Indigenous background (Australian Bureau of Statistics, 2013a), as do older adults residing in more rural locations than urban areas. Of a sample of 102 older adults (mean age 77 years) from a rural area of NSW, 49% had three or more chronic conditions and were admitted to hospital a mean of 4.1 times in the past year. Despite all respondents reporting having a GP, only 38% had a written GP care plan, and around a third (31%) of this sample reported psychological distress of a moderate to severe level (Longman et al., 2012). Additionally, incarcerated individuals are another subgroup of older adults who are growing rapidly (348% from 2002 to 2018) (Ginnivan et al., 2018). It is therefore essential that health care services consider subgroups of the older adult population that may be disproportionately impacted by poor health and develop strategies to identify these patients and support them to access and use health services appropriately. Whilst there are barriers to providing health care services to a diverse older adult population in Australia, diversity can also be embraced and celebrated within older adults.

Box 13.10 Reflection—Incarceration of older people

Health professionals, particularly mental health professionals (e.g., psychologists, social workers, mental health nurses), dentists and oral health professionals, GPs, nurses and pharmacists often need to work with people who have been incarcerated. Older prisoners have accelerated ageing, which is attributable to a range of factors including lifestyle before incarceration (e.g., substance abuse, inadequate nutrition), in addition to the effects of the prison environment (e.g., stress, environment designed for younger offenders) on exacerbating age-associated illnesses (Carlisle, 2006). The older prisoner population has been classified into four main groups in relation to their offence history, with the experience of incarceration differing for each group (Aday, 2006):

- First-time prisoners who are incarcerated at an older age
- Ageing recidivist offenders who enter and exit prison throughout their lifetime, returning to prison at an older age
- Prisoners serving a long sentence who grow old while incarcerated
- Prisoners sentenced to shorter periods of incarceration late in life

(Baidawi et al., 2011)

Box 13.11 Case study—An integrated diabetes care and prevention program

The Wollondilly Diabetes Program is an integrated diabetes care and prevention service that was introduced in an inner-regional, local government area of South Western Sydney

(Simmons et al., 2018). The majority of users of this service are older adults with type 2 diabetes. Prior to introduction of the service, there were no secondary care centres, no endocrinology services, limited allied health professional services and a low ratio of GPs to people (1:2750) within the area. Access to diabetes care therefore was a challenge, particularly for older people with mobility and/or transport limitations. The program introduced clinical services (including case conferencing and group education) and peer support groups to improve patient management of diabetes to the inner-regional area. Other health promotion and peer support groups were initiated, focused on the prevention of diabetes, as well as diabetes screening roadshows to identify those at highest risk or with undiagnosed diabetes. Particularly important for older adults, this program has provided access to diabetes prevention and management support through the provision of services in a local community centre, general practices, in existing public groupings, such as churches and health promotion groups, and through the use of a local council mobile bus service to take health promotion and screening activities to residents.

Towards a health care system to support Australia's ageing population

Interventions have been developed and tested to modify and support the health care system across primary, secondary and private levels to assist in caring for the growing ageing population in Australia (McPake & Mahal, 2017). These include the restructuring of general practice governance from the Divisions of General Practices to Medicare Locals in 2011, and later to Primary Health Networks in 2015, the introduction of the *"Transition Care"* program in 2005, which was aimed at supporting older adults' transition into residential or community care, and reducing the length of stay in hospitals, in addition to various reforms in private health insurance in 1997–2002 (McPake & Mahal, 2017).

Health care systems require further adaptation and reform to effectively support the challenges associated with the rising ageing population. Many of the chronic conditions experienced by older adults, such as coronary heart disease, are largely preventable (Australian Institute of Health and Welfare, 2018b). By encouraging and supporting older adults to maintain healthy lifestyle behaviours, including participation in regular physical activity and adequate dietary consumption, chronic conditions will be better managed and may reduce exacerbation of the conditions.

Box 13.12 Reflection—Exploring social determinants of health in older adults

Put yourself in the shoes of a health care professional. An older person has attended your service for a regular health check, and you are concerned about their mental health. Think about the social determinants of their health. What questions would you ask about this person's life to help you identify appropriate support that is culturally safe and age-appropriate to improve and maintain their health? What steps might you take to ensure this older person is supported with culturally relevant information, services and/or resources? Who else, other than the older person, might you need to consult? What cultural, ethnic, social, religious, geographic, gender and sexual orientation factors are important to consider?

Box 13.13 Reflection—A health-promotion approach

The 1986 Ottawa Charter (World Health Organisation, 1986) was created to frame the development of health-promotion interventions. The Charter describes five action areas in health promotion: building healthy public policy, creating supportive environments, re-orienting health services (to focus on prevention of ill health and promotion of health), strengthening community action and developing personal skills. Prevention of falls, improving and maintaining musculoskeletal function, prevention of cognitive decline and prevention of diseases, including CVD, diabetes, cancer and respiratory conditions, are all priority areas of health need in older Australians. For each of these areas of health need, identify

- What health promotion interventions have previously been implemented in Australia to attempt to address prevention of falls in older people? You can find information on the health promotion falls prevention programs for older people via the Australian Government Department of Health's national stocktake: https://www1.health.gov.au/internet/main/publishing.nsf/Content/phd-injury-falls-stocktake-cnt.htm
- What strategies from the Ottawa Charter do these interventions relate to?
- What interventions do you think could be introduced to target these health issues? Justify your choice.

Conclusion

Australia's population is ageing, with the number of people age 65 years and over expected to reach 6.8 million by 2040 (Australian Bureau of Statistics, 2013c). This chapter introduced the multifactorial components of ageing, including physical and mental health complications, changes in social dynamics and the effects on the health care system. This was discussed in the context of the social determinants of health, including cultural, ethnic, religious, social, geographic, gender, and sexuality factors. Key concepts were examined, including ageism, elder abuse, loneliness and social exclusion, health literacy and caregiver burden. Finally, the shifting requirements of the health care system and its workforce has been unpacked. It is essential for health care professionals to be aware of the diversity in Australia's ageing population in order to promote culturally safe health care that is accessible, appropriate and relevant for older people and their families.

Box 13.14 Reflection—Chapter summary

- What individual factors influence a person's needs as they age?
- What are the mental health issues faced by older people?
- What Australian legislation is in place to protect the rights of older people?
- What is caregiver burden?
- What are some of the professional roles and requirements for health care professionals working with older people?

Questions for discussion:

- How does cultural, social, ethnic, geographic, sexual orientation and gender diversity affect an individual's journey into older age?
- What are the major health and wellbeing complications that emerge in older age?
- What strategies could be used to reduce social isolation and loneliness and improve the health and wellbeing in older people?
- How does health literacy affect older people and their engagement with health care?

What are some of the complexities faced by the health care system because of Australia's ageing population?

Questions for reflection:

- What are your individual factors, and how will they influence your needs as you age?
- How might older people that you know be affected by social isolation and loneliness?
- What strategies will you use to mitigate health and wellbeing complications as you grow older?
- What are your personal expectations for the health care system in relation to your health needs as you age?
- What are your professional responsibilities with regards to working with older people?
- What are your personal values, and how will you live by them when working with older people?

Useful website resources

Aged Care Quality and Safety Commission. Guidance and Resources for Providers to support the Aged Care Quality Standards: https://www.agedcarequality.gov.au/sites/default/files/media/Guidance_%26_Resource_V11.pdf

Australian Association on Gerontology (AAG): https://www.aag.asn.au/

Australian Commission on Safety and Quality in Health Care: National Statement on Health Literacy: Taking Action to Improve Safety and Quality: https://www.safetyandquality.gov.au/wp-content/uploads/2014/08/Health-Literacy-National-Statement.pdf

Australian Department of Health: Ageing and Aged Care: https://agedcare.health.gov.au/

Australian Department of Health: Australia's Physical Activity and Sedentary Behaviour Guidelines: http://www.health.gov.au/internet/main/publishing.nsf/Content/health-pubhlth-strateg-phys-act-guidelines

Australian Human Rights Commission: A Future Without Violence: Quality, safeguarding and oversight to prevent and address violence against people with disability in institutional settings: https://www.humanrights.gov.au/sites/default/files/document/publication/AHRC_report_VAPWD_2018.pdf

Australian Law Reform Commission: Elder Abuse—A National Legal Response: https://www.alrc.gov.au/publication/elder-abuse-a-national-legal-response-alrc-report-131/

Council on the Ageing (COTA): https://www.cota.org.au/

Dementia Australia: https://www.dementia.org.au/

Royal Commission into Aged Care Quality and Safety: https://agedcare.royalcommission.gov.au/

References

Aday, R. H. (2006). Ageing prisoners. In B. Berkman, and S. D'Ambruoso (Eds.), *Handbook of social work in health and ageing*. Oxford University Press. https://doi.org/10.1093/acprof:oso/9780195173727.003.0019.

Aged Care Quality and Safety Commission. (2018). *Guidance and resources for providers to support the aged care quality standards*. https://www.agedcarequality.gov.au/sites/default/files/media/Guidance_%26_Resource_V9.pdf.

Alzheimer's Australia NSW, & Deloitte Access Economics. (2014). *Dementia prevalence in NSW by SED (state electoral district)*, Alzheimer's Australia.

Atkins, J., Naismith, S. L., Luscombe, G. M., & Hickie, I. B. (2015). Elderly care recipients' perceptions of treatment helpfulness for depression and the relationship with help-seeking. *Clinical Interventions in Aging*, *10*, 287–295.

Australian Bureau of Statistics. (2010). *Disability, ageing and carers, Australia: Summary of findings, 2009* (no. 4430.0). https://www.abs.gov.au/AUSSTATS/abs@.nsf/allprimarymainfeatures/E36A0C8CC46057B9CA257C21000D8846?opendocument.

Australian Bureau of Statistics. (2012a). *Australian health survey: First results, 2011–12* (no. 4364.0.55.001). https://www.abs.gov.au/ausstats/abs@.nsf/lookup/4364.0.55.001main+features12011-12.

Australian Bureau of Statistics. (2012b). *Caring in the community, Australia: Summary of findings* (no. 4436.0). https://www.abs.gov.au/ausstats/abs@.nsf/mf/4436.0.

Australian Bureau of Statistics. (2013a). *Australian demographic statistics*. (no. 3101.0). https://www.abs.gov.au/ausstats/abs@.nsf/Previousproducts/3101.0Main%20Features3Jun%202013?opendocument&tabname=Summary&prodno=3101.0&issue=Jun%202013&num=&view=

Australian Bureau of Statistics. (2013b). Disability, ageing and carers, Australia: Summary of findings, 2012 (no. 4430.0). https://www.abs.gov.au/ausstats/abs@.nsf/Lookup/A813E50F4C45A338CA257C21000E4F36?opendocument.

Australian Bureau of Statistics. (2013c). *Population projections, Australia, 2012* (no. 3222.0). https://www.abs.gov.au/ausstats/abs@.nsf/Previousproducts/3222.0Main%20Features12012%20(base)%20to%202101?opendocument&tabname=Summary&prodno=3222.0&issue=2012%20(base)%20to%202101&num=&view=

Australian Bureau of Statistics. (2015). *Australian demographic statistics* (no. 3101.0). https://www.abs.gov.au/ausstats/abs@.nsf/Previousproducts/3101.0Main%20Features1Jun%202015?opendocument&tabname=Summary&prodno=3101.0&issue=Jun%202015&num=&view=

Australian Bureau of Statistics. (2016). *Census, unpublished data generated using ABS tablebuilder*. https://www.abs.gov.au/websitedbs/d3310114.nsf/home/about+tablebuilder.

Australian Bureau of Statistics. (2017a). *Australian demographic statistics* (no. 3101.0). https://www.abs.gov.au/ausstats/abs@.nsf/Previousproducts/3101.0Main%20Features1Jun%202017?opendocument&tabname=Summary&prodno=3101.0&issue=Jun%202017&num=&view=

Australian Bureau of Statistics. (2017b). *Census of population and housing: Reflecting Australia—stories from the census, 2016* (no. 2071.0). https://www.abs.gov.au/ausstats/abs@.nsf/Lookup/by%20Subject/2071.0~2016~Main%20Features~Ageing%20Population~14.

Australian Bureau of Statistics. (2017c). *Census, unpublished data generated using ABS tablebuilder*. https://www.abs.gov.au/websitedbs/d3310114.nsf/home/about+tablebuilder.

Australian Bureau of Statistics. (2018a). *Census of population and housing: Estimating homelessness, 2016*. https://www.abs.gov.au/statistics/people/housing/census-population-and-housing-estimating-homelessness/latest-release.

Australian Bureau of Statistics. (2018b). *Disability, ageing and carers, Australia: Summary of findings, 2018*. https://www.abs.gov.au/statistics/health/disability/disability-ageing-and-carers-australia-summary-findings/latest-release#:~:text=In%202018%20there%20were%204.4,years%20and%20over%20had%20disability.

Australian Commission on Safety and Quality in Health Care. (2014). *National statement on health literacy: Taking action to improve safety and quality*. https://www.safetyandquality.gov.au/sites/default/files/migrated/Health-Literacy-National-Statement.pdf.

Australian Government Department of Health. (2020). *Aged care diversity framework action plans.* https://www.health.gov.au/resources/collections/aged-care-diversity-framework-action-plans.

Australian Government the Treasury. (2007). *Intergenerational report 2007.* https://treasury.gov.au/publication/intergenerational-report-2007-2.

Australian Human Rights Commission. (2013). *Fact or fiction? Stereotypes of older Australians, Research Report, 2013.* https://www.humanrights.gov.au/our-work/age-discrimination/publications/fact-or-fiction-stereotypes-older-australiansresearch.

Australia Institute of Health and Welfare. (2012). *Cancer incidence projections: Australia 2011–2020.* https://www.aihw.gov.au/getmedia/a79de4a1-49f5-4c93-bc59-4d181430aa69/14096.pdf.aspx?inline=true.

Australian Institute of Health and Welfare. (2012). *Dementia in Australia.* https://www.aihw.gov.au/getmedia/199796bc-34bf-4c49-a046-7e83c24968f1/13995.pdf.aspx?inline=true.

Australian Institute of Health and Welfare. (2013). *Depression in residential aged care 2008–2012.* https://www.aihw.gov.au/getmedia/7ad35fb2-bc14-4692-96b1-c15d73072319/16256.pdf.aspx?inline=true.

Australian Institute of Health and Welfare. (2014a). Ageing and the health system: Challenges, opportunities and adaptations. In Australian Institute of Health and Welfare (Ed.), *Australia's health 2014* (pp. 256–270). https://www.aihw.gov.au/getmedia/d2946c3e-9b94-413c-898c-aa5219903b8c/16507.pdf.aspx?inline=true.

Australian Institute of Health and Welfare. (2014b). Australia's health 2014. https://www.aihw.gov.au/getmedia/d2946c3e-9b94-413c-898c-aa5219903b8c/16507.pdf.aspx?inline=true.

Australian Institute of Health and Welfare. (2014c). Chronic disease—Australia's biggest health challenge. In Australian Institute of Health and Welfare (Ed.), *Australia's health 2014* (pp. 94–104). https://www.aihw.gov.au/getmedia/d2946c3e-9b94-413c-898c-aa5219903b8c/16507.pdf.aspx?inline=true.

Australian Institute of Health and Welfare (2015a). *Mortality and life expectancy of Indigenous Australians 2008 to 2012.* https://www.aihw.gov.au/getmedia/b0a6bd57-0ecb-45c6-9830-cf0c0c9ef059/16953.pdf.aspx?inline=true.

Australian Institute of Health and Welfare. (2015b). Risk factors, disease and death.

Australian Institute of Health and Welfare. (2016). *Australia's health 2016.* https://www.aihw.gov.au/getmedia/9844cefb-7745-4dd8-9ee2-f4d1c3d6a727/19787-AH16.pdf.aspx.

Australian Institute of Health and Welfare. (2018a). *Alcohol, tobacco and other drugs in Australia.* https://www.aihw.gov.au/reports/alcohol/alcohol-tobacco-other-drugs-australia/contents/introduction.

Australian Institute of Health and Welfare. (2018b). *Australia's health 2018.* https://www.aihw.gov.au/getmedia/7c42913d-295f-4bc9-9c24-4e44eff4a04a/aihw-aus-221.pdf.aspx?inline=true.

Australian Institute of Health and Welfare. (2018c). *Older Australia at a glance.* https://www.aihw.gov.au/getmedia/2cb104f4-c6d1-4728-9be3-a418840588de/Older-Australia-at-a-glance.pdf.aspx?inline=true.

Australian Institute of Health and Welfare. (2019). *Government spending on aged care.* https://www.gen-agedcaredata.gov.au/Topics/Government-spending-on-aged-care.

Australian Tax Office. (2015). 10 Poorest Suburbs in Sydney.

Baidawi, S., Turner, S., Trotter, C., Browning, C., Collier, P., O'Connor, D., & Sheehan, R. (2011). Older prisoners: A challenge for Australian corrections. *Trends & Issues in Crime and Criminal Justice, 426*, 1–8. https://www.aic.gov.au/sites/default/files/2020-05/tandi426.pdf.

Banks, G. (2008). Health costs and policy in an ageing Australia [Speech]. 2018 Health Policy Oration 2008, Australian National University, Canberra. https://www.pc.gov.au/news-media/speeches/cs20080328/cs20080701-agedhealthpolicy.pdf.

Birkenshaw, M. (1988). *Social marketing for health.* World Health Organisation. https://apps.who.int/iris/handle/10665/62146.

Bunce, D., Batterham, P. J., Mackinnon, A. J., & Christensen, H. (2012). Depression, anxiety and cognition in community-dwelling adults aged 70 years and over. *Journal of Psychiatric Research, 46*(12), 1662–1666. https://doi.org/10.1016/j.jpsychires.2012.08.023.

Carlisle, D. (2006). So far, so bleak: Increasing numbers of older prisoners in a prison estate, designed essentially for fit young men, pose a problem for health service providers. *Nursing Older People, 18*(7), 19–23. https://doi.org/10.7748/nop.18.7.19.s14.

Centre for Western Sydney. (2019a). *Data and visualisations.* https://www.westernsydney.edu.au/cws/gws_research.

Centre for Western Sydney. (2019b). *Greater Western Sydney region highest level of schooling*. https://profile.id.com.au/cws/schooling.

Chesser, A. K., Keene Woods, N., Smothers, K., & Rogers, N. (2016). Health literacy and older adults: A systematic review. *Gerontology & Geriatric Medicine, 2*, 1–13. https://doi.org/10.1177/2333721416630492.

Chiao, C.Y., Wu, H. S., & Hsiao, C.Y. (2015). Caregiver burden for informal caregivers of patients with dementia: A systematic review. *International Nursing Review, 62*(3), 340–350. https://doi.org/10.1111/inr.12194.

Colombo, F., Llena-Nozal, A., Mercier, J., & Tjadens, F. (2011). *Help wanted? Providing and paying for long-term care*. OECD Publishing. https://doi.org/10.1787/9789264097759-en.

Cooper, C., Tandy, A. R., Balamurali, T. B., & Livingston, G. (2010). A systematic review and meta-analysis of ethnic differences in use of dementia treatment, care, and research. *American Journal of Geriatric Psychiatry, 18*(3), 193–203. https://doi.org/10.1097/JGP.0b013e3181bf9caf.

Cosco, T. D., Howse, K., & Brayne, C. (2017). Healthy ageing, resilience and wellbeing. *Epidemiology and Psychiatric Sciences, 26*(6), 579–583. https://doi.org/10.1017/S2045796017000324.

Cox, T., Hoang, H., Goldberg, L. R., & Baldock, D. (2019). Aboriginal community understandings of dementia and responses to dementia care. *Public Health, 172*, 15–21. https://doi.org/10.1016/j.puhe.2019.02.018.

Daly, J. M., Bay, C. P., Levy, B. T., & Carnahan, R. M. (2015). Caring for people with dementia and challenging behaviors in nursing homes: A needs assessment geriatric nursing. *Geriatric Nursing, 36*(3), 182–191. https://doi.org/10.1016/j.gerinurse.2015.01.001.

Dementia Australia. (2018). Dementia prevalence data 2018–2058. https://www.dementia.org.au/information/statistics/prevalence-data.

Department of Health. (2017). *Australia's physical activity and sedentary behaviour guidelines*. https://www1.health.gov.au/internet/main/publishing.nsf/content/F01F92328EDADA5BCA257BF0001E720D/$File/brochure PA Guidelines_A5_18-64yrs.PDF

Department of Human Services. (2018). *Medicare Australia statistics, MBS Group by patient demographics reports*. http://medicarestatistics.humanservices.gov.au/statistics/mbs_group.jsp.

Ding, D., Grunseit, A. C., Chau, J.Y., Vo, K., Byles, J., & Bauman, A. E. (2016). Retirement—A transition to a healthier lifestyle? Evidence from a large Australian study. *American Journal of Preventive Medicine, 51*(2), 170–178. https://doi.org/10.1016/j.amepre.2016.01.019.

ELDAC. (2019). *Australia's ageing culturally and linguistically diverse population*. https://www.eldac.com.au/tabid/5779/Default.aspx.

Essue, B., Mirzaei, M, Leeder, S. R., & Colagiuri, R. (2007). *Epidemiology of diabetes, the serious and continuing illness policy and practice study (SCIPPS)*. The Menzies Centre for Health Policy.

Farrer, L., Leach, L., Griffiths, K. M., Christensen, H., & Jorm, A. F. (2008). Age differences in mental health literacy. *BMC Public Health, 8*(125), 1–8. https://doi.org/10.1186/1471-2458-8-125.

Federation of Ethnic Communities' Councils of Australia. (2015). Review of Australian research on older people from culturally and linguistically diverse backgrounds. http://fecca.org.au/wp-content/uploads/2015/06/Review-of-Australian-Research-on-Older-People-from-Culturally-and-Linguistically-Diverse-Backgrounds-March-20151.pdf.

Ferrante, J. M., Chen, P. H., Crabtree, B. F., & Wartenberg, D. (2007). Cancer screening in women: Body mass index and adherence to physician recommendations. *American Journal of Preventive Medicine, 32*(6), 525–531. https://doi.org/10.1016/j.amepre.2007.02.004.

Forbes, M. K., Crome, E., Sunderland, M., & Wuthrich, V. M. (2017). Perceived needs for mental health care and barriers to treatment across age groups. *Aging and Mental Health, 21*(10), 1072–1078. https://doi.org/10.1080/13607863.2016.1193121.

Galenkamp, H., & Deeg, D. J. H. (2016). Increasing social participation of older people: Are there different barriers for those in poor health? Introduction to the special section. *European Journal of Ageing, 13*(2), 87–90. https://doi.org/10.1007/s10433-016-0379-y.

Garrido, S., Steiner, G. Z., & Russo, N. (2018). People with dementia: The challenges for data collection with a vulnerable population. *SAGE Research Methods Cases*, 1–12. https://doi.org/10.4135/9781526439024.

Gerst-Emerson, K., & Jayawardhana, J. (2015). Loneliness as a public health issue: The impact of loneliness on health care utilization among older adults. *American Journal of Public Health, 105*(5), 1013–1019. https://doi.org/10.2105/AJPH.2014.302427.

Ginnivan, N. A., Butler, T. G., & Withall, A. N. (2018). The rising health, social and economic costs of Australia's ageing prisoner population. *Medical Journal of Australia, 209*(10), 422–424. https://doi.org/10.5694/mja18.00266.

Hall, J., Karch, D. L., & Crosby, A. E. (2016). *Elder abuse surveillance: Uniform definitions and recommended core data elements for use in elder abuse surveillance.* https://www.cdc.gov/violenceprevention/pdf/EA_Book_Revised_2016.pdf.

Haralambous, B., Dow, B., Tinney, J., Lin, X., Blackberry, I., Rayner, V., Lee, S. M., Vrantsidis, F., Lautenschlager, N., & Logiudice, D. (2014). Help seeking in older Asian people with dementia in Melbourne: Using the cultural exchange model to explore barriers and enablers. *Journal of Cross Cultural Gerontology, 29*(1), 69–86. https://doi.org/10.1007/s10823-014-9222-0.

Harris, A., & Sharma, A. (2018). Estimating the future health and aged care expenditure in Australia with changes in morbidity. *PLoS ONE, 13*(8), 1–10. https://doi.org/10.1371/journal.pone.0201697.

Health Workforce Australia. (2012). *Health workforce 2025: Doctors, nurses and midwives.* https://submissions.education.gov.au/forms/archive/2015_16_sol/documents/Attachments/AustralianNursing and Midwifery Accreditation Council (ANMAC).pdf.

Henderson, S., & Kendall, E. (2011). Culturally and linguistically diverse peoples' knowledge of accessibility and utilisation of health services: Exploring the need for improvement in health service delivery. *Australian Journal of Primary Health, 17*(2), 195–201. https://doi.org/10.1071/PY10065.

Holt-Lunstad, J., Smith, T. B., Baker, M., Harris, T., & Stephenson, D. (2015). Loneliness and social isolation as risk factors for mortality: A meta-analytic review. *Perspectives on Psychological Science, 10*(2), 227–237. https://doi.org/10.1177/1745691614568352.

Inouye, S. K., Studenski, S., Tinetti, M. E., & Kuchel, G. A. (2007). Geriatric syndromes: Clinical, research, and policy implications of a core geriatric concept. *Journal of the American Geriatrics Society, 55*(5), 780–791. https://doi.org/10.1111/j.1532-5415.2007.01156.x.

Jessup, R. L., Osborne, R. H., Beauchamp, A., Bourne, A., & Buchbinder, R. (2017). Health literacy of recently hospitalised patients: A cross-sectional survey using the health literacy questionnaire (HLQ). *BMC Health Services Research, 17*(52), 1–12. https://doi.org/10.1186/s12913-016-1973-6.

Kane, R. L. (2005). What's so good about aging? *Research in Human Development, 2*(3), 115–132. https://doi.org/10.1207/s15427617rhd0203_2.

Kardamanidis, K., Lim, K., Cunha, C. D., Taylor, L. K., & Jorm, L. R. (2007). Hospital costs of older people in New South Wales in the last year of life. *Medical Journal of Australia, 187*(7), 383–386. https://doi.org/10.5694/j.1326-5377.2007.tb01306.x.

King, M., Usherwood, T., Brooker, R., & Reath, J. (2016). *Supporting primary health care providers in Western Sydney areas of socio-economic disadvantage.* Australian Primary Health Care Research Institute.

Lambert, S. D., Bowe, S. J., Livingston, P. M., Heckel, L., Cook, S., Kowal, P., & Orellana, L. (2017). Impact of informal caregiving on older adults' physical and mental health in low-income and middle-income countries: A cross-sectional, secondary analysis based on the WHO's Study on global AGEing and adult health (SAGE). *BMJ Open*, 7, 1–14. https://doi.org/10.1136/bmjopen-2017-017236.

Levy, S. R., & Macdonald, J. L. (2016). Progress on understanding ageism. *Journal of Social Issues, 72*(1), 5–25. https://doi.org/10.1111/josi.12153.

Longman, J. M., Rolfe, M. I., Passey, M. D., Heathcote, K. E., Ewald, D. P., Dunn, T., Barclay, L. M., & Morgan, G. G. (2012). Frequent hospital admission of older people with chronic disease: A cross-sectional survey with telephone follow-up and data linkage. *BMC Health Services Research, 12*, 373. https://doi.org/10.1186/1472-6963-12-373.

Maker, Y., & Mcsherry, B. (2018). Regulating restraint use in mental health and aged care settings: Lessons from the Oakden scandal. *Alternative Law Journal, 44*, 29–36. https://doi.org/10.1177/1037969X18817592.

Marengoni, A., Angleman, S., Melis, R., Mangialasche, F., Karp, A., Garmen, A., Meinow, B., & Fratiglioni, L. (2011). Aging with multimorbidity: A systematic review of the literature. *Ageing Research Reviews, 10*(4), 430–439. https://doi.org/10.1016/j.arr.2011.03.003.

McBride, K. A., Fleming, C. A. K., George, E. S., Steiner, G. Z., & MacMillan, F. (2019). Double discourse: Qualitative perspectives on breast screening participation among obese women and their health care providers. *International Journal of Environmental Research and Public Health*, *16*(4), 534. https://doi.org/10.3390/ijerph16040534.

McPake, B., & Mahal, A. (2017). Addressing the needs of an aging population in the health system: The Australian case. *Health Systems & Reform*, *3*(3), 236–247. https://doi.org/10.1080/23288604.2017.1358796.

Noguchi, N., Blyth, F. M., Waite, L. M., Naganathan, V., Cumming, R. G., Handelsman, D. J., Seibel, M. J., & Le Couteur, D. G. (2016). Prevalence of the geriatric syndromes and frailty in older men living in the community: The Concord health and ageing in men project. *Australasian Journal on Ageing*, *35*(4), 255–261. https://doi.org/10.1111/ajag.12310.

O'Loughlin, K., Browning, C., & Kendig, H. (2016). *Ageing in Australia: Challenges and opportunities*. Springer. https://doi.org/10.1007/978-1-4939-6466-6.

Ong, A. D., Uchino, B. N., & Wethington, E. (2016). Loneliness and health in older adults: A mini-review and synthesis. *Gerontology*, *62*, 443–449. https://doi.org/10.1159/000441651.

Phongsavan, P., Grunseit, A. C., Bauman, A., Broom, D., Byles, J., Clarke, J., Redman, S., Nutbeam, D., & Project, S. (2013). Age, gender, social contacts, and psychological distress: Findings from the 45 and Up study. *Journal of Aging and Health*, *25*(6), 921–943. https://doi.org/10.1177/0898264313497510.

Pinquart, M., & Sörensen, S. (2003). Differences between caregivers and noncaregivers in psychological health and physical health: A meta-analysis. *Psychology and Aging*, *18*(2), 250–267. https://doi.org/10.1037/0882-7974.18.2.250.

Private Healthcare Australia. (2019). *Supporting an ageing Australia*. https://www.privatehealthcareaustralia.org.au/have-you-got-private-healthcare/why-private-health-insurance/ageing-australia/.

Pyke, K. D., & Bengtson, V. L. (1996). Caring more or less: Individualistic and collectivist systems of family eldercare. *Journal of Marriage and Family*, *58*(2), 379–392. https://doi.org/10.2307/353503.

Salive, M. E. (2013). Multimorbidity in older adults. *Epidemiologic Reviews*, *35*, 75–83. doi:10.1093/epirev/mxs009.

Sarkisian, C. A., Lee-Henderson, M. H., & Mangione, C. M. (2003). Do depressed older adults who attribute depression to old age believe it is important to seek care? *Journal of General Internal Medicine*, *18*(12), 1001–1005. https://doi.org/10.1111/j.1525-1497.2003.30215.x.

Segel-Karpas, D., Ayalon, L., & Lachman, M. E. (2018). Loneliness and depressive symptoms: The moderating role of the transition into retirement. *Aging Mental Health*, *22*(1), 135–140. https://doi.org/10.1080/13607863.2016.1226770.

Shanley, C., Boughtwood, D., Adams, J., Santalucia, Y., Kyriazopoulos, H., Pond, D., & Rowland, J. (2012). A qualitative study into the use of formal services for dementia by carers from culturally and linguistically diverse CALD communities. *BMC Health Services Research*, *12*(354), 1–11. https://doi.org/10.1186/1472-6963-12-354.

Sharpe, L., McDonald, S., Correia, H., Raue, P. J., Meade, T., Nicholas, M., & Arean, P. (2017). Pain severity predicts depressive symptoms over and above individual illnesses and multimorbidity in older adults. *BMC Psychiatry*, *17*(166), 1–8. https://doi.org/10.1186/s12888-017-1334-y.

Simmons, D., Jani, R., MacMillan, F., Derek-Smith, K., Pham, A., Fernandes, B., Zarora, R., Alexander, R., Khoo, C., & Dench, A. (2018). The Wollondilly diabetes programme: A developing model of diabetes integrated care. *International Journal of Integrated Care*, *18*(39), 1–8. doi:10.5334/ijic.s1039.

South Western Sydney Local Health District. (2016). Year in review 2015/16. https://www.swslhd.health.nsw.gov.au/pdfs/2016_review.pdf.

South Western Sydney Local Health District. (2017). *Towards 2021*. https://www.swslhd.nsw.gov.au/planning/.

South Western Sydney Local Health District, & Medicare Local. (2014). *Population health needs assessment of the communities of South Western Sydney and the Southern Highlands*. https://www.swslhd.health.nsw.gov.au/pdfs/SWSML_PopHNA.pdf.

Steiner, G. Z., Al-Dabbas, M. A., Bailey, P., Chang, E., Garrido, S., George, E. S., Henshaw, F. R., Hohenberg, M. I., Liu, K., MacRitchie, J., Mears, J., & Wilson, L. A. (2018). *Ageing white paper*. Western Sydney University. https://www.westernsydney.edu.au/__data/assets/pdf_file/0009/1483884/Ageing_White_Paper_FINAL.pdf.

Steiner, G. Z., Ee, C., Dubois, S., MacMillan, F., George, E. S., McBride, K. A., Karamacoska, D., Mcdonald, K., Harley, A., Abramov, G., Andrews-Marney, E. R., Cave, A. E., & Hohenberg, M. I. (2020). We need a one-stop-shop: Co-creating the model of care for a multidisciplinary memory clinic with community members, GPs, aged care workers, service providers, and policy-makers. *BMC Geriatrics*, *20*(49), 1–14. https://doi.org/10.1186/s12877-019-1410-x.

United Nations Department of Economic and Social Affairs. (2017). *World Population Ageing*. https://www.un.org/en/development/desa/population/publications/pdf/ageing/WPA2017_Highlights.pdf.

van Gaans, D., & Dent, E. (2018). Issues of accessibility to health services by older Australians: A review. *Public Health Reviews*, *39*(1), 1–16. https://doi.org/10.1186/s40985-018-0097-4.

Vickrey, B. G., Strickland, T. L., Fitten, L. J., Adams, G. R., Ortiz, F., & Hays, R. D. (2007). Ethnic variations in dementia caregiving experiences. *Journal of Human Behavior in the Social Environment*, *15*(2–3), 233–249. https://doi.org/10.1300/J137v15n02_14.

Wang, X. X., Lin, W. Q., Chen, X. J., Lin, Y. Y., Huang, L. L., Zhang, S. C., & Wang, P. X. (2017). Multimorbidity associated with functional independence among community-dwelling older people: A cross-sectional study in Southern China. *Health and Quality of Life Outcomes*, *15*(1), 1–9. https://doi.org/10.1186/s12955-017-0635-7.

Willis, R. (2012). Individualism, collectivism and ethnic identity: Cultural assumptions in accounting for caregiving behaviour in Britain. *Journal of Cross-Cultural Gerontology*, *27*(3), 201–216. https://doi.org/10.1007/s10823-012-9175-0.

Wohler, Y., & Dantas, J. A. (2017). Barriers accessing mental health services among culturally and linguistically diverse (CALD) immigrant women in Australia: Policy implications. *Journal of Immigrant and Minority Health*, *19*(3), 697–701. https://doi.org/10.1007/s10903-016-0402-6.

World Health Organisation. (1986). Ottawa charter for health promotion: First international conference on health promotion, Ottawa, 21 November 1986. https://www.who.int/healthpromotion/conferences/previous/ottawa/en/.

World Health Organisation. (2017). *Mental health of older adults*. https://www.who.int/news-room/fact-sheets/detail/mental-health-of-older-adults.

World Health Organisation. (2018). *Ageing and health*. https://www.who.int/news-room/fact-sheets/detail/ageing-and-health.

World Health Organisation. (2020). *Elder Abuse*. https://www.who.int/ageing/projects/elder_abuse/en/.

Yon, Y., Mikton, C. R., Gassoumis, Z. D., & Wilber, K. H. (2017). Elder abuse prevalence in community settings: A systematic review and meta-analysis. *The Lancet Glob Health*, *5*, e147–e156. https://doi.org/10.1016/S2214-109X(17)30006-2.

Yon, Y., Ramiro-Gonzalez, M., Mikton, C. R., Huber, M. & Sethi, D. (2019). The prevalence of elder abuse in institutional settings: A systematic review and meta-analysis. *European Journal of Public Health*, *29*(1), 58–67. https://doi.org/10.1093/eurpub/cky093.

Zhu, R. (2016). Retirement and its consequences for women's health in Australia. *Social Science & Medicine*, *163*, 117–125. https://doi.org/10.1016/j.socscimed.2016.04.003.

Zunzunegui, M. V., Minicuci, N., Blumstein, T., Noale, M., Deeg, D., Jylha, M. & Pedersen, N. L. (2007). Gender differences in depressive symptoms among older adults: a cross-national comparison: The CLESA project. *Social Psychiatry and Psychiatric Epidemiology*, *42*, 198–207. https://doi.org/10.1007/s00127-007-0158-3

Part IV

Culturally safe teaching and learning

14 The future of culture, diversity and health in Australia

Culturally safe teaching and learning

Tinashe Dune, Kim McLeod and Robyn Williams

Learning outcomes

After engaging with the teaching and learning strategies presented in this chapter, students should be able to:

1. Describe how the social determinants of health and intersectionality influence health and wellbeing in diverse Australian contexts.
2. Outline the circumstances and health needs of a range of marginalised Australians including (but not limited to); Aboriginal and/or Torres Strait Islander peoples; Australians of culturally, religious or linguistically diverse backgrounds; sexually diverse Australians; ageing Australians and Australians living with disability.
3. Explore the experiences of health, wellbeing, health services and health outcomes from diverse perspectives.
4. Establish an understanding of what is meant by cultural safety as well as its significance and relationship with professional skills and behaviour in Australia.
5. Demonstrate critical and self-reflection in relation to their role in supporting culturally safe health care provision and practice as a future health professional.

Key terms

Curriculum: The totality of student experiences that occur in the educational process. The term often refers specifically to a planned sequence of instruction, or to a view of the student's experiences in terms of the educator's or school's instructional goals.
Learning activity: The things learners and educators do, within learning events, that are intended to bring about the desired learning outcomes
Learning assessment: A method to measure how much of the knowledge and skills a learner has acquired during a course of study. There are two types of assessments, formative and summative.
Learning: The process of acquiring new, or modifying existing, knowledge, behaviours, skills, values or preferences.
Pedagogy: The approach to teaching, including the theory and practice of learning, and how this process influences, and is influenced by, the social, political and psychological development of learners.
Self-awareness: The capacity to become the object of one's own attention. In this state one actively identifies, processes and stores information about the self.
Self-reflection: A genuine curiosity about the self, where the person is intrigued and interested in learning more about his or her emotions, values, thought processes and attitudes.

Teaching: The concerted sharing of knowledge and experience, which is usually organised within a discipline and, more generally, the provision of stimulus to the psychological and intellectual growth of a person by another person or artefact.

Chapter summary

This final chapter provides a cultural safety curriculum model to assist tertiary health discipline educators to create content and assessment tasks that support the development of a culturally safe health workforce. The chapter also provides educators with interprofessional activities that help students develop the required capacities and skills in line with national accreditation expectations. In this chapter readers, will find multimedia links to provide students with examples of culturally safe practice (for example, developing self-awareness, enacting cultural responsiveness, culturally safe communication), case studies to assist with tutorial discussions or to be used as assessment tasks. This chapter consolidates and expands on the learning outcomes within each chapter into demonstrable and assessable outputs aligned with national cultural safety requirements. This will also allow students to indicate the ways in which they have worked towards each cultural safety requirement and in what areas they seek to continue their cultural safety journeys.

A model for cultural safety teaching and learning in Australia

Learning about diversity and difference can be exciting and invigorating but can also be challenging and confronting. This may be the case for those who have had little opportunity to engage deeply and holistically with people who are different from themselves or for those whose professional experiences or organisational cultures were not diversity oriented. In order to engage students in the process of learning about, and then enacting, cultural safety, the following elements are required. Importantly, these steps occur simultaneously, in a cyclical fashion, and are not easily separated from each other. These principles include (Table 14.1)

The rationale and impact of the aforementioned principles are discussed below and examples of learning activities and learning assessments are provided to guide students' development of cultural safety. Initially, following this sequence in chronological order is suggested however adapting the curriculum as needed is encouraged. Expansion, reduction or adjustment of the activities and assessments below is welcomed as it allows educators to respond to needs of learners and other health related curricula. However, it is suggested that the foundational principles, as noted above, are maintained to ensure all aspects of cultural safety learning and teaching are addressed.

Table 14.1 Principles of cultural safety teaching and learning

Principle 1: Consistent self-awareness and self-reflection.
Principle 2: Reflecting on social constructions, social determinants of health and intersectionality.
Principle 3: Exploring diversity and difference in experiences and expectations of health and wellbeing.
Principle 4: Becoming familiar with the principles of cultural safety.
Principle 5: Understanding the importance of cultural safety and its relevance to health policy and advocacy.
Principle 6: Engaging in culturally safe health care practice.
Principle 7: Applying principles for cultural safety with diverse populations.
Principle 8: Evaluating the impact of cultural safety in practice.

Principle 1: Consistent self-awareness and self-reflection

To learn about cultural safety, students are first required to develop self-awareness and begin the process of critical self-reflection with themselves and their own cultures, upbringings and beliefs. In each chapter, there are a range of reflection-focused activities that guide students to thinking about the meaning of the concepts presented and how they might play out in the students' own lives. The development of these skills is integral across all health professions and central to the learner's ability to adapt and respond to a constantly shifting set of expectations and experiences across local, national and international arenas.

It is important to distinguish the difference between self-awareness and self-reflection. While they are related processes with self-reflection being dependent upon the student's ability to engage with self-awareness, they are different processes. On the one hand, self-awareness is

> the capacity of becoming the object of one's own attention. In this state one actively identifies, processes, and stores information about the self … One becomes self-aware when one reflects on the experience of perceiving and processing stimuli … Self-awareness represents a complex multidimensional phenomenon that comprises various self-domains and corollaries.
>
> (Morin, 2011, p. 808)

On the other hand, self-reflection "represents a genuine curiosity about the self, where the person is intrigued and interested in learning more about his or her emotions, values, thought processes, attitudes, etc. This type of introspection mostly leads to positive consequences" (Morin, 2011, p. 809).

With this distinction reiterated, let's expand on Reflection Box 1.1 from Chapter 1 to demonstrate how students can engage with self-awareness and then self-reflection.

Box 1.1 Reflection—Understanding identity and social determinants

Answer the following questions to begin exploring your identity and the social determinants that have an impact on your health and wellbeing.

1. Where were you born?
2. Where were your parents born?
3. Where were your ancestors from?
4. Where do you live? Is it urban or rural?
5. What language(s) do you speak?
6. Do you follow a religion? If yes, which one?

This Reflection Box helps students to develop basic self-awareness related to elements of their identity. For many students, the answers to these questions will be easy to produce. While for others several of these questions may elicit distress because the answers are either unclear or are related to difficult experiences. It is therefore important for students to become aware of their experiences as diverse from those of others.

Table 14.2 Learning activity—Developing self-awareness and self-reflection

Self-Awareness Questions	*Self-Reflection Questions*	*Critical Self-Reflection Questions*
Where were you born?	How might your country of birth be a benefit (or not) to you?	If you were born somewhere else how might that change the trajectory of your life?
Where were your parents born?	What does your parents' country of birth mean for you?	Do you identify more with one parent's country of origin? If so, why does it matter to you?
Where were your ancestors from?	How might your ancestry impact your daily life and experiences?	Is your ancestry related to power and control or subjugation and oppression? Both? Neither? What does this mean for you, your family or your community?
Where do you live? Is it urban or rural?	How might were you live impact the way you grew up?	If you lived somewhere else, how would your life be different?
What language(s) do you speak?	Does speaking another language (or not) have benefits?	If you were not taught to speak more than one language, how might this change who you are?
Do you follow a religion? If yes, which one?	Does following this religion (or no religion) make life easier or harder for you? How so?	How might it be to follow a religion that is socially marginalised?

Learning activity

The following Learning Activity aims to guide students towards not only being aware of themselves but also reflecting on their experiences and in the context of their interactions with the world around them. The term *critical self-reflection* extends on this concept by encouraging students to critique and deconstruct what they find through the process of self-reflection (Table 14.2).

Box 14.1 Learning assessment—Assessing self-awareness and self-reflection

Assessment Instructions

Step 1 (Self-Awareness): List and define three aspects of your identity. For example,

- Race—I identify as Black.
- Gender—I identify as a woman.
- Nationality—I have multiple nationalities (Zimbabwean, Canadian and Australian)

Step 2 (Self-Reflection): Reflect on how these aspects of identity impact on your daily experiences in society. For example,

- Being Black means that I am more likely to experience racial discrimination in countries where the majority of people do not look like me.
- Being a woman means that I am more likely to get paid less than a man in the same role as me.

- Having multiple nationalities means that I have multiple opportunities to easily move around the world (e.g., for travel, work or study) without having to apply for visas or encounter significant international restrictions.

Step 3 (Critical Self-Reflection): Provide an explanation for how and why your self-reflections in Step 2 are significant to you. Each explanation for each aspect of your identity should be at least 100 words. Here is an example of one aspect of my identity:

Being Black is significant to me because it is the primary lens through which others perceive me. Although much of who I am is not based on my skin colour, when others meet me it is the first thing that they see. This is especially the case given that people with my skin colour and of African descent are a minority population in Australia. This may result in people's first impressions of me being based on what they have learnt, experienced, read or seen about Black people. As a result, I feel that I visibly stand out, and that sometimes makes me feel uncomfortable—especially when people stare.

Learning assessment

To engage students in actively developing this process and to assess their progress, the following Learning Assessment instructs students to explore, critique and report on their reflections.

Importantly, the aim of this Learning Assessment is not about the production of a "correct" answer but the demonstration of developing awareness and reflection. With that in mind, the assessment is not to be marked based on the accuracy (or not) of the statements produced (as this is somewhat subjective), but instead a mark should be provided based on the student's effort at demonstrating their introspective thinking processes. To gauge the development of self-awareness and self-reflection over time, the preceding Learning Assessment can be submitted by students at multiple points across their learning journey. That might be before and after their cultural safety training or even their course. It could also be administered several times throughout a teaching semester.

Feedback

Whether the assessment is delivered once or multiple times, educator feedback should be focused on asking more questions to encourage students to further reflect on their submissions. For instance, feedback on Step 3 (Critical Self-Reflection) might include the following.

Box 14.2 Feedback—Self-awareness and self-reflection

Dear Tinashe,

Your critical reflection on the experience of being Black demonstrates insight into your social experience and its impact on your wellbeing (e.g., hyper-visible and sometimes uncomfortable). You mention that other elements of your identity may be overlooked by others. What might some of these elements be and what importance do they hold for you? What impressions might others perceive of you because of your skin colour? You mention these impressions are based on what others have learnt, experienced, read or seen about Black people. Where might these learnings come from, and how are they perpetuated or challenged? Looking forward to reading about your reflections on these questions in your next submission.

Important in the feedback provided to students in this assessment is the educator's focus on the process of introspection and the provision of encouragement for the student to introspect further. This supportive feedback is important, as the experience of self-awareness and self-reflection can provoke feelings of discomfort and distress in some students (Olson, 2013). Supportive feedback reduces the likelihood of disengagement, although for some students, significant frustration with learning about and enacting principles for cultural safety is part of their process towards developing foundational cultural competencies (Marjadi et al., 2020). Supportive feedback also encourages the production of a learning environment where students feel safe and therefore more willing to invest themselves into the process of learning about cultural safety.

Principle 2: Reflecting on social constructions, social determinants and intersectionality

With the basics of self-awareness and self-reflexive practice emerging, students can engage with Principle 2, where they begin to critique social constructions, explore the impact of social determinants of health and understand the relevance of intersectionality. Chapters 1, 2 and several others integrate these concepts and provide students with the opportunity to begin deconstructing these socially defined elements of identity and being. Drawing on Chapter 2, Reflection Box 2.3 provides an opportunity to integrate these concepts into their growing capacity for cultural and diversity awareness—another step towards cultural safety.

Box 2.3 Reflection—Understanding culture

On a piece of paper, reflect on your own culture(s):

- What cultural groups do you belong to?
- Which do you identify with?

Write down all the cultural groups/identities you can think of and how these might impact on your health and wellbeing.

Going back to the case study in Box 2.2 (Chapter 2):

- What are some of the cultural groups/identities that Deng was a part of?
- How might these cultural groups shape Deng's health and wellbeing?

This Reflection Box encourages students to delve further into their own identities and to describe what cultural constructions influence their identity and experiences. This Reflection Box also engages student to think about how social constructions (culture) influence social determinants (race, nationality, religion) and the intersections of these (multiple cultural identities) on the student's health and wellbeing. If a student has not reflected on these elements of their identity before, or in this way, they may be unsure of where to start or how to move towards critically reflecting on their experiences. As such, the case study on Deng Adut discussed throughout Chapter 2 provides students with some distance from themselves and an important opportunity to reflect on the experiences of others. In doing so, the skill of reflection is strengthened, allowing the student to more comfortably approach reflecting on themselves with more scrutiny.

Table 14.3 Learning activity—Reflecting on social constructions, social determinants and intersectionality

Reflection Questions	*Social Construction Questions*	*Social Determinants Questions*	*Intersectionality Questions*
What cultural groups do you belong to? Which do you identify with? Write down all the cultural groups/identities you can think of.	What are some stereotypes or expectations of people of your cultural group? How is your cultural (group) or identity perceived by others?	What are some characteristics or collective experiences of your cultural group? Do these characteristics or collective experiences make life easier or harder?	Within your cultural group are there different sub-groups? Perhaps by age or gender? What expectations are there for sub-groups within your cultural group? How might these expectations make life easier or harder for you?

*Before proceeding, choose one of your cultural identities that matters to you. Consider the following questions in relation to the one cultural group you have decided to reflect on.

Learning activity

After students have responded to Reflection Box 2.3, they can expand on their reflections by critiquing the social constructions, social determinants of health and intersectionality that influence their identities and experiences with the following Learning Activity (Table 14.3).

Learning assessment

Now that students have had the opportunity to investigate their culture in more detail, they can further develop their understanding by reflecting on how their health and wellbeing is affected. Further students can be assessed on their ability to reflect on how the circumstances of others impact their health and wellbeing and how this may be similar to or different from themselves.

In this Learning Assessment, students are expected to know what key terms like *identity*, *culture*, *social constructions*, *social determinants* and *intersectionality* are. While they may still be grasping

Box 14.3 Learning assessment—Reflecting on social constructions, social determinants and intersectionality: Impacts on health and wellbeing

Assessment Instructions

Step 1 (Self-Awareness): Write down all of the cultural groups/identities that you identify with. For example,

- I identify as Aboriginal of the Gamilaroi nation.
- I also have Scottish and Irish ancestry.
- My nationality is Australian.

Step 2 (Reflecting on Social Constructions): What social constructions exist about these cultural identities? Let's review the first cultural identity, for example,

- On the one hand, Aboriginal people are often perceived as being from low socio-economic backgrounds, involved in criminal activity, to have substance abuse and mental health problems and to be involved in domestic violence. On the other hand, where opportunity exists, they are perceived to only excel at athletic or creative endeavours, with most of the well-known Aboriginal people being rugby superstars, Australian Football League players or prolific dot painting artists, singers, actors or models. The majority of Aboriginal people are therefore socially constructed as problems with a few exceptions focused primarily on narrow categories of achievement.

Step 3 (Reflecting on Social Determinants): To illustrate the social determinants, across multiple levels that factor into your identity and experiences, visually represent them using a picture(s) or a drawing(s). Label each element, and include a few words to describe its relevance to your experience, identity or wellbeing. For example, see Figure 14.1.

Step 4 (Reflecting on Intersectionality): How might the social constructions you described earlier and the aforementioned social determinants impact on your health and wellbeing? How do they all interact to influence your health outcomes? For example, with regards to being Aboriginal, the social constructions about being Aboriginal and my other social determinants impact on my health and wellbeing at a more mental than physical level. Most of my social determinants make me totally average. However, being average is perceived of as unusual for an Aboriginal person. This means that people question my Indigeneity, with some saying that I am not really Aboriginal because I grew up in a metropolitan area, with both my parents, who have uni degrees, worked full time and provided me with all the love and opportunities I needed to thrive in life. People also think of me as less Aboriginal because I am not as dark skinned as my mother. This makes me feel frustrated and angry because I feel that I always have to explain and prove that I am Aboriginal. However, because I am lighter skinned, I have experienced more privileges than some of my other relatives. While everyone in the family laughs about it, I sometimes feel like the odd one out and am self-conscious about it. So, for me my identities intersect in ways that have an impact on my mental and cultural wellbeing.

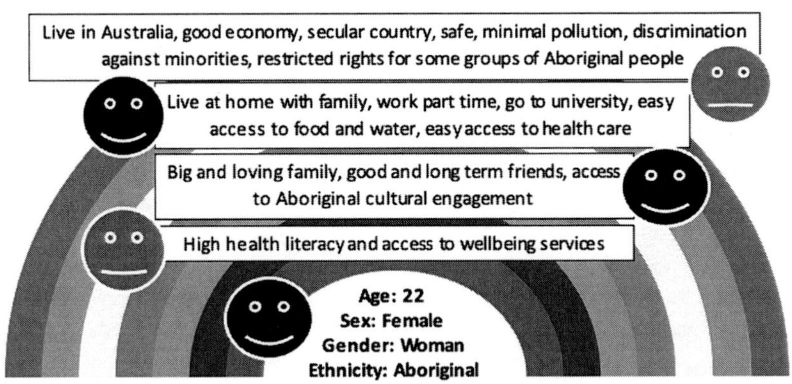

Figure 14.1 Example of student self-reflection on social determinants of health

the gist of the more theoretically informed terms, they should have some foundational understandings before attempting this Learning Assessment. This can include having read and completed the reflection activities from Chapters 1 and 2. To ensure students have engaged with appropriate scholarly literature, educators may ask students to provide references within each Step of the Learning Assessment.

Marking of this Learning Assessment should be focused on the student's emerging ability to accurately articulate, through self-reflexive examples, how the aforementioned constructs function in their everyday life. Accurate in this context means that students' examples describe the concepts as they are defined in Chapters 1 and 2 (for instance). Educators can therefore assess whether a student's response at Step 3 (Reflecting on Social Determinants), for example, is in line with scholarly models of social determinants of health and whether the student has provided examples of social determinants at each level of the model. In this way marks are attributed to the students' ability to accurately bring the concepts to life.

Feedback

This Learning Assessment, like many within cultural safety learning and teaching, require the student to tap into and articulate a certain level of vulnerability. Educators should be careful to provide students with supportive feedback to encourage further introspection. Additionally, feedback that helps the students to unpack their reflections and to begin thinking about how their experiences differ from others is helpful, as this will be required in the next Principle of Cultural Safety Teaching and Learning. Feedback on Step 4 (Reflecting on Intersectionality) might include the following:

Box 14.4 Feedback—Reflecting on intersectionality

Dear Naya,

Your reflections demonstrate great willingness to reflect on your experiences and comfort with sharing your reflections of discomfort. This is an important skill to hone with your development of culturally safe health practice. Your reflections about intersectionality provides examples of how being Aboriginal and how social constructions influence your experiences of mental and cultural wellbeing. In Step 3 you indicated your age, gender and sex; however, these were not included in your discussion on intersectionality. I would be interested to know how these elements intersect with your Indigeneity, socioeconomic status and family environment. It would also be helpful to know if and how your identities intersect with your lifestyle factors.

Such feedback highlights the strengths of the student's work but also indicates areas requiring further reflection and analysis. This form of constructive critique encourages the student to engage in further introspection in the consistent and cyclical fashion required of a burgeoning understanding of cultural safety and its implications for oneself and others.

Principle 3: Exploring diversity and difference in experiences and expectations of health and wellbeing

With a growing understanding of the self and the ability to apply the concepts at the foundation of cultural safety, students can begin to explore diversity and difference. Following the reflections on Deng Adut in Chapter 2, students should now be aware of difference and can now focus on extending that awareness to an increased capacity to interpret the impact of difference on health and wellbeing. In Chapter 3, students are introduced to diversity in what health and wellbeing means to themselves and others. While the permutations of constructions of health and wellbeing are endless, Chapter 3 summarised the foundational aspects of the biomedical, Eastern and Indigenous models of health. Reflection Box 3.2 engages students to think about how their experiences of health are socially constructed and the impact this has on their wellbeing.

Box 3.2 Reflection—Understanding health

How do you define health?
Point of consideration: answer the following questions before you proceed:

1. How do you define health?
2. Where does your own understanding of "health" come from?
3. How do you explain the concept of "health" to other people?
4. Think about whether "health" is something we have or something we do or both?
5. What are its essential components?
6. Who decides on these components?
7. What is a healthy person?
8. What does a person need to have to make them healthy?
9. How do we learn about "health", and how might this influence our understandings of "wellbeing"?

This Reflection Box covers a range of concepts presented across Chapters 1, 2 and 3. In this Reflection Box students are asked to become aware of what influences their own health, how they learnt about that, what it means to them and how they participate in various health behaviours or practices. These reflections can inform students' exploration of health in line with the foundational concepts of cultural safety.

Learning activity

To expand on students' capacity to delve into the social, political and economic aspects of health and wellbeing, as both sources of social constructions and as social determinants, the following Learning Activity is suggested.

Learning assessment

To assess students' ability to meaningfully extend their reflections to the experiences of others, they should be encouraged to interact with others whose values are not the same as their own.

Box 14.5 Learning activity—Exploring diversity and difference in experiences and expectations of health and wellbeing

Reflection Questions

1. How do you define health?
2. Where does your own understanding of "health" come from?
3. How do you explain the concept of "health" to other people?
4. Think about whether "health" is something we have or something we do or both?
5. What are its essential components?
6. Who decides on these components?
7. What is a healthy person?
8. What does a person need to have to make them healthy?
9. How do we learn about "health", and how might this influence our understandings of "wellbeing"?

Social Determinants Question

1. What social determinants of health influence your responses? Consider social determinants at all levels (e.g., individual, interpersonal, community and societal).

Exploring Diversity and Difference Question

Reflecting on the answers from another student:

1. How are your answers different?
2. If you lived in a country very different from Australia, how might your answers be different from those of a student who has only lived in Australia?

This can be a confronting task but an important step towards engaging with cultural safety. Within her cultural competence framework, Campinha-Bacote (2002) calls this step cultural encounters. While cultural safety extends past the acquisition of competence, engaging with different others can be a powerful catalyst for self-awareness and self-reflection. If students are appropriately prepared for the experience of exploring difference and provided with guided opportunities to debrief, this can be a very powerful learning experience (Table 14.4).

Criteria for this Learning Assessment can include the requirement of scholarly literature to support statements made throughout. The assessment can also be expanded or condensed to meet the needs of educators and students. Marking for this Learning Assessment can focus on the student's reflections on their cultural encounter as well as their reflections on how models of health align with or conflict with one another. At this third step, more academic expectations and robust criteria can be applied to the ways that educators grade the assessment. This reinforces for students the importance of increasing awareness through engagement with appropriate scholarly sources and providing accurate assessments of models of health and how they support or reduce experiences of health and wellbeing outcomes.

Table 14.4 Learning assessment—Exploring diversity and difference in experiences and expectations of health and wellbeing

Assessment Instructions	
Step 1 (Self-Awareness): Identify someone you know who you feel comfortable talking to about their perspectives on health and wellbeing. This person should be different from you in relation to at least one social determinant (e.g., age, sex, gender, ethnicity, education, political beliefs, religious beliefs, etc.). This person can be a member of your family, a friend, another student or a workmate.	
Step 2 (Exploring Diversity and Difference): Ask this person questions from Reflection Box 3.2 so you can understand how their understandings and experiences influence their expectations of health and wellbeing. Provide a transcript of the discussion as an appendix to your assessment.	
Step 3 (Self-Reflection): Prepare a table to compare your answers to Reflection Box 3.2 and those of your interviewee. Next, identify which model of health best aligns with your own responses and those of your interviewee. Describe the model(s) identified support your own health and wellbeing as well as that of your interviewee. For example, responses to Question 7 of Reflection Box 3.2 might include,	
Question 7. What is a healthy person?	
My Response A healthy person is someone who is able to experience wellbeing in all aspects of their life. This includes being able to be with people who are supportive, having access to healthy food, different forms of exercise and safety from abuse, discrimination or inequality. This perspective best aligns with the biopsychosocial model, which indicates that biological health is supported by psychological and social wellbeing.	*Interviewee Response* A healthy person is someone who is in touch with their spiritual wellbeing. Prayer and your religious faith community is central to being mentally and physically well. God provides and takes care of us in all ways and shows us how to live to protect our wellbeing. This perspective also aligns with the biopsychosocial model because this model appreciates the role of spirituality as a central element of wellbeing.
Step 4 (Exploring Diversity and Difference): Compare the models identified in Step 3, and reflect on how it aligns or conflicts with the biomedical model—Australia's primary model of health and wellbeing. How might this impact your health and wellbeing as well as that for your interviewee? For example, • The biomedical model aligns with the biological aspect of the biopsychosocial model. However, the biomedical model does not respond thoroughly towards supporting and preventing mental health concerns. The biomedical model may also cause mental and social health concerns by embracing policies and procedures that discriminate against people from minority backgrounds. This includes people of a minority religious group or whose faith is vilified. As such, my interviewee may suffer poor health consequences because the biomedical model does not adequately accommodate for spiritual health as a means for ensure holistic wellbeing.	

Feedback

To support student willingness to continue engaging with different others, feedback can focus on the depth of the interview presented by the student. Reviewing the interview transcript can be a task assigned to students with the aim of identifying where they could have asked more questions or discussed various aspects of social constructions and/or social determinants. Based on the responses given in the Learning Assessment, feedback can be focused on seeking more specificity around experiences of health and wellbeing of their interviewee. For instance, see Box 14.6.

By providing feedback on the students' process of engaging with different others to explore diverse perspectives of health and wellbeing, they are encouraged to prioritise the principles of cultural safety. Importantly, the process of engaging in cultural encounters is central to the outcomes of cultural safety, which provide a space for health professionals/practitioners to self-reflect and hone their capacity to adapt to a variety of people and environments.

Box 14.6 Feedback—Exploring diversity and difference in experiences and expectations of health and wellbeing

Dear Shivani,

Your reflections on the ways that the biomedical model influences your health and that of your interviewee demonstrates increasing capacity to explore and critique the role of difference in health. You mention that some biomedical health policies support disadvantage for certain communities. A specific example that could be related to your own or the experience of your interviewee would have strengthened your submission. Further discussion about how your interviewee's health may be hindered by the biomedical model would help to demonstrate your understanding of the various models of health. Your interview transcript provides answers to these queries and demonstrates a high level of skill in exploring these sensitive issues with different others.

Principle 4: Becoming familiar with the principles of cultural safety

To orient students to the application of their knowledge to health practice, they must become familiar with the principles of cultural safety. In particular students will need to be provided with clear definitions for cultural safety and understand how cultural safety is different from other forms of cultural support frameworks or philosophies. In Chapter 4 these distinctions are made in depth. To assist students in their understanding of cultural safety, Reflection Box 4.1 highlights the differences between cultural safety and cultural competence.

Box 4.1 Reflection—Conceptual confusion

There is limited literature referring to the inconsistent use of and confusion about cultural safety terminology. Many terms including cultural awareness, cultural appropriateness, cultural sensitivity, cultural competency, and cultural safety are often used interchangeably, even though they do not share the same meaning. This conceptual confusion and inconsistent use of terminology is reflected in much of the literature on Indigenous health, cultures, and health care.

Consider the definition of cultural competence, for example: a set of congruent behaviours, attitudes and policies that come together in a system, agency or among professionals and enable that system, agency or those professionals to work effectively in cross-cultural situations (National Health and Medical Research Council, 2005, p. 6).

How is this definition different from cultural safety?

Who is the focus of cultural competence, and why might that be problematic? The health professional or the health consumer?

Understanding the distinctions between cultural competency and cultural safety is important, as it allows students to move past a focus on the acquisition of skills to a more nuanced engagement with that health and health care means to services users. This process of discovery should be the focus of trying to understand the role of cultural safety in health care.

Learning activity

Once students understand the difference in cultural support terminology, they can investigate how these terms manifest in real life. To continuously develop their ability to be self-aware and to self-reflect, the following Learning Activity implores them to apply their new knowledge to themselves.

Box 14.7 Learning activity—Becoming familiar with the principles of cultural safety

Define the following cultural support concepts
Cultural awareness:
Cultural sensitivity:
Cultural responsiveness:
Cultural appropriateness:
Cultural competence:
Cultural safety:
If you needed to engage with a health care professional which of the preceding terms would best support your health, and why?,
Student Response:

This Learning Activity encourages students to begin distinguishing for themselves the differences between cultural support terminology. By researching and producing statements that define each concept, students will compare and contrast each and then determine which focus they would like their own health care professional to engage with. This reflection on what the student would want helps them to become more aware about the feeling of having the support you need to be healthy and the reasons why that is impactful. Importantly, students do not have to indicate cultural safety as their preferred cultural support experience. What is integral, and they are thinking about the distinctions between concepts and then reflecting on their own experiences and thoughts.

Learning assessment

To engage students in the process of linking their new understandings of cultural safety to their own experiences and the experiences of others, assessing the ability to translate knowledge is key. This skill is central to cultural safety, which requires that students are able to adapt their approaches in ways that support health and wellbeing outcomes. To gauge this developing ability students can engage with the following Learning Assessment.

Box 14.8 Learning assessment—Becoming familiar with the principles of cultural safety

Assessment Instructions

Step 1 (Becoming familiar): Research the cultural support terminology used by your professional codes of conduct/practice.

- What terminology do they use? Cultural competence, cultural awareness, cultural safety etc.?
- How do they define this term (e.g., cultural awareness)?
- If they do not provide a definition, provide a definition for this terminology.

Step 2 (Principles of Cultural Safety): How is the definition they use different from or similar to cultural safety as described in Chapter 4 of this textbook?

Step 3 (Self-Reflection): Based on your responses to Steps 1 and 2, have a discussion with another student, and answer the following questions in relation to yourself and your peer. Be sure to include relevant details about social determinants of health and intersectionality in your responses.

- How might the terminology used in your codes of conduct (e.g., cultural awareness) apply to a situation where you need health care support?
- How might the principles of cultural safety apply to a situation where you need health care support?
- How might the terminology used in your codes of conduct (e.g., cultural awareness) apply to a situation where your peer needed health care support?
- How might the principles of cultural safety apply to a situation where your peer needed health care support? An example response for this last point could be:

My partner for this assessment is a 20-year-old male of Caucasian race, Australian nationality and European ancestry. He identifies as a gay man and as Christian. If he needed to see the doctor for a refill on his asthma medication, cultural safety would be important as it would ensure that his identity as a gay man did not cause the health care professional to be prejudiced or discriminatory towards him. The health professional will be aware that people from gender or sexuality diverse identities experience unfair treatment in all areas of life and will avoid doing the same in their practice. My student partner has indicated that because he is not hyper-feminine, some health practitioners do not consider that he might be gay and have made comments about how masculine he "seems" and that they would never have known. If the health professional was engaged with a culturally safe approach, they would not diminish, demean or disempower his identity by presuming him to be heterosexual and asking questions or making comments that are irrelevant to his need to get a script for his asthma medication.

Important to this assessment is the consistent inclusion of other principles of cultural safety teaching and learning that encourage the student to keep diversity and multiple factors related to health in mind. Grading can focus on the student's ability to reflect on diverse social determinants and the impact these might have on themselves and their peer. References to scholarly literature may be required to ensure that students are linking their growing knowledge from the curriculum with existing evidence related to particular social determinants, principles of cultural safety and expectations of their profession when engaging with difference.

Feedback

As the Learning Assessments get more personal, students who have not engaged in shared reflective practice before may begin feeling more and more uncomfortable, especially around topics related to privilege and power dynamics. Feedback focused on acknowledging this developing skill, being comfortable with being uncomfortable, is central to students' ability to trust their capacity for experiences and encounters that disrupt their perceptions and values. Feedback may include the following.

> **Box 14.9 Feedback—Becoming familiar with the principles of cultural safety**
>
> Dear Kim,
>
> The reflections you have produced demonstrate a growing ability to understand different cultural support terminology and identify how cultural safety is different. You have been able to demonstrate how the principles of cultural safety can support engagement with health consumers. The presentation of social determinants related to your peer was helpful to contextualising your partner's experiences with health care providers. It would be interesting to know how your peer's Christianity was perceived or supported in health care encounters and the outcome of this intersectional social determinant on his health and wellbeing. For future assessments more focus on intersections would provide more depth to this well-developed submission.

Feedback to students can also respond to the accuracy of the terminology used in their Learning Assessment or the application of cultural safety principles to themselves of their peer(s). Importantly, students should be increasingly encouraged to think about the impact of cultural safety on health and wellbeing in real life. This will help them develop the ability to understand and critique policies and programming that seek to support cultural safety.

Principle 5: Understanding the importance of cultural safety and its relevance to health policy and advocacy

As students immerse themselves with the principles of cultural safety, assisting them in developing an understanding of the relevance of cultural safety to health and wellbeing is needed. Chapter 5 engages students to learn more about how cultural safety is linked to policies that contribute to health services, programs, management and health professional accreditation. Further, Chapter 5 discusses the role of health care professionals and providers in health and wellbeing advocacy. While not all students will take on formal advocacy roles in their future careers, each health encounter whether with a patient directly or with colleagues outside of health is an opportunity for advocacy that supports cultural safety for all stakeholders. Reflection Box 5.4 expands on concepts from Chapter 5 to help students' reflection on how cultural safety is embedded (or not) in the health environments that they have encountered.

> **Box 5.4 Reflection—Considering cultural safety**
>
> Consider the cultural safety definition just given, and think about the last time you were in a health care centre, perhaps a doctor's surgery or a hospital.

- How have you seen cultural safety principles embedded in the system?
- Was there recognition of cultural diversity and the capacity to meet the needs of people who are not of the dominant culture?

If you have worked in a health care institution (or plan to), you might like to consider how these features might translate into policy.

In Chapter 5 students are being asked to identify where cultural safety fits into existing systems and processes and how that relates to policy. Health care policies and practice guidelines are unknown to many students. By engaging students in reflecting on systems, they can begin to see how cultural safety is not simply based on interactions between individuals but is also relevant to working within systems that may not be inherently designed to accommodate for diversity and difference.

Learning activity

Given that students may not have had an opportunity to see how health care systems are built or how they run behind the scenes, engaging them to reflect on these processes is crucial. Often students perceive cultural safety as a process of gaining competency. Much of this perception is linked to their limited exposure to the health system as an insider of that system. The following Learning Activity can help students to learn how to look for and identify where cultural safety exists not only in "practice" but also in systems.

Box 14.10 Learning activity—Understanding the importance of cultural safety and its relevance to health policy and advocacy

Reflection Questions

Consider the cultural safety definition given and think about the last time you were in a health care setting like a doctor's surgery, hospital or allied health visit.

1. How have you seen cultural safety principles embedded in the system?
2. Was there recognition of cultural diversity and the capacity to meet the needs of people who are not of the dominant culture?
3. If you have worked in a health care institution (or plan to), you might like to consider how these features might translate into policy.

Self-Awareness and Self-Reflection Questions

When you were last in a health care setting:

1. What images or information stood out to you?
2. What made your experience a positive or a negative one?
3. How might your answers link to principles for cultural safety?

Cultural Safety and Health Policy/Advocacy Questions

Reflecting on your last visit to a health care setting:

1. What policies do you think helped you to have a positive experience?
2. What policies may have hindered you from having a positive experience?
3. How might these policies link to principles for cultural safety?

By drawing on personal experiences, students can reflect on how policies impact on their health and wellbeing outcomes. From Chapter 5 they would have been introduced to critiques on policy as not all are designed to support cultural safety. Importantly, cultural safety links to much bigger and global ideals about health and wellbeing as evidenced by the *Universal Declaration of Human Rights* (United Nations, 1948).

Learning assessment

To expand students' perspectives about cultural safety and its application to policy and advocacy, linking to human rights is recommended. For some students the "why?" of cultural safety may be unclear when reviewing the principles and policies alone. However, with the additional reflection on human rights there is some additional clarity about the role cultural safety plays in advocating for holistic health and wellbeing for all people. Further, reviewing human rights provides an opportunity for students to reflect on the universality of the declaration over time. In particular, students should consider the used of gendered terminology and why such terms have not been updated in line with contemporary perspectives on gender (equality). To gauge students' growing capacity to make these links, the following Learning Assessment is suggested.

Box 14.11 Learning assessment—Understanding the importance of cultural safety and its relevance to health policy and advocacy

Assessment instructions

Step 1 (Relevance of Health Policy): Review the New South Wales (NSW) Health Code of Conduct (https://www1.health.nsw.gov.au/pds/ActivePDSDocuments/PD2015_049.pdf) and then sort the following statements according to whether they are human rights or items/excerpts from the New South Wales Code of Conduct. For example,

- Everyone has the right to a standard of living adequate for the health and wellbeing of himself and of his family, including food, clothing, housing and medical care and necessary social services, and the right to security in the event of unemployment, sickness, disability, widowhood, old age or other lack of livelihood in circumstances beyond his control. (Is this a human right or an item/excerpt from the NSW Health Code of Conduct?
- Everyone ... should expect to be treated, and must treat others, with respect, dignity and fairness. High standards of workplace practice and conduct improve ... morale. They also produce more effective working relationships and enhanced patient outcomes. In particular, bullying and/or harassment will not be tolerated. (Is this a human right or an item/excerpt from the NSW Health Code of Conduct?

Step 2 (Relevance of Health Policy): Check your answers by referring to the United Nations Universal Declaration of Human Rights (https://www.un.org/en/udhrbook/index.shtml#6) and the NSW Health Code of Conduct.

Step 3 (Understanding Health Policy): Reflect on how three articles from the United Nations Universal Declaration of Human Rights are linked to items form the NSW Health Code of Conduct.

Step 4 (Relevance of Health Policy and Advocacy): Find a news story about someone who has recently had a positive and/or negative experience with a health service, professional or system.

- From the story identify the relevant social determinants and intersectional aspects of the person's identity or experience/s.
- Identify at least one human right and at least one NSW Health Code of Conduct item that were violated or highlighted in the story.
- If the outcomes were positive, how might you advocate for others so that the positive outcomes can be experienced by others?
- If the outcomes were negative, how might you advocate for the person in the news story to have had a better health experience?
- How does your plan for advocacy align with the principles of cultural safety? An example response might be:

The person in the news story was not able to access a practitioner who spoke their language, which caused significant delay in the treatment of their health issue. If I encountered a patient who was not able to speak English, I would ask for help to find an interpreting service to make interactions with that patient easier for all involved. I would ask the receptionist of the health care service to make a note on the patient's file indicating that an interpreter is required for all appointments so that one can be arranged before their arrival. During their appointment I would ask the interpreter to provide the number for the interpreting service to the patient. This would ensure that if the patient needed further support at other health appointments, they would have the information they needed to access an interpreter for those appointments. This approach for advocacy aligns with cultural safety as it seeks to provide equitable access to health services not just equal access to health services. By adapting my practice, informing others about how to support patients in need of an interpreter and ensuring the patient has the information they need to have agency over their health encounters, cultural safety is supported.

Through this Learning Assessment students identify and articulate meaningful links between human rights, cultural safety policy and advocacy as well as earlier concepts, including social determinants of health and intersectionality. Marking of this Learning Assessment could focus on the students' ability to accurately identify social determinants from the news story and the role of human rights terminology in ensuring the rights of the consumer. Marking can also reflect on students' ability to consider diverse human rights or policy items from a national or state-wide health policy or code of conduct relevant to the students' and educators' location. Educators can assess the advocacy elements within the Learning Assessment in relation to the student's ability to provide a detailed account of how they could advocate for the person in the news story. They can also be assessed on how their plan for advocacy extends past the clinical or interpersonal setting and into the community

Feedback

To provide opportunity for development, feedback can focus on identifying areas where the student did or did not appropriately link human rights or policy. Feedback can also be provided in relation to the students' ability to identify the social determinants and intersectional elements relevant to the person in their news story. Feedback should also be given about the student's reflections on how cultural safety is aligned with their approach to advocacy. Sample feedback is shown in Box 14.12.

Box 14.12 Feedback—Understanding the importance of cultural safety and its relevance to health policy and advocacy

Dear Robyn,

The advocacy approach you propose demonstrates an understanding of the individual, professional, organisational health care levels that need to be addressed in order to support access to health care services. You have identified that the person in the news story has a disability. I wonder how that experience might impact on the way the client may or may not be supported to engage with health care systems. The alignment of your advocacy approach to principles of cultural safety are articulated well and indicate a growing understanding of the role of the health care professional in supporting cultural safety outcomes.

With feedback that guides students to continuously think about the complex nature of diversity and difference they gain insight into how they perceive health experiences. Importantly, students are called to reflect on their role in advocating for culturally safe health practices in diverse and flexible ways.

Principle 6: Engaging in culturally safe health care practice

Developing knowledge about cultural safety and relevant policies in relation to Australian, state, organisational and professional guidelines allows students to move into learning how to translate these understandings into practice. At this point of their learning students may again feel frustration and confusion about the multidimensional and complex nature of engaging with people from diverse backgrounds and the expectation upon them to provide a health experience that the client deems appropriate and beneficial. Chapter 6 discusses these contentions and encourages students to reflect on their thoughts and feelings in this regard. Additionally, Chapter 6 draws students into considering specific examples and potential strategies. Reflection Box 6.9 uses the example of health literacy to that effect.

Box 6.9 Reflection—Culturally safe practice

Many health programs focus on the delivery of health care, education and information to groups of people who have limited health access and/or literacy in a particular health area.

1. Make a list of some elements of programs that successfully support marginalised communities to increase their health and wellbeing.

Watch the PHC Case Study—Culture and care in Australia video: https://www.youtube.com/watch?v=cC94MsIsje0

2. Does this program support some of the elements you noted in Question 1?
3. How does this program put cultural safety into practice?

As discussed in Chapter 6, there are diverse and various elements that could be included in health literacy programming, as an example, and certainly dozens more across each type of health support initiative from research to clinical practice. Importantly, students should be encouraged to think in innovative ways and include ideas that may or may not feature in this book. Again, this leads students to think outside of the rigidity of their immediate pedagogical engagement and towards thinking about how principles of cultural safety manifest in the real world.

Learning activity

Students learning about cultural safety often lament that culturally safe practice "is not my job". Notably, students have the sense that a narrow set of individuals with specific titles are in the business of culturally safe health care practice and that they and their profession are coincidental bystanders. The following Learning Activity therefore seeks to engage students to consider the relationship between their professional role and culturally safe practice (Table 14.5).

While health literacy is a broad term, it provides enough range for students to produce a variety of responses and see that diverse approaches can produce similar results. This reiterates the value of their individual and professional differences and their ability to complement the role and skills of others. As can be seen throughout this pedagogical guide, self-reflection is central to students' ability to project what might be helpful when working with diverse people and communities.

Learning assessment

Working in collaboration with other health professionals and importantly with diverse people and individuals is a central aspect to engaging in culturally safe health care practice. To support this practice while students are learning about cultural safety, using a Learning Assessment that assists them in developing their interprofessional and/or multidisciplinary skills is encouraged. Importantly, working as a team can assist students to better understand the professional role of

Table 14.5 Engaging in culturally safe health care practice

With a peer from a different health discipline or area of interest complete the following:

Reflection Question	*Self-Reflection Question*	*Culturally Safe Health Care Question*
Make a list of some elements of programs that successfully support communities to increase their health literacy.	What role could you play in supporting some of the elements you listed?	How might the current Australian health care system support or hinder your ability to support the health literacy elements you have discussed?

other health professionals and be better able to refer appropriately or provide developmental opportunities for others in the future across professions.

Box 14.13 Learning assessment—Engaging in culturally safe health care practice

Assessment Instructions

Step 1 (Culturally Unsafe Health care Practices): Review the following case study of ageing Indigenous peoples' experiences of seeking culturally safe aged care supports—Indigenous Australians call for more culturally appropriate aged care facilities: https://www.youtube.com/watch?v=-Eg1CtQHy6k

Step 2 (Reflecting on culturally safe health care practice): In a small group of students from health disciplines or areas of interest different from yours, complete the following tasks in relation to the listed video:

- Why did the interviewees feel that the current aged care system is culturally unsafe? Reflect on power, distrust, discrimination and racism (for example).
- Outline why each issue perpetuates a culturally unsafe health care system for ageing Indigenous Australians and their families.
- If your team was working with one of the older people in the video, what would each of you do to address the concerns held by families seeking to enrol their loved ones into an aged care facility? Reflect on the role of trust, respect and collaboration (for example).
- Consider the social determinants of one of an older family member. How would their experience of aged care be similar to or different from those presented in the video? What privileges does their identity provide them (or not)? An example response from one student for this point might be as follows.

My grandfather is a Vietnamese refugee who fled following the Vietnam War. When he arrived in Australia in 1976, he did not speak much English and experienced significant racism and discrimination from White Australians. He still has a strong accent but speaks English fluently and became a very successful and self-made businessman. Now that he has retired and is rather elderly, my parents and family are taking care of him. He has a range of chronic illnesses including emphysema from years of smoking. Our family has not once thought to enrol him to an aged care facility although his care is getting harder and harder to manage for us all. There are many similarities between my grandfather and the ageing Indigenous people in the case study. However, some major differences include that he is a migrant like all non-Indigenous people, he has a large family who take care of him and do not take his money and he has strong connections to his culture and language, which has been stolen from Indigenous people.

Grading for this task can focus on the students' ability to provide a robust breakdown and application of a range of cultural safety principles. Students' perspectives on how they would support a culturally safe approach should include accurate statements and not including elements of other cultural support terminology (e.g., cultural competence). As students engage with this Learning Assessment, they may be inclined to begin discussing their role in terms of skills and competencies that they would use "on" the clients. Grading criteria can advise students that they should avoid conflating terms and focusing on how they can do or help and instead on how their actions or engagement can produce a culturally safe experience as defined by the client/s.

Feedback

Feedback that encourages students to develop their understanding of the difference between cultural competence (for example) and cultural safety is needed as they begin to reflect on how cultural safety can be "practiced". Importantly, it cannot nor should it be applied as a tick box exercise. Diverse responsive from students may provide a significantly culturally safe approach. Feedback can remind students of where they may have reiterated simplified lists presented in other literature. Feedback on the preceding example of reflecting on social determinants could include the following.

> **Box 14.14 Feedback—Engaging in culturally safe health care practice**
>
> Dear Son,
>
> Thank you for sharing this summary about your grandfather and his experiences of migrating to Australia. You have outlined significant social determinants that demonstrate your understanding of the diverse impact these elements have on your grandfather's experience and intersectionality. You have indicated how your grandfather's experience is different with some clear examples. I would suggest you review the video, which indicated that the family youth did not perceive their asking older relatives for money as "taking" or as "abuse". It sounds like your grandfather was able to engage in business and develop a strong financial base for his family. You also mention that your family has ensured that your grandfather is cared for at home. How might these resources and opportunities be different for older Indigenous people and their relatives? You have indicated that there are similarities but have not indicated what these similarities are. Further indication of these similarities would have improved the comprehensiveness of your response.

By this point in the students' learning journey, feedback can include corrective elements that encourage the student to reflect back on their words as well as the information they were asked to engage with. Many Australian students may have been taught or learnt about difference in such a way that problematises the ways that those who are different from them live their lives. Feedback can therefore provide clarity around the factual elements of the case study (for example) while also encouraging the students' ability to reflect on how their perceptions impact on the delivery of culturally safe health care.

Principle 7: Applying principles for cultural safety with diverse populations

Cultural safety teaching and learning provides students with the foundations of how to apply the principles of cultural safety to engagement and interactions with diverse populations. As reiterated throughout the textbook, the "cultural" in cultural safety is a reflection of everything we are and everything we do and think. With this in mind, Chapters 7–13 provide students with the opportunity to reflect on various manifestations of Australian culture across a diverse range of population groups. Across the Principles of Cultural Safety Teaching and Learning indicated earlier (1–6), there are many Reflection Boxes and Learning Activities that support student understandings of cultural safety and its relevance to oneself and diverse experiences. It is suggested that students engage with those tasks in depth before proceeding with Principle 7. With this in mind, Principle 7 focuses on providing educators and students with an integrated Learning Assessment that asks students to consolidate their knowledge and consider its application across diverse populations.

Learning assessment

Many health students express frustration that their education and training did not provide them with the opportunity to learn how to present their new set of knowledge and skills in ways that employers want to hear. Remarkably, only a limited number of tertiary students have ever responded to selection criteria for a potential job or been taught how to effectively do so (Moore & Morton, 2017). This crucial skill can result in unnecessary delays to students' commencement of paid work in their field. Job applications require individuals to consolidate large chunks of knowledge, content and experience into one or two pages of text in response to the selection criteria questions. To assess students' ability to appropriately and/or accurately integrate their knowledge of cultural safety into a tangible form, the following Learning Assessment asks them not only to respond to a hypothetical job as a "Cultural Liaison" but also to do so in reference to their specific health discipline. This reinforces for students that cultural safety is relevant across all areas of the Australian health care system and their profession in particular.

While definitions vary depending on context and population groups, a Cultural Liaison links people and communities (often from minority and marginalised groups) to services, supports or resources. Cultural Liaisons need to have a background in working with individuals from diverse sociocultural groups in a capacity related to the employer's areas of service. Cultural Liaisons may also have tertiary or vocational training in a discipline area related to the employer's areas of service. Cultural Liaisons may be from the same sociocultural, ethnic or religious group as the communities they are hired to support but may also be from backgrounds different to their client groups. Job posting for Cultural Liaisons often seek candidates with some of the following skills that are linked to cultural safety.

Box 14.15 Skills required for Cultural Liaisons jobs

1. Knowledge about different cultural communities, and the issues they face in becoming part of the larger community.
2. Respect for all people, regardless of their social, cultural, religious, sexuality differences.
3. Enjoy working with individuals and families from a variety of backgrounds.
4. A keen interest in helping individuals with diverse experiences integrate into the larger community.
5. The desire to assist others through collaboration to support improved health and wellbeing outcomes.
6. A client-centered approach to engaging with individuals and communities.
7. The ability to effectively and appropriately translate the needs of individuals and communities to the service and vice versa.

In mainstream health services and practice the term *cultural safety* is not always used in the context of seeking employees or in regular delivery of services. As a result, students may not see how being a Cultural Liaison is of relevance to their learning about and applying cultural safety. Again, they may perceive such work to be within the purview of social workers and other community support workers. The following Learning Assessment ensures that students can begin to make meaningful connections between their discipline and cultural safety as well as learn how to articulate these links convincingly.

Box 14.16 Learning assessment—Applying principles for cultural safety with diverse populations

Assessment Instructions

Step 1: Clearly identify the specific course in which you are enrolled (i.e., Nursing, Medicine, Paramedicine, Health Promotion, Dental, Podiatry, Sport and Exercise Science, Public Health, etc.).

Step 2: Find your specific discipline codes of conduct/practice guidelines. For many students these can be found via The Australian Health Practitioner Regulation Agency (Ahpra) or through their accrediting association website.

Step 3: With your specific profession in mind, respond to the selection criteria in relation to a position as a Cultural Liaison within your discipline area for a state health service. Be sure to include examples from any part of your life (does not need to be health-service related) to support your responses. Students may begin by writing:

To whom it may concern:

My name is Sango Yarran, and I am applying for the role of Cultural Liaison within the Physiotherapy Department for NSW Health. I have provided responses to the selection criteria in support of my interest and expertise in fulfilling this role.

1. What have you learnt from your professional training that makes you the best candidate for the role of Cultural Liaison? (approx. 100–150 words)
2. Demonstrate your understanding of the relevance and relationship between social determinants, human rights, cultural safety and health and wellbeing outcomes. (approx. 200–250 words)
3. With reference to specific items within your professional codes of conduct/practice guidelines, demonstrate your knowledge of the relationship between these items and the principles of cultural safety. (approx. 250–300 words)
4. Identify, with practical examples and links to your professional codes of conduct/practice guidelines, how you would support and/or enact culturally safe health practice with an individual or community different to yourself. (approx. 300–400 words)
5. Demonstrate an understanding of the barriers and facilitators to culturally safe practice for both staff in your profession and health consumers. (approx. 200–250 words)
6. Given your disciplinary expertise and understanding of cultural safety, explain how your ability to self-reflect supports your ability to provide culturally safe care within the role of Cultural Liaison. (approx. 200 words)

Provide a list of references, both in-text and below, that demonstrate your scholarly knowledge in relation to cultural safety. (8–10 references should be included).

Grading on this Learning Assessment should focus on the students' ability to integrate their knowledge in prose that is cohesive instead of appearing as a list of definitions or dot points. Marking should also focus on students' ability to present a diverse range of contexts and social determinants, including nuanced presentations of diverse social, ability, religious, sexuality and cultural groups. Students who only focus on ethnic or cultural heritage or consistently present diversity through a problematised lens will likely provide examples of culturally safe health practice that are in fact competency or awareness based and limited to activities like: the provision of interpreters or posters with different languages and the provision of gender-specific health services. Academic writing is also evaluated in this assessment, with marks being given or lost due to grammatical and syntax errors. This is rather important in this Learning Assessment, which students can presume should be at the quality expected of a job application going to a state-level health service. To ensure the academic quality of student responses, they should include in-text references to reputable scholarly sources as well as a reference list at the end of the Learning Assessment.

Feedback

By this point of their learning, students should be rather well versed in the principles of cultural safety and their professional policies. They may, however, still struggle to move away from a skill and competencies focused way of supporting holistic health and wellbeing. As such, feedback can focus on the students' presentation of ideas in accurate and appropriate ways and their use of academic sources to support their claims. Feedback on this kind of Learning Assessment has included the following.

Given the importance of cultural safety in health care, feedback should be critical but also provide insight into specific areas for further development. Reiterating to students that cultural safety is a journey and not a destination can assist students, and especially those whose feedback is accompanied by a less than desirable grade. At this point of cultural safety teaching and learning, foundational understanding should be clearly articulated while application and process reflections may still need development such that students are able to consider the impact of their practice on a range of health experiences and outcomes.

Box 14.17 Feedback—Applying principles for cultural safety with diverse populations

Dear Juan,
Based on your submission, the following feedback has been given for each criterion:

1. This section could have been more succinct and emphasised more on the specific skills from your Paramedicine training that could be transferred to the role. The response could have incorporated references or examples to strengthen this section. Instead the section focused only on personal characteristics in support of your expertise for this role.
2. You have done well in providing concrete examples (although not referenced) of how social determinants, health outcomes and cultural safety are related within Indigenous population; however, your response did not address human rights.
3. The response indicates understanding of cultural awareness, knowledge and skill. However, the response has not addressed cultural safety as it is focused on cultural

competence. You have, however, presented good practical examples with diverse and intersectional cases (e.g., Jewish, gay and with cerebral palsy) to demonstrate how social constructs influence perceptions and health practice.

4. The response does not clearly demonstrate knowledge of professional guidelines and provide clear links with cultural safety. It does, however, demonstrate an understanding of cultural safety and generally how guidelines contribute to cultural safety.
5. You have provided good examples of barriers and facilitators to culturally safe practice for health consumers but have not addressed these factors for staff within Ambulance service, where you will be a Cultural Liaison.
6. The response has not really addressed the selection criteria here as there is limited indication of the role of self-reflection and cultural safety to demonstrate why you are the best person for the role.
7. References were used sparingly, and more was needed to support the statements in-text.

Overall this was a fair attempt; however, the writing could be improved by removing information not relevant to the questions, and by being more succinct. Prior to the next assessment, please review the readings to familiarise yourself with the principles of cultural safety with particular focus on the role of self-reflection and applying cultural safety to better understand diverse sociocultural groups.

Principle 8: Evaluating the impact of cultural safety in practice

This final Principle of Cultural Safety Teaching and Learning is not really final at all as it occurs throughout Principles 1 to 7. Within each Principle, students will be reflecting on the impact of culturally safe practice and increasingly reviewing their role in that process. However, students may ask, "I am not actually in my profession so how can I see or report on the impacts of culturally safe practice?" If we recall that culture includes all aspects of our existence and that health and wellbeing is experienced (or not) in every moment of life, then students can evaluate the impact of culturally safe practice anytime and anywhere. In fact, with some minor adjustments, students can complete every one of the preceding tasks with friends and family with different and thought-provoking answers at various points in time. As such, drawing on Reflection Box 1.4 from Chapter 1, self-awareness and self-reflection are at the core of cultural safety.

Box 1.4 Reflection—The role of health professionals in promoting cultural safety

If cultural safety is about the client/patient/consumer, does cultural safety apply to the people who provide health care?

What social determinants and social constructions about health workers might influence their experience of working in a culturally safe environment?

What social determinants and social constructions about health workers might influence their ability to provide care that is culturally safe?

If students can keep these questions in their minds throughout their cultural safety teaching and learning (and beyond), they can consistently evaluate their experiences, perceptions and histories as well as their role and their actions in the production or destruction of culturally safe environments. Self-reflection is highlighted from the beginning and throughout this final chapter and rightfully closes with the same. Whether evaluation is formal or informal, the ability to evaluate the impact of culturally safe practice as experienced by others is completely dependent upon the students' ability to develop the capacity for critical self-evaluation across their past, present and future.

Conclusion

In this chapter, Principles for Cultural Safety Teaching and Learning for Australian tertiary health students was presented. Through a diverse array of Reflection Boxes, Learning Activities, Learning Assessments and Feedback frameworks, tertiary health discipline educators can further develop tasks that support the development of a culturally safe health workforce. Engaging students in this way seeks to ensure that the students and their journey remain central to their development of culturally safe health practice and the ability to see their role as change-makers (for better and for worse) in the health setting and also in their everyday lives and interactions with others. In the words of Former President of South Africa,

> What counts in life is not the mere fact that we have lived. It is what difference we have made to the lives of others that will determine the significance of the life we lead.
>
> -Nelson Mandela

References

Campinha-Bacote, J. (2002). The process of cultural competence in the delivery of healthcare services: A model of care. *Journal of Transcultural Nursing, 13*(3), 181–184. https://doi.org/10.1177/10459602013003003.

Marjadi, B., Mapedzahama, V., Rogers, G., Donnelly, M., Harris, A., Donadel, D., Jakstas, E., Dune, T. M., Lo, W., Michael, S., McKnight, T., Hennessy, A., Ganapathy, V. A., & Pacey, F. (2020). Medicine in context: Ten years experience in diversity education for medical students in Greater Western Sydney, Australia. *GMS Journal for Medical Education, 37*(2), 1–17. https://doi.org/10.3205/zma001314.

Moore, T., & Morton, J. (2017). The myth of job readiness? Written communication, employability, and the skills gap in higher education. *Studies in Higher Education, 42*(3), 591–609. https://doi.org/10.1080/03075079.2015.1067602.

Morin, A. (2011). Self-awareness part 1: Definition, measures, effects, functions, and antecedents. *Social Personality and Psychology Compass, 5*(10), 807–823. https://doi.org/ 10.1111/j.1751-9004.2011.00387.x.

National Health and Medical Research Council. (2005). *Cultural competency in health: A guide for policy, partnerships and participation.* Commonwealth of Australia. https://www.nhmrc.gov.au/about-us/publications/cultural-competency-health#block-views-block-file-attachments-content-block-1.

Olson, E. D. (2013). Why blame me? Interpreting counselor student resistance to racially themed course content as complicity with white racial hegemony [Doctoral Dissertation, University of New Mexico]. University of New Mexico Digital Repository. https://digitalrepository.unm.edu/educ_ifce_etds/10/.

United Nations. (1948). *Universal declaration of human rights.* https://www.ohchr.org/EN/UDHR/Documents/UDHR_Translations/eng.pdf

Glossary

Ableism Refers to attitudes and beliefs that infer ableness as superior and disability as inferior.

Aboriginal The first peoples of this land now called Australia are the Aboriginal peoples; however, they also have other names that they use to refer to themselves: Goori, Koori, Arrernte, Kamilaroi, Yungl, Yaegl and so on.

Aboriginal Community Controlled Health Organisations (ACCHOs) A non-profit incorporated Aboriginal Community Controlled Organisation, which provides wholistic and culturally appropriate Primary Health care and Aboriginal health-related services to the community it serves. An ACCHO is governed by an Aboriginal board of management elected by a local Aboriginal community membership.

Aboriginal Health & Medical Research Council of NSW (AHMRC of NSW) Aboriginal Health & Medical Research Council of NSW was established in 1985. Members are ACCHOs led by their respective Aboriginal Communities to deliver comprehensive and culturally appropriate primary health care services.

Aboriginal Medical Service (AMS) First established in 1971 in Redfern (Redfern AMS). There are now around 140 Aboriginal Medical Services across Australia.

Accessibility Mobility, environmental, information, communication and sensory access needs met with minimal effort or stress on the part of the individual with disability.

Ageing The process of growing old.

Ageism Discrimination or prejudice based on age.

Agency Individuals' capacities to take actions, which can be constrained by social structures.

Artefact of measurement A widely disproved explanation discussed in the historic *Black Report,* which suggests health inequalities are merely a statistical anomaly.

Assimilation Processes of adopting the cultural practices of the dominant group in a society, often encouraged, sometimes enforced, by the majority group.

Asylum The right to international protection within a particular country. An "asylum seeker" describes someone who is seeking such protection but whose claim for refugee status has not yet been determined.

Australian Health Practitioner Regulation Agency (Ahpra) The national association of 15 professional boards that regulate and enforce standards in health.

Australian Institute of Aboriginal and Torres Strait Islander Studies (AIATSIS) An independent government statutory authority for research, collection and publication. A premier resource for Aboriginal and Torres Strait Islander peoples learning and record-keeping.

Behavioural factors An explanation, accounting for approximately 20% of disparities in health outcomes, discussed in the *Black Report,* which attributes health inequalities to individual lifestyle choices.

Bias Refers to generally negative feelings and evaluations of individuals because of their group membership (prejudice), overgeneralised beliefs about the characteristics of group members (stereotypes) and inequitable treatment (discrimination).

Biomedical model of health and wellbeing The biomedical modal of health and wellbeing focuses on biological factors. In this model, health is conceptualised as the absence of disease or illness.

Biopsychosocial models of health and wellbeing An interdisciplinary **model** that looks at the interconnection between biology, psychology, and socio-environmental factors.

Caregiver burden A multidimensional response to the psychological, emotional, physical, social and financial stress of caring for a family member who is elderly, disabled or ill.

Chronic conditions Health conditions lasting 3 months or more.

Cisgender A term used to describe individuals whose gender identity and expression matches the biological sex with which they were presumed at birth.

Client-centred care Health care where a person's cultural values, needs and preferences are placed at the forefront of their ongoing medical care.

Collaboration Working together to achieve greater impacts than can occur in isolation.

Colonisation A process of subjugating a people to gain access to their territory and its resources.

Cultural determinants of health Ethnic, religious, racial, but also class and sexuality differences that underpin behavioural patterns and social experiences leading to divergent health outcomes across minority and majority groups.

Cultural diversity The presence of many different cultural or ethnic groups within a society.

Cultural identity Affinity with and sense of belonging to a culture or cultural group.

Culturally safe health care practice Health care that aims to be guided by the recipient of the health care, noting in particular what they consider to be important and appropriate practices and beliefs, and respecting these.

Cultural safety An environment that is spiritually, socially and emotionally safe, as well as physically safe for people; where there is no assault challenge or denial of their identity, of who they are and what they need.

Culturally and linguistically diverse (CALD) A term adopted in Australia to describe people with a cultural heritage differing from that of the Anglo-Australian majority. This term includes diversity in terms of country of birth, preferred language, English proficiency, and other ethnocultural characteristics such as year of arrival in Australia, religious affiliations, and birthplace of parents.

Culturally sensitive care Care that reflects the ability to be appropriately responsive to the attitudes, feelings or circumstances of groups of people that share a common and distinctive racial, national, religious, linguistic or cultural heritage.

Culture The evolved human capacity to classify and represent experiences with symbols and to act imaginatively and creatively. Cultures are differentiated by the distinct ways that people, who live differently, classify and represent their experiences.

Culture clash Conflict or tension arising between individuals attributable to dissimilarities in cultural values and practices.

Culture shock A sense of disorientation or unfamiliarity when experiencing a new cultural environment.

Curriculum The totality of student experiences that occur in the educational process. The term often refers specifically to a planned sequence of instruction, or to a view of the student's experiences in terms of the educator's or school's instructional goals.

Death bed visions The experience of a person who is dying. They see loved ones and family members who have already died.

Dementia Cognitive impairment that interferes with everyday functioning.

Disability Disability is an umbrella term for impairments, activity limitations and participation restrictions. This text occasionally uses the phrase "people with disability", which is an example of person-first language and appropriate for professional writing. The text occasionally uses the phrase "disabled people" as an example of identity-first language. The phrase "disabled people" recognises the experience of disability as a core part of identity, equal to being identified as a gay woman or an African woman.

Discrimination Occurs when a person is excluded from benefits generally available to other members of a society because of a perceived difference or a stigmatised identity.

Diversity Degree of variation of cultures, identities and other social and economic factors within a given society.

Elder abuse A single or repeated act, or lack of appropriate action, occurring within any relationship where there is an expectation of trust that causes harm or distress to an older person.

Endemic A disease that is consistently present within a population.

Ethnicity A category or group of people who identify with each other, usually on the basis of presumed similarities such as common language, geography, ancestry, history, society, culture and/or social treatment.

Ethnocentrism Evaluation of other cultures according to preconceptions originating in the standards and customs of one's own culture.

Eurocentrism A cultural phenomenon that views the histories and cultures of non-Western societies from a European or Western perspective.

Femininity A socially constructed set of attributes, behaviours, and characteristics considered "typical" or "appropriate" for girls and women.

Fundamental social causes of health inequalities A theory that explains health inequalities by emphasising access to material and immaterial resources to mitigate the effects should disease occur.

Gender A socially constructed characterisation of people based on their roles, attitudes, behaviours, attributes and opportunities. There are many ways in which an individual may choose to define their gender, including those who identify as being agendered or non-binary (neither a man nor a woman).

Gender binary A classification system consisting of two genders, male and female, and underpins the social foundations of Australian society and many other societies globally.

Gender diverse A term used to describe individuals whose gender identity does not necessarily align with their presumed sex.

Gender diversity An umbrella term that is used to describe gender identities that demonstrate a diversity of expression beyond the binary framework.

Gender dysphoria In medical discourse, gender dysphoria refers to distress arising from incongruence between with one's internal sense of gender, the sex they were presumed at birth and/or their body.

Gender expression Outward gender presentation and behaviour that may communicate gender to others.

Gender fluidity A spectrum of gender identities that are not exclusively masculine or feminine—identities that are outside the gender binary.

Gender identity A person's internal view of their gender—that is, one's innermost sense of themselves as a gendered person. A person's gender identity may or may not correspond with their sex presumed at birth. Gender identity often influences the name and pronouns people use.

Gender sensitivity An iterative process by which people demonstrate awareness and responsiveness to the influence of gender on behaviour and wellbeing. A gender-sensitive clinician appreciates and positively responds to the differences, inequalities and varying needs of individuals of differing gender identities.

Health advocacy Means providing care to health care consumers that includes the promotion of health and access to services.

Health care system The system in which the purpose of all the services and activities are to promote, restore or maintain health.

Health literacy The ability to obtain, process and understand basic health information and services in order to make appropriate health decisions.

Hegemony The social dominance of one group over another, supported by legitimising norms and the subordination of other social groups or identities.

Heteronormativity Everyday interactions, practices and policies that construct individuals as heterosexual.

Homophobia and biphobia Negative beliefs, prejudices and stereotypes that exist about people who are not heterosexual.

Identity Identity is a person's conception and expression of their individuality or group affiliations.

Immigrational/emigrational experiences of health The experiences of health over the course of immigration/emigration, including increases/decreases in vulnerability to health diseases and conditions or the development and occurrence of health problems.

Impairments Refers specifically to biological or psychological characteristics that impact on how a person functions.

Institutional discrimination A form of racism expressed in the practice of social and political institutions. It effects racial minorities but is also a term used to describe the discrimination experienced by people of minority such as, but not limited to, ethnic, cultural, sexual orientation, gender identity and religious groups. It is reflected in disparities regarding wealth, income, criminal justice, employment, housing, health care, political power and education, among other factors.

Institutional racism A form of racism expressed in social and political institutions that devalue and ignore people of a racial minority

Intersectionality The interconnected nature of social categorisations such as race, class and gender as they apply to a given individual or group, regarded as creating overlapping and interdependent systems of discrimination or disadvantage.

Invasion An occasion when a country and its army uses force to enter and take control of another country.

Learning The process of acquiring new, or modifying existing, knowledge, behaviours, skills, values or preferences.

Learning activity The things learners and educators do, within learning events, that are intended to bring about the desired learning outcomes.

LGBTIQA+ An evolving acronym that stands for lesbian, gay, bisexual, transgender, intersex, queer/questioning, asexual and other terms (such as non-binary and pansexual) that people use to describe experiences of their gender, sexuality and physiological sex characteristics.

Masculinity A socially constructed set of attributes, behaviours and characteristics considered "typical" or "appropriate" for boys and men.

Methodological agnosticism A way of thinking that makes no judgement on the truth or falsity of religious beliefs and practices, but that still allows the individual to have their own views on these matters. Their practice is agnostic, although the health care worker themselves may not be an agnostic.

Midstream factors Intermediary determinants of health, such as material resources, psychosocial and behavioural factors.

Migration The movement of people from one place to another with the intention of settling.

National Aboriginal Community Controlled Health Organisation (NACCHO) The peak body representing 143 Aboriginal Community Controlled Health Organisations (ACCHOs) across the country on Aboriginal health and wellbeing issues. It has a history extending back to a meeting in Albury in 1974.

Natural selection An explanation supported by only modest evidence discussed in the *Black Report,* which suggests health inequalities are the result of the downward social mobility of people with poor health.

Neoliberalism An extreme form of capitalism characterised by a political and economic ideology supporting economic growth through the privatisation of public goods and services, and most recently, through new strategies of relying on insecure and precarious forms of labour.

Non-binary When a person's gender identity does not align with binary gender, male/female. Non-binary people may identify as gender fluid, trans masculine, trans feminine, agender, bigender, gender queer and a multitude of other such terms.

Non-Western models of health and wellbeing Non-Western models of health and wellbeing embrace more than just the disease or illness an individual may experience. These models also focus on developing a deep connection to the regions philosophical and spiritual values.

Nonreligion People who do not identify with any particular religion. This includes Atheists (who reject religion), agnostics (who are not sure about religion), people who are just not very interested in religion and people who are "spiritual but not religious".

Othering Practices of division and exclusion that can result when cultural groups cast outside groups as morally inferior.

Partnership Two or more individuals or groups or coming together to achieve a common purpose.

Pathogenic Conditions or factors that pose a risk to health.

Pedagogy The approach to teaching including the theory and practice of learning, and how this process influences, and is influenced by, the social, political and psychological development of learners.

Penal colony A type of prison, especially one that is far away from other people, as Australia was set up by the British.

Prejudice A preconceived belief regarding another individual based upon their membership, affiliation or affinity with a particular group or cultural identify.

Primary health care model The entry level to the health system and, as such, is usually a person's first encounter with the health system.

Psychosocial explanation A theory that points to the higher levels of stress and anxiety experienced by those in lower positions within a social hierarchy in explaining persisting health inequalities.

Race A socially constructed grouping of humans based on shared physical categories generally viewed as distinct by a society.

Racism Any cognition, affective state, or behaviour that advances the differential treatment of individuals or groups due to their racial, ethnic, cultural, or religious background.

Refugee An individual who is forced to leave their country of origin and is unable to return due to the threat of persecution or harm. Refugees have been formally recognised under the *1951 Convention Relating to the Status of Refugees.*

Religion Ritual practices, typically as part of a community, that draw on symbols and beliefs that guide how people behave and relate.

Religious diversity The variety of religious and not religious people in Australia. Australia's changing religious diversity includes the rising numbers of people who are not religious; the decline of traditional Christianity and the increasing ethnic diversity within Christianity; the growing numbers of Buddhists, Muslims, Hindus and Sikhs, mostly as a result of migration; the growth of Pentecostals; and the rise of alternative spiritualities such as the New Age and meditation.

Residential aged care Care options and accommodation for older people who are unable to live independently in their own homes.

Respect An essential component of a high-performance organization. It helps to create a healthy environment in which clients feel cared for as individuals, and members of health care teams are engaged, collaborative and committed to service. Within a culture of respect, people perform better, are more innovative and display greater resilience. On the contrary, a lack of respect stifles teamwork and undermines individual performance. It can also lead to poor interactions with clients. Cultivating a culture of respect can truly transform an organization, and leaders set the stage for how respect is manifested. (James, 2018)

Salutogenic Conditions or factors that promote health.

Self-awareness The capacity to become the object of one's own attention. In this state one actively identifies, processes and stores information about the self.

Self-reflection A genuine curiosity about the self, where the person is intrigued and interested in learning more about his or her emotions, values, thought processes and attitudes.

Sex The term *sex* can have different meanings in different contexts. Sex can refer to a person's physical characteristics, including their genitals and reproductive organs, or to their assigned or legal status. Sex can also refer to engaging in sexual activities.

Sexuality Encompasses who a person may be attracted to romantically and sexually.

Social and medical gender affirmation Social affirmation is when a person makes changes in appearance and social situations to reflect their gender. This may include changes to hairstyle and clothing, name and pronoun changes, and use of different bathrooms/gendered facilities. They may choose to do this all at once, or only in specific social circles such as with close family and friends. Medical affirmation could include hormone therapy to help develop secondary physical characteristics of gender (such as voice deepening or development of breast tissue) or gender affirmation surgery so that genitalia reflects the person's gender.

Spirituality The individual experience of ritual practices, symbols and beliefs that guide behaviour and relationships. Individual spirituality may be part of a person's participation in a religious group, or may be completely separate from organised religion.

Social construct A perception of an individual, group, or idea that is "constructed" through cultural or social practice.

Social democracy: A state, party or sovereignty that enacts policies to redistribute wealth, support primary health care and prioritise illness prevention through collaboration across sectors.

Social determinants of health Conditions in which people are born, grow, work, live and age, and the wider set of forces and systems shaping the conditions of daily life. These forces and systems include economic policies and systems, development agendas, social norms, social policies and political systems.

Socio-economic status A term describing a person's or group's social standing, typically assessed using a combination measure of income, occupation and education.

Social gradient of disease The graded relationship between social position and health outcomes, with those at the bottom experiencing the worst health outcomes, those in the middle experiencing better health outcomes, and those at the top experiencing the best health outcomes.

Social isolation The state of lack of contact, or minimal contact between an individual and society.

Social justice A political and philosophical theory that broadens the concept of justice beyond those embodied in the principles of civil or criminal law, economic supply and demand, or traditional moral frameworks. Social justice tends to focus more on just relations between groups within society as opposed to the justice of individual conduct or justice for individuals.

Social structure The way social systems are organised and work to shape individual behaviour and life chances.

Stigma Defined as the co-occurrence of labeling, stereotyping, separation, status loss and discrimination in a context in which power is exercised.

Structural/materialist explanation The reason for health inequalities that gets the most support in the *Black Report*: differences in living and working conditions, material and economic resources.

Structural racism The way social systems are organised to favour the majority group and exclude, subjugate or disadvantage minority groups.

Structural violence The harm inflicted through social systems designed to limit opportunities and capabilities, particularly for those in minority groups.

Teaching The concerted sharing of knowledge and experience, which is usually organised within a discipline and, more generally, the provision of stimulus to the psychological and intellectual growth of a person by another person or artefact.

Torres Strait Islanders Torres Strait Islanders are a seafaring peoples, whose traditional countries are in the Torres Strait, off the Australian mainland's northernmost point. The region has over 270 islands in the strait of ocean between the northern tip of Queensland, Cape York, and the south-east coast of Papua New Guinea.

Transgender Refers to people whose gender is not aligned with the gender presumed for them at birth.

Transphobia Negative beliefs, prejudices and stereotypes that exist about transgender/trans and gender diverse people.

Trust Refers to people's expectations, typically for goodwill, advocacy and competence (and/or good outcome). As such, it is future-directed; although past experiences and other forms of knowledge influence the degree of current trust in another, measuring trust itself requires measuring the beliefs of the person who trusts about the trustee's behaviour. Patient or client trust in their health care professional is central to clinical practice. Clients must be able to trust health professionals with their health and to work in their best interest and outcome. Trust in the health care professional is a central factor in effective treatments and fundamental for patient-centered care.

Upstream factors Health determinants that can be intervened in well before they pose a risk to health, such as socio-policies related to education and income.

Whiteness Whiteness and White privilege are ways of conceptualising racial inequalities that focuses as much on the advantages that whites accrue as on the disadvantages that people of colour experience. Unlike theories of overt racism or prejudice, which suggest that people actively seek to oppress or demean other racial groups, theories of White privilege assert that the experience of Whites is viewed by Whites as normal rather than advantaged. Whites as a group hold social advantages rather than experiencing a "normal" state of existence.

Wholistic Placing a "w" in front of holistic makes us reflect that the process, design and collaboration would look at the whole approach—not a hole that the approach could fall or sink into. It would be circular in its wholeness, which conceptualises the way we have grown up and the cycle of life, including our connection to land and Country.

Index

Page numbers in *italics* refer to figures and those in **bold** refer to tables.

For Product Safety Concerns and Information please contact our
EU representative GPSR@taylorandfrancis.com Taylor & Francis
Verlag GmbH, Kaufingerstraße 24, 80331 München, Germany